Health and Medicine in the circum-Caribbean, 1800–1968

Routledge Studies in the Social History of Medicine

Edited By David Cantor, *National Institutes of Health, Bethesda, Maryland, USA*

For a full list of titles in this series, please visit www.routledge.com

Health and Medicine in the circum-Caribbean, 1800–1968

Edited by Juanita De Barros, Steven Palmer and David Wright

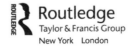

Routledge
Taylor & Francis Group
New York   London

First published 2009
by Routledge
711 Third Avenue, New York, NY 10017

Simultaneously published in the UK
by Routledge
2 Park Square, Milton Park, Abingdon, Oxfordshire OX14 4RN

First issued in paperback 2014

Routledge is an imprint of the Taylor and Francis Group, an informa business

© 2009 Taylor & Francis

Typeset in Sabon by IBT Global.

Library of Congress Cataloging in Publication Data

A catalog record has been requested for this book.

ISBN 978-0-415-96290-2 (hbk)
ISBN 978-1-138-86754-3 (pbk)
ISBN 978-0-203-88020-3 (ebk)

Contents

Figure and Tables

Tables

Figure

Acknowledgements

The editors would like to thank several individuals who have provided assistance and support for this book. We would first like to thank David Cantor, the editor responsible for Studies in the Social History of Medicine series, who has guided the edited volume from its inception. Two anonymous referees contributed excellent comments on individual chapters and the monograph as a whole. The editors of Routledge/Taylor & Francis—Max Novick and Erica Wetter—have been generous and patient in their support of this volume. Typesetting assistance was kindly provided by Barbara-Ann Bartlett and Shawn Day of the History of Medicine Unit at McMaster University, a unit supported through the AMS/Hannah Endowment. Additional editorial assistance was provided by Nathan Flis of Linacre College, University of Oxford. We would also like to thank Terence Johnson, of IBT Global, who coordinated the copyediting and composition of the book, and Noeline Bridge who constructed an excellent index. All but one chapter of this book are original research essays that have not appeared previously in any publication. David Sowell's chapter appeared, in part, in an internal university journal; permission to reprint parts of the chapter has been granted by the author. Chapter 9, originally written in French, was translated into English by David Wright. Finally, we would like to thank our authors for their patience and their excellent contributions to this novel collection.

Introduction

*Juanita De Barros, Steven Palmer,
and David Wright*

The diverse territories of the Caribbean share a complex and fascinating
history borne of the ways European colonialism combined with slavery,
indentureship, migrant labour, and plantation agriculture. The large African-descended populations of the islands in the Caribbean Sea and the
encircling mainland territories of the Americas—originally shipped in to
work on the estates and, in many cases, outnumbering those of European
descent—created hybrid social expressions and configurations that were
nowhere more evident than in the area of health and medicine. The arrival
of several hundred thousand indentured workers between roughly 1840
and World War I brought South Asians and Chinese into these medical
systems, adding to their cultural complexity.[1] In some areas of the Spanish
mainland, including the Yucatán peninsula, indigenous populations maintained strong and distinct medical systems that intermingled with African and popular Hispanic medical practices, while in Cuba (and to some
extent, Puerto Rico) an increasing influx of Spanish labourers starting in
the 1870s rejuvenated popular European humoural and folk medical traditions that had long informed the healing cultures of rural Latin America.[2]
Superimposed over this complex terrain of popular health care was a Western European family of medical institutions, discourses, and practitioners
generated as part of the apparatus of colonial power, and remaining (sometimes uneasily) in the service of colonial and post-colonial governments
even after emancipation and the acquisition of different degrees of local
sovereignty.[3] The history of medical care in the Caribbean therefore draws
our attention to the transfer of cultural practices from Africa and Asia; the
process of creolization in the African and Asian diasporas; the persever-
ance of indigenous and popular medicine; and the emergence of distinct
forms of Western medical professionalism, science, and practice.

Working both in the estate hospitals (where they functioned nominally
under white colonial oversight) and in the slave quarters, healers with African roots played important roles in the community of the enslaved, ministering to its physical and spiritual ills with creole religious–medical practices
such as *obeah*, voodoo, and *santería*. In the French and Spanish Caribbean, where colonial state licensing boards regulated the medical trades,

free black and coloured men and women began to enter the domain of official medicine well prior to the end of slavery, mostly as barber–surgeons and midwives. In the English colonies during the period of slavery, some free, mixed-race men acquired medical training in Great Britain, returning home to practice medicine in their islands despite encountering considerable discrimination from colonial authorities.[4] Following the abolition of slavery in the British Empire, the prior occupation of the slave infirmary medic continued under the informal "black doctors" and, increasingly, healers of African ancestry began to join the formal medical systems that were established throughout the region in the nineteenth and early twentieth centuries, as estate nurses, doctors, and midwives.[5]

Just as Africans, Asians, and their descendents attempted to deal with disease and ill health by turning to traditional and creolized forms of medical practice, so too did the European and Euro-American populations. They aimed to protect their own health and ensure white survival in this often-inhospitable region; however, like colonizer populations elsewhere, they also wanted to make sure that the labouring population was healthy enough to work on the estates.[6] Medical workers in the Caribbean confronted diseases of old- and new-world provenance, but the history of plantation agriculture and tied labour helped determine their nature. Although elite-produced discourses tended to emphasize this aspect of Caribbean medical history, disease—combined with poor working and living conditions—afflicted the masses of the population with poor health and shortened their lives. The end of slavery did not see much improvement in this regard. Indeed, sources describe the late nineteenth- and early twentieth-century urban and rural areas inhabited by the non-white masses as unsanitary. Poor public health conditions, as well as the lifestyle of plantation agriculture and the resource extraction industries the inhabitants were destined to work in, resulted in the spread of disease among these groups, who found themselves the target of racist science and scientific racism.

Health and Medicine in the circum-Caribbean, 1880–1968 is the first volume to examine this unique modern history of health and medicine in the region as a whole. Although several important essay collections have explored the history of colonial and post-colonial health and medical practice, they have excluded the Caribbean islands and their mainland entourage. Those edited by David Arnold, Roy MacLeod, and Milton Lewis focused on colonial Asia and Africa, with both Latin America and the Caribbean strikingly absent.[7] Nor is there a single chapter on the Caribbean in edited volumes on race and medicine, plural medicine, or colonies and identity.[8] The Hispanic Caribbean has hardly figured in the recent renaissance in the Latin American history of medicine and public health. Much of the dynamism of this new historiography has come from its exploration of scientific excellence on the periphery, and its questioning of metropolitan paradigms equating tropical medicine with Western European imperialism, but ironically scholars have tended to concentrate on the 'core of the periphery'—Mexico City, Lima, Buenos Aires, and the urban nodes of Brazil.[9] The brief special issue of *Caribbean Quarterly* edited by Juanita De Barros and Sean Stilwell remains the only attempt to pull together some of the emerging scholarship on the history of medicine in the Caribbean, but its focus is primarily on the British West Indies.[10] Despite many good intentions, the historiographies of the French, British, and Hispanic Caribbean rarely rub elbows, let alone incorporate work on other parts of the region with distinct colonial traditions. The thirteen original research essays collected here, featuring scholarship on the nineteenth- and twentieth-century French, English, Spanish, Dutch, and Danish Caribbean, are thus exceptional in their range. They also reveal the breadth and richness of subjects and methodological approaches that concern this growing community of scholars who frame classic topics in ways that reflect the new social and cultural history of medicine and the new political history of public health.

Health and medicine in colonial environments is one of the most active, contested, and fascinating areas of the history of medicine. It is also one of the newest. As Shula Marks argued in her Presidential Address to the Society for the Social History of Medicine in 1992, it was only in the late 1980s that the subject began to spawn a dynamic and critical historiography. During the 1990s, scholarship slowly moved away from narrow, triumphalist accounts of imperial medicine and the battle against tropical diseases toward interdisciplinary inquiries into the way medical practice, discourses, and professions informed the colonial project.[11] The history of medicine and empire is now robust and dynamic, with substantial literatures on the Indian subcontinent, South Africa, and Canada.[12] Though Caribbean cases are conspicuously lacking in this new historiography, its foundations were laid by works of fundamental importance on disease and demography in the colonial Atlantic world.

It is probably fair to say that the first generation of scholars engaged in the social history of colonial medicine in the Atlantic world devoted themselves to several core themes, the first (and arguably most famous) of which was a demographic analysis of the spread of, and battle against, infectious diseases precipitated by Contact. The literature on the 'Columbian Exchange' by such renowned historians as Alfred Crosby and William McNeill set the stage for a passionate and politically charged debate over the demographic decline (and in some cases collapse) of indigenous peoples in the Caribbean and the mainland Americas.[13] Historians of the eighteenth century focused predictably on the impact of the Atlantic Slave Trade. Enslaved Africans transported African pathogens to Caribbean plantations, resulting in epidemic diseases such as yellow fever, which influenced imperial power relations in this, the original "white man's grave". So great was the demographic and epidemiological impact of slavery that Kenneth Kiple and Kriemhild Conee Ornelas characterized the disease environment of the Caribbean as largely an "Africanized" one.[14]

In the ensuing debate, dozens of historians used case studies of regions to chart the extraordinary social, ecological, and political impact of infectious diseases.[15] What is clear is that the epidemiological impact varied enormously, depending upon the geographical place of contact (tropical, temperate,[16] and circumpolar[17]), the types of infectious disease, the duration of contact (often due to the proximity of aboriginal peoples to coastal trading areas), and the impact of European contact on trade patterns and indigenous residential patterns. These historical case studies were often carried out by geographers and historically inclined medical anthropologists and leaned heavily on quantitative analysis and population modeling.[18] The crux of the debate lay in how one 'counted', and equally, the degree to which one could extrapolate whole populations from burial sites of often a few dozen individuals or fragmentary contemporary European population estimates. The debate over whether Amerindian society represented the 'virgin soil' hypothesized by Crosby and McNeill has been even more contentious.

The last two decades have witnessed an evolution from quantitative, epidemiological analyses to studies focused more and more on medical discourses and their relationship to the apparatus of empire.[19] Diseases were no longer something 'out there'—objective entities that were independent of social, cultural, and political forces. Rather, they became central to the imperial problematic. As Warwick Anderson points out, the clash between Europeans and tropical climes produced multiple tensions and a central conundrum: Why and how could racially superior Europeans succumb to tropical diseases? How could white man's dominion over the tropical world be justified if whites were unable to triumph over tropical disease?[20] Indeed, the very terms 'tropics', 'tropical medicine', and 'tropical diseases' were concepts heavily imbued with political and ideological imperatives. Mark Harrison has eloquently argued that the nineteenth-century Western medical world fixated on the nexus of race and climate. More specifically, debate centred on whether diseases were 'different' in the tropical or (temperate) colonial milieux, and, if so, whether Europeans could adapt or 'acclimatize' over time to the new disease environment.[21] Such concerns were behind the rise of Schools of Tropical Medicine in Britain and gave urgency to the work of the Pasteur Institute in France. In an important contribution to the rise of the cultural history of medicine, scholars have demonstrated how the medico-scientific battles over disease classification (and eradication) were culturally and psychologically intertwined with imperial success. Thus the germ theory of disease (or competing germ theories of disease) became allegorical for the eradication, or at least assimilation, of non-European cultures, practices, and peoples.

In the British Caribbean, Kiple, Richard Sheridan, Michael Craton, and K.O. Laurence began the task of examining such subjects as the history of slave health and medical care, the epidemiology of the plantation complex, the role played by European physicians during the period of slavery, and the health of indentured South Asians.[22] In the French West Indies, historians have been motivated by important French-language works on the history of slave medical practices and on epidemic disease in the nineteenth century (especially those of Pierre Pluchon and Dominique Taffin, respectively). The St Domingue revolution has attracted some scholarly attention; David Geggus' earlier work on the impact of yellow fever on the outcome of the revolution, and Karol K. Weaver's more recent book on the role of slave healers in the revolution demonstrate the utility of using this particular conflict as a source for medical history.[23] Cuban historiographical concerns have dominated the field in the Spanish Caribbean, with the priority dispute between Carlos Finlay and the Reed Commission over the discovery of the yellow fever vector provoking a rich body of work about the role of imperialism in the production, validation, and use of science.[24]

The essays collected in this volume build on this important, earlier work, extending the study of such subjects as the history of slave health and medical care; the presence (and ongoing vitality) of African-derived medical practices; the relationship between tied labour systems and disease; the construction of racial identities through medical practices; and the intersection between imperialism, neo-imperialism, and the history of medicine. At the same time, this collection marks the shift to a new historiographical register. First of all, it shows that contemporary historians of medicine in the Caribbean are more inclined to cross linguistic and nation–state boundaries and take into consideration work and analytical trends in other parts of the Caribbean, Latin America, and indeed, Africa and Asia. Complementing this is a willingness to trace Caribbean actors as they migrate intraregionally—that is, as opposed to the macro-regional studies of disease epidemiology characteristic of an earlier generation involved in mapping the implications of the Atlantic exchange of peoples through European conquest and the slave trade, historians are now interested in doing more discrete, micro-level tracing of the health implications of West Indian and Puerto Rican workers in other parts of the Caribbean.

Reflecting trends in the discipline of history as a whole, the following pages reveal an increasing interest in cultural and social domains of medical experience. For example, these chapters show the emerging influence of environmental history on the field, one that is bound to get stronger as this promising analytical approach grows in importance. In keeping with the theme of this book series, the patient's view remains as elusive as ever in the historical sources, but when it is found, the authors make sure it is in full view. The instinct to incorporate history from below is perhaps more clearly in evidence in a greater awareness of the dynamics and tensions of power: the chapters that follow place emphasis on the contestation of subjects to forms of medicalization and the controls of public health, and on the politics of professionalization, not simply as an expression of colonial power, but also of the power of a local elite against colonial or neo-colonial control. Here, a distinct Caribbean perspective emerges within the historiography of medicine and imperialism, since as in the Americas more widely, "Western medicine," having arrived with the conquest and taken strong root at many levels of society, could not so easily be considered an alien, colonizing imposition in the nineteenth century in the way it was in many Asian and African colonial contexts.

There is a correspondingly clear influence from Foucauldian understandings of the impact of institutions and professional perceptions in constructing categories of race and gender through the way they pathologize subjects. The essays collected here also display the greater sensitivity of historians to the cultural history of race, describing and analyzing Caribbean concatenations of racist science, scientific racism, and the construction of race by science. Perhaps most significant and novel is the emergence of gender as a crucial category of historical analysis, no longer simply in its demographic implications, but as it is woven into the fabric of institutional control, expressed in the social policy priorities of colonial and post-colonial states, and lived, and as its definitions and boundaries are contested by women actors. Many of the authors in this collection incorporate gender into their consideration of Caribbean health and medicine, exploring not only the significance of gender ideologies in informing policy decisions, but also the nature of women's involvement in Caribbean health-care systems, both as patients and as health workers, particularly in the field of maternity and infant work.

Medical professionalization, discourses, and practice were not simply about power structures or elites, they were also about a subtler process of 'colonizing the body', to borrow a turn of phrase from one of the most influential historians of colonial medicine, David Arnold.[25] As several of the chapters in this volume attest, women's bodies became important sites of economic and political contestation in post-emancipation Caribbean society.[26] This book is replete with examinations of this complex phenomenon, particularly as it pertained to the contested professional and cultural terrain of midwifery and childbirth. On one level, the now well-rehearsed battle between medical men and (female) midwives that played itself out in nineteenth-century Europe was fought, in part, in the islands of the Caribbean. There, however, one must add the complicating factors of race and slavery to the mix. In general, slave and (later) emancipated Afro-Caribbean women in the nineteenth-century Caribbean tended to use networks of Afro-Caribbean 'midwives' and wisewomen. These midwives occupied a variety of statuses; some were even in the official employment of plantation owners. The emergence of (Western-trained) obstetrical specialists was very limited during this period, for obvious financial and cultural reasons. 'Men of science', who in the British Caribbean were often graduates of Scottish medical schools and who positioned themselves as *accoucheurs* to the elite, and experts in 'complicated deliveries', were simply too expensive for plantation owners or most families. Yet in some cases, hybrid systems of midwifery did emerge, such as the Danish system of licensed midwives on the island of St Croix. As Niklas Thode Jensen demonstrates, between 1803 and 1848 the Danish colonial administration established a hierarchical structure of royal (licensed) midwives of European training and ancestry. These royal midwives had as their duties, amongst other things, the training of enslaved plantation midwives. The struggle to reform birthing practices in Danish St Croix was a classic expression of colonial planter-state care. Anticipating the consequences of the abolition of the slave trade, and seeing emancipation on the horizon, the need for hale, free-born bodies for a future free market in labour imposed itself alongside the maturation of a new model of state medicine.

Tara Iniss shows us the other side of the equation—the expansive traditions of popular midwifery stretching across the English Caribbean, across slavery and emancipation, and across and back to African practices that remained vital into the twentieth century. During the era of slavery, plantation owners regularly employed slave 'midwives' or slave 'nurses' to care for parturient mothers. With the end of slavery, real and feared labour shortages (which would be partly relieved by indentured labourers from India and China) became a preoccupation of the plantation oligarchy. Ensuring a ready and healthy future supply of workers, therefore, was in their own financial interest. In this manner, we can understand the importance of the Baby Saving Leagues in British Guiana and elsewhere, the subject of Juanita De Barros' contribution to this book. Women's participation in Caribbean medical institutions grew significantly in the twentieth century, particularly in the fields of public health and maternity. De Barros uses a case study of the British Guiana Baby Saving League to trace the evolution of infant welfare work in early twentieth-century British Guiana, linking its development to wider British policies in the region, themselves informed by an imperial discourse of reproduction, race, and gender. With the cooption of Afro-Caribbean women of the middle ranks, the Baby Saving Leagues sought to marginalize folk practices of childbirth, to bring women into the realm of Western male medical practices, and to extend the hegemony of a growing middle-class professional elite, as well as the dominance of Western intellectual traditions, all in the guise of 'saving babies' and securing the economic future of the colony. In short, the imposition of Western childbirth practices was an attempt to 'civilize' non-white healers (and mothers) and stabilize the sources of labour (in both senses of the word).

Women's and children's bodies also became targets of disease production and control. In Denise Challenger's chapter in this volume, it is vividly demonstrated that the Barbadian colonial regime invested considerable sums in an institutional archipelago of carceral institutions, including a lunatic asylum and a repressive Lock (or syphilis) hospital.[27] The Contagious Diseases Act was used across the British Empire to constrain women's behaviour and sexuality through the ostensibly medical goal of controlling the epidemic of syphilis.[28] Challenger examines the adoption of the Act in Barbados in particular as a way of controlling Afro-Caribbean female sexuality, of disciplining the female body. When it was found that they could not be rescued by the new salvation of medicine, these vulnerable, tough women—who were symbols of the unregulated sexuality of females of colour—had to be locked away and punished. Clearly the transmission of venereal disease (particularly syphilis) was of immense public health and political importance, given the large number of ports, the ubiquity of stationed military personnel, and the absence (before the 1940s) of any effective anti-venereal treatment.

April Mayes's chapter on prostitution in early twentieth-century, US-occupied Dominican Republic explores a different kind of official response to the "problem" of prostitution, but one that also points to the continuing relevance of colonialism (albeit in a neo-imperial form) in the region in the twentieth century. Some countries, like the Dominican Republic, preferred to establish areas where prostitutes and their customers could congregate. The operation of such semi-regulated 'tolerance zones', where American soldiers could frequent brothels that were physically and symbolically kept away from respectable Dominican society, precipitated a struggle between municipal officials (who supported the tolerance zones as a way of exerting some control over the spread of venereal disease) and the US military governor (who eventually signed a decree to make prostitution illegal). For the US military government, new sanitation laws were a means of exerting imperial governance under the guise of 'public health'. Mayes argues that the struggle over the imposition (and nature) of public health measures was, in part, a proxy for the resistance to American governance itself. The control and eradication of syphilis thus represents a fascinating case study of the intersection of colonialism, culture, sexuality, gender, and race.

In her stress on the role of medical men in the construction of these regulations governing prostitutes, Mayes points to the emergence of professional medical classes in the late nineteenth and early twentieth centuries and their contribution to contemporary ideas about race, nationality, and gender. Several chapters in this volume illustrate how different elites used medical discourses of race to position themselves (sometimes successfully, sometimes not) in the shifting political sands of post-emancipation and post-colonial Caribbean nations. Thus, *criollos* (those native born, but claiming pure white European ancestry) in Cuba and elsewhere attempted to use the language of medicine to reinvent themselves as native-born elites, above the Afro-Caribbean, 'coloured', and indigenous masses, but also distinct from (and more legitimate than) the retreating European-born colonial elites. Steven Palmer's chapter shows that doctors working the plantation circuits of Cuba during its nineteenth-century sugar boom were part of stressed and often forced encounters, pitting the suffering bodies of labourers brought to the region from elsewhere against the vital managerial needs of a local elite. Their power was often an expression of plantation wealth, and a colonial state with a distinct set of health-care models propping up its power. In this circuitry, a new *criollo* medical edifice was constructed, one that allowed Cuban-born elites or, in some cases, transplanted drifters of the Atlantic world to transform their access to masses of slave bodies into a great island clinic that could produce a native scientific discourse and professional opportunity in the growing medical metropolis of Havana. David Sowell shows us a distinct Hispanized medical universe on the other side of the Yucatán channel, where Mayan healers rivaled their elite Mexican counterparts. He explores the contested nature of medical authority, notably the competition among the different groups of health workers in the Yucatán, and the efforts of formally trained physicians to construct a privileged professional status.

In investigating physicians' class and professional status in US-dominated Puerto Rico, Nicole Trujillo-Pagan demonstrates that, although Puerto Rico's physicians participated in the kinds of public health activities their counterparts carried out elsewhere in the region and were motivated by similar ideas about the 'civilizing' role of physicians in social reform, the particular context of US neo-colonialism informed the nature of state–physician relations. Her chapter reveals an unsuccessful attempt by *criollo* physicians to distance themselves from the American colonial structure and establish themselves above unregulated medical practitioners. Pushed aside by the US military forces, they reluctantly yielded to the inevitable and gave up their vision of an independent *criollo*-led Puerto Rican medical community to become an adjunct group of the American Medical Association. Thus, medical professions, medical discourses, and medical practices were crucial to jockeying for position within incipient Caribbean nationalism and emerging nationhood, attenuated to one degree or another by the new imperial presence of the United States.[29]

The emergence of tropical medicine is one example of a field and nexus of institutions that had a strong role in shaping the new medical universe of the twentieth-century Caribbean. The power of tropical medicine was magnified by the establishment and work of the Rockefeller Foundation, whose influence over Latin America and the Caribbean loomed large.[30] Over the last few decades, the public health campaigns to control or eradicate certain diseases, developed after 1914 by the Foundation's International Health Board, have undergone increasingly critical scrutiny. This recent scholarship has highlighted the geopolitical, ideological, and racial factors involved in which diseases would be targeted, how the eradication programs would proceed, and whether the programs were ultimately successful or not. Rosemarijn Hoefte's contribution focuses on the Rockefeller eradication program for ankylostomiasis (or hookworm disease) in early twentieth-century Suriname which, the Foundation believed, would assist with establishing the broader structural foundations of public health in that country. In Suriname, as in British Guiana and Trinidad, the Rockefeller Foundation was heavily involved in efforts to ameliorate perceived public health problems suffered by Asian and Javanese plantation labourers. The economic rationale behind the introduction of public health measures and this emphasis on the health of workers continued to be salient even as the region's economies changed and the plantation sector declined in economic importance.

Hoefte's chapter also introduces us to the unusual story of an elite Surinamese-born woman, Grace Schneiders-Howard, who promoted the work of the Rockefeller Foundation in early twentieth-century Suriname. Despite her undoubted eccentricities, Schneiders-Howard was impelled by the same kind of civilizing impulse that encouraged other women (and indeed, other members of the local middle and professional classes) to participate in the social welfare field. As the public health infrastructure expanded in the British Caribbean in the 1930s, so did the variety and extent of medical work performed by women, as Debbie McCollin shows in her chapter. She, like many of the authors in this collection, does not limit her exploration of health workers to those who were the recipients of formal training and state recognition. McCollin emphasizes the importance of mothers, grandmothers, and other female relatives who were on the "frontline" of Trinidad and Tobago's informal health-care system.

Several chapters in this volume resonate with the debate about the physical vulnerability (or robustness) of both white and non-white peoples in the context of such changing economic circumstances. As Jacques Dumont demonstrates, ideologies of race and, in particular, negative views of the region's African-descended population, informed medical thinking and state policies in the early twentieth century. Dumont explores French medical representations of non-white French West Indian troops in the context of the First World War, arguing that a "racialized perception" contributed to conclusions about the poor state of their physical and moral health. Dumont demonstrates how French medical practitioners conceptualized the inability of *créole* conscript soldiers from Guadeloupe and the Antilles to adapt to the temperate climate of France on the eve of the First World War. France, as it were, was the "black man's grave" for troops from the Antilles. French doctors used medico-scientific indexes of 'fitness' to buttress conceptions of racial inferiority of coloured troops and occlude discussion of the public health problems back in the Caribbean, problems that had been exacerbated by French colonialism. On the other hand, racialized medical science could also be marshalled to support arguments in favour of greater racial immunity. As David McBride demonstrates in his chapter on bauxite mining in post-WWII Jamaica, it was widely believed by scientists in the 1950s that Afro-Jamaicans had a greater degree of protection from the environmental toxins that resulted from this early stage of aluminium production. He also shows the continuing inclination of foreign medical and scientific authorities to point to race and climate as causative factors. Only after decades of epidemiological and environmental distortion did research demonstrate clearly that Jamaicans working in or near the huge mines exhibited elevated levels of cancer.[31]

There are several intriguing themes raised in the following chapters that are worth mentioning as possible areas for more intense historical inquiry in the future. Somewhat ironically, considering their status as staple entitles in the history of health and medicine, one area ripe for more research is the rise of formal medical institutions.[32] As alluded to in several chapters in this volume, the Caribbean had a complement of such large institutions—for example, one for the mentally ill in Barbados—that have not received any sustained attention. This is in contrast to the enormous literature on the history of madness and psychiatry in other colonies (or former colonies), including India, South Africa, Canada, New Zealand, Australia, and Quebec.[33] Although the danger is always to place too much emphasis on elite institutions and medical practitioners, trends in medical historiography have revealed how institutional records can also be used to shed light on lay and folk practices, as well as extramural care and treatment.

Second, many contributors allude to the social, political, cultural, and medical impact of the movement of labour (slave, indentured, 'free') betwixt and between colonies of the Caribbean (and, to a lesser extent, to the coastal regions of the mainlands of South, Central, and North America). The circulation of informal and formally trained health practitioners between countries and (often lost) to the richer industrialized world has received less scrutiny. Although the movement of medical practitioners between jurisdictions is not new, the post-WWII era saw a heightened problem, despite (or perhaps because of) the creation of the medical school at the University of West Indies. The change in immigration laws in the 1950s and 1960s (to relieve labour shortages in Britain, the United States, and Canada) would also occasion a remarkable leakage of nurses and doctors to those countries, the beginnings of the health human resource "brain drain" that has haunted many Caribbean and 'developing' countries in the second half of the twentieth century. The socialist orientation of the Cuban revolution, meanwhile, led to the exodus of the Caribbean's largest community of medical professionals in the space of a few years in the early 1960s, most of them ending up in the United States. Research on the post-WWII era needs to explore the impact of the globalization of health human resources on medical care in the Caribbean, as well as the intriguing counter-currents flowing to and from Cuba that have been the subject of much more impassioned rhetoric than careful study.

Our collection terminates in the 1960s, a watershed moment in the history of health and medicine in the Caribbean. On the one hand, in the British colonial universe, many of these islands won their outright independence, and the impact of this achievement on the fate of medical professionals and institutions, fields such as tropical medicine, and the health of national communities—a tantalizing glimpse of which can be found in McBride's chapter—remains high on the agenda of historians who must now turn with greater seriousness to the second half of the twentieth century. Second, especially beginning in the 1950s, US-based medical institutions, programs, and science begin to achieve clear dominance in the region, as the influence of the former colonial metropoles waned. This is a radical shift that requires close and systematic comparative attention. Finally, of course, after 1960, a counter-hegemonic strain in health and medicine emerges boldly in the revolutionary project of Cuba, which develops a practical and ideological specialty in primary care and undertakes to train vast numbers of health-care workers, not only from and for Cuba, but from and for other Caribbean countries as well.[34] The responses to this development, again led by the United States (though with a strong, complementary, and alternative presence of international health organizations), and structured by a Cold War discourse on health, played a large, but as yet little-studied, role in the development of modern public health and community medicine infrastructure and programs throughout the Caribbean. There is no shortage of work to be done. We hope, however, that the chapters presented here already suggest the multinational, cross-cultural, and interdisciplinary spirit and methods that must animate those who broach the next phase of research on the history of health and medicine in the Caribbean.

NOTES

1. The study of healing and healers of Asian origin is in need of much more attention; among the few works to treat the subject are Clem Seecharan, *'Tiger in the Stars': The Anatomy of Indian Achievement in British Guiana 1919–29* (London: Macmillan Caribbean Publishers, 1997); Brian L. Moore, *Cultural Power, Resistance, and Pluralism: Colonial Guyana, 1838–1900* (Montreal and Kingston, Jamaica: University of West Indies Press and McGill-Queen's University Press, 1995), 155–240 and 265–94; and Miguel Angel Sabater Reyes, "Los primeros médicos chinos en Cuba," *Boletín del Archivo Nacional* (Cuba) 11 (1988): 23–9.

2. Carlos Viesca Treviño, "*Curanderismo* in Mexico and Guatemala: Its Historical Evolution from the Sixteenth to the Nineteenth Century," in *Mesoamerican Healers*, ed. Brad R. Huber and Alan R. Sandstrom (Austin: University of Texas Press, 2001), 47–64. For an interesting reiteration of Foster's famous Spanish genealogy of indigenous Mexican humoural medicine, see Luz María Hernández and George M. Foster, "Curers and their Cures in Colonial New Spain and Guatemala: The Spanish Component," in *Mesoamerican Healers*, 19–45. Also, see Steven Palmer, *From Popular Medicine to Medical Populism: Doctors, Healers, and Public Power in Costa Rica, 1800–1940* (Durham, NC: Duke University Press, 2003); and David Sowell, *The Tale of Healer Miguel Perdomo Neira: Medicine, Ideologies, and Power in the Nineteenth-Century Andes* (Wilmington, DE: Scholarly Resources, 2001). On the intermingling of different folk forms of medicine in Cuba, see Lydia Cabrera, *La medicina popular de Cuba: medicos de antaño, curanderos, santeros y paleros de hogaño* (Miami: Ediciones Universal, 1984). On classic Mayan medicine, see Sandra Orellana, *Indian Medicine in Highland Guatemala: The Pre-Hispanic and Colonial Periods* (Albuquerque: University of New Mexico Press, 1987).

3. See, for example, Sean Quinlan, "Colonial Bodies, Hygiene and Abolition-
ist Politics in Eighteenth-Century France," *History Workshop Journal* 42
(1996): 107–125; Anya Jabour, "Slave Health and Health Care in the British
Caribbean: Profits, Racism and the Failure of Amelioration in Trinidad and
British Guiana, 1824–1834," *Journal of Caribbean History* [Barbados] 28
(1994): 1–26; Nadine Joy Wilkins, "Doctors and Ex-Slaves in Jamaica 1834–
1850," *Jamaican Historical Review* 17 (1991) 19–30; Wilkins, "The Medical
Profession in Jamaica in the Post-Emancipation Period," *Jamaica Journal* 21
(1988–1989) 27–32; Philip N. Alexander, "John H. Rapier, Jr and the Medi-
cal Profession in Jamaica, 1861–1862 [Part One]," *Jamaica Journal* 24 (1993):
37–46; Luis J. Oliver, "Breve historia de la sanidad en Puerto Rico durante
el periodo colonial español y la participación de la Iglesia en el proceso [A
Brief History of Public Health in Puerto Rico during the Spanish Colonial
Period and of the Participation of the Church in the Process]," *Horizontes*
[Puerto Rico] 36 (1992–1993): 127–156; Dominique Taffin, "A Propos d'une
Epidemie de Cholera: Science Medicale, Société Créole et Pouvoir Colonial
à la Guadeloupe (1865–1866) [Medical Science, Creole Society, and Colo-
nial Power in Guadeloupe: The Case of the Cholera Epidemic, 1865–1866],"
Asclepio [Spain] 44 (1992): 215–221; Juanita De Barros, "Sanitation and
Civilization in Georgetown, British Guiana," in ed. Juanita De Barros and
Sean Stilwell, special issue, Colonialism and Health in the Tropics, *Caribbean
Quarterly* 49, no. 5 (2003): 65–86; José G. Rigau-Pérez, "The Introduction
of Smallpox Vaccine in 1803 and the Adoption of Immunization as a Government Function in Puerto Rico," *Hispanic American Historical Review*
69 (1989): 393–423; Rigau-Pérez, "Strategies That Led to the Eradication
of Smallpox in Puerto Rico, 1882–1921," *Bulletin of the History of Medicine* 59 (1985): 75–88; José Ronzón, *Sanidad y modernización en los puertos
del alto Caribe, 1870–1915* (México: Universidad Autónoma Metropolitana,
2004); Juanita De Barros, *Order and Place in a Colonial City: Patterns of
Struggle and Resistance in Georgetown, British Guiana 1889–1924* (Kingston and Montreal: McGill-Queens University Press, 2003); and Alexandra
Minna Stern, "Yellow Fever Crusade: U.S. Colonialism, Tropical Medicine,
and the International Politics of Mosquito Control, 1900–20," in *Medicine
at the Border: Disease, Globalization and Security, 1850 to the Present*, ed.
Alison Bashford (London: Palgrave, 2006), 41–59.
4. See, for example, Bridget Brereton, *A History of Modern Trinidad, 1783–
1962* (Kingston, Jamaica: Heinemann Educational [Caribbean] Books,
1981), 64–66.
5. Among the many works that treat this subject, for the French West Indies,
see Pierre Pluchon, *Vaudou sorciers empoisonneurs de Saint-Domingue à
Haïti* (Paris: Karthala, 1987); Karol K. Weaver, "The Enslaved Healers of
Eighteenth-Century Saint Domingue," *Bulletin of the History of Medicine*
76 (2002): 429–460; C. Bougerol, "Medical Practices in the French West
Indies: Master and Slave in the 17th and 18th Centuries," *History and
Anthropology* 2 (1985): 125–143; and James E. McLellan, *Colonialism and
Science: Saint Domingue in the Old Regime* (Baltimore, MD: Johns Hop-
kins University Press, 1992). For the Spanish Caribbean context, see Yolanda
Texera Arnal, "Médicos y cirujanos pardos 'en condición de por ahora' en
la provincia de Venezuela, siglo XVIII," *Colonial Latin American History
Review* 8, no. 3 (1999): 321–338; and Stephan Palmié, *Wizards and Scien-
tists: Explorations in Afro-Cuban Modernity and Tradition* (Durham, NC:
Duke University Press, 2002), 39–289. On the English Caribbean, see Juanita
De Barros, "'Setting Things Right': Medicine and Magic in British Guiana,

1803–1834," *Slavery and Abolition* 25 (April 2004): 28–50; Juanita De Barros, "'Spreading Sanitary Enlightenment': Race, Identity, and the Emergence of a Creole Medical Profession in British Guiana," *Journal of British Studies* 42 (2003): 483–504; Richard Sheridan, *Doctors and Slaves: A Medical and Demographic History of Slavery in the British West Indies, 1680–1834* (Cambridge: Cambridge University Press, 1985); Moore, *Cultural Power, Resistance, and Pluralism,*17–154; Brian L. Moore and Michele A. Johnson, *Neither Led Nor Driven: Contesting British Cultural Imperialism in Jamaica, 1865–1920* (Kingston, Jamaica: University of the West Indies Press, 2004), 1–13, 205–244, and 271–325; and Michael Craton, "Death, Disease and Medicine on Jamaican Slave Plantations: the Example of Worthy Park, 1767–1838," *Histoire Sociale/Social History* [Canada] 9 (1976): 237–255.

6. Philip Curtin, *Death by Migration: Europe's Encounter with the Tropical World in the Nineteenth Century* (Cambridge: Cambridge University Press, 1989), 40–129.

7. David Arnold, ed., *Imperial Medicine and Indigenous Societies* (Manchester: Manchester University Press, 1988); Milton Lewis and Roy McLeod, eds., *Disease, Medicine, and Empire: Perspectives on Western Medicine and the Experience of European Expansion* (New York: Routledge, 1988).

8. Waltraud Ernst and Bernard Harris, eds., *Race, Science and Medicine, 1700–1960* (London: Routledge, 1999); Ernst, ed., *Plural Medicine, Tradition and Modernity, 1800–2000* (London: Routledge, 2002); Bridie Andrews and Mary Sutphen, eds., *Medicine and Colonial Identity* (London: Routledge, 2003).

9. Diego Armus, ed., *Disease in the History of Modern Latin America: From Malaria to AIDS* (Durham, NC: Duke University Press, 2003); Armus, ed., *Avatares de la medicalización en América Latina, 1870–1970* (Buenos Aires: Lugar Editorial, 2005); Armus and Gilberto Hochman, eds., *Cuidar, controlar, curar: ensayos históricos sobre saúde e doença na América Latina e Caribe* (Rio de Janeiro: Editoria Fiocruz, 2004); Marcos Cueto, ed., *Missionaries of Science: The Rockefeller Foundation and Latin America* (Bloomington: Indiana University Press, 1994). Cueto's collection of articles on the activities of the Rockefeller Foundation, and Armus' recent collection on disease in the history of modern Latin America, address the core Hispanic and Portuguese cultures of the mainland. While the other recent edited collections—one on medicalization by Armus and another on illness and health by Armus and Hochmann—go further afield, only one essay by Steven Palmer (on the Caribbean peregrinations of the Cuban spiritist and healer, Carlos Carbell) in the former volume, and one by Paul Farmer (on AIDS in contemporary Haiti) reproduced in the latter volume, fall in the Caribbean domain. Perhaps the most relevant study for Caribbeanists due to its attentiveness to the creole medical science that emerged through the attention of Europhile physicians to local medical conditions among a Bahian population of predominantly African origin, is the work of Julyan Peard, *Race, Place, and Medicine: The Idea of the Tropics in Nineteenth-Century Brazilian Medicine* (Durham, NC: Duke University Press, 1999).

10. De Barros and Stilwell, eds., *Colonialism and Health in the Tropics.*

11. Shula Marks, "What is Colonial about Colonial Medicine?" *Social History of Medicine* 10 (1997): 205–220.

12. The literature on health and medicine is now vast, particularly with the rise of a substantial literature on the history of health and medicine in colonial India, South Africa, Canada, and Australia. This section will focus mainly on the Atlantic World, though it will draw parallels, from time to time, with the experience in other colonial environments.

13. Alfred Crosby, *The Columbian Exchange: The Biological Consequences of 1492* (Westport, CT: 1972) and William McNeill, *Plagues and Peoples* (Garden City, NY: 1976), esp. chapter 5, "Transoceanic Exchanges, 1500–1700," 205–241. For literature that clearly sees this as an epidemiological 'holocaust', see R. Thornton, *American Indian Holocaust and Survival: A Population History since 1492* (Norman: Oklahoma University Press, 1987) and David Stannard, *American Holocaust: Columbus and the Conquest of the New World* (Oxford: Oxford University Press, 1992).

14. Kenneth Kiple and Kriemhild Conee Ornelas, "Race, War and Tropical Medicine in the Eighteenth-Century Caribbean," in *Warm Climates and Western Medicine: The Emergence of Tropical Medicine, 1500–1900*, ed. David Arnold (Amsterdam-Atlanta: Rodopi, 1996), 66.

15. Jay R. Mandle, "The Decline in Mortality in British Guiana, 1911–1960," *Demography* 7 (1970): 301–315; Noble David Cook, *Demographic Collapse: Indian Peru, 1520–1620* (New York: Cambridge University Press, 1981); José Rigau-Pérez, "Smallpox Epidemics in Puerto Rico During the Pre-Vaccine Era," *Journal of the History of Medicine and Allied Sciences* 37 (1982): 423–438; Donald Joralemon, "New World Depopulation and the Case of Disease," *Journal of Anthropological Research* 38 (1982): 108–127; H. Roy Merrens and George D. Terry, "Dying in Paradise: Malaria, Mortality, and the Perceptual Environment in Colonial South Carolina," *Journal of Southern History* 50, no. 4 (1984): 533–550; K. David Patterson, "Yellow Fever Epidemics and Mortality in the United States, 1693–1905," *Social Science and Medicine* 34 (1992) 855–865; Daniel Relf, "Contact Shock in Northwestern New Spain, 1518–1764," in *Disease and Demography in the Americas*, ed. J.W. Verano and D.H. Ubelaker. (Washington, DC: Smithsonian Institution Press, 1992), 265–276; Suzanne Austin Alchon, *Native Society and Disease in Colonial Ecuador* (Cambridge: Cambridge University Press, 1992); and W. George Lovell, "'Heavy Shadows and Black Night': Disease and Depopulation in Colonial Spanish America," *Annals of the Association of American Geographers* 82 (1992): 426–443.

16. See John F. Taylor, "Sociocultural Effects of Epidemics on the Northern Plains: 1734–1850," *Western Canadian Journal of Anthropology* 7 (1977): 55–81; Robert Larocques, "L'introduction de maladies européenes chez les autochtones des XVIIe et XVIIIe siècles," *Recherches amérindiennes au Québec* 12, no. 1 (1982): 13–24; Bruce Trigger, *Natives and Newcomers: Canada's 'Heroic Age' Reconsidered* (Kingston, Jamaica: McGill-Queen's University Press, 1985); J. F. Decker, 'Tracing Historical Diffusion Patterns: The Case of the 1780–82 Smallpox Epidemic among the Indians of Western Canada,' *Native Studies Review* 4 (1988): 1–24. For an excellent discussion on this topic from a Canadian perspective, see James Waldram, D. Ann Herring, and T. Kue Young, *Aboriginal Health in Canada: Historical, Cultural, and Epidemiological Perspectives* (Toronto: University of Toronto Press, 1995), 43–64.

17. See T. K. Young, *Health Care and Cultural Change: The Indian Experience in the Central Subarctic* (Toronto: University of Toronto Press, 1988).

18. For an American example, see T. Whitmore, *Disease and Death in Early Colonial America: Simulating Amerindian Depopulation* (Boulder, CO: Westview Press, 1992).

19. Sheldon Watts, *Epidemics and History: Disease, Power and Imperialism* (New Haven, CT: Yale University Press, 1997), 3–14.

20. Warwick Anderson, "Disease, Race, and Empire," *Bulletin for the History of Medicine* 70 (1996): 63.

21. Mark Harrison, "'The Tender Frame of Man': Disease, Climate, and Racial Difference in India and the West Indies," *Bulletin for the History of Medicine* 70 (1996): 68–93.
22. Philip N. Alexander, "John H Rapier, Jr and the Medical Profession in Jamaica, 1861–1862," [Part One]," *Jamaica Journal* 24 (1993): 37–46; Barry Higman, *Slave Populations of the British Caribbean, 1807–1834* (Kingston: The Press University of the West Indies, 1995); Barry Higman, *Slave Population and Economy in Jamaica, 1807–1834* (Cambridge: Cambridge University Press, 1979); Rosemarijn Hoefte, *In Place of Slavery: A Social History of British Indian and Javanese Laborers in Suriname* (Gainesville: University Press of Florida, 1998); Kenneth Kiple, *The Caribbean Slave: A Biological History* (New York: Cambridge University Press, 1984); K. O. Laurence, *A Question of Labour: Indentured Immigration into Trinidad and British Guiana 1875–1917* (Kingston, Jamaica: Ian Randle Publishers, 1994); Mark Harrison, "The Tender Frame of Man"; Brian T. Higgins and Kenneth Kiple, "Cholera in Mid-Nineteenth Century Jamaica," *Jamaican Historical Review* 17 (1991): 31–47; David Killingray, "'A New Imperial Disease': The Influenza Pandemic of 1918–1919 and Its Impact on the British Empire," in Colonialism and Health in the Tropics, eds. Jaunita De Barros and Sean Stilwell, special issue, *Caribbean Quarterly* 49, no. 4 (2003): 30–49; Kenneth Kiple, "Cholera and Race in the Caribbean," *Journal of Latin American Studies* 17 (1985): 157–177; Kenneth Kiple and Virginia Kiple, "Deficiency Diseases in the Caribbean," in *Caribbean Slave Society and Economy*, ed. Hilary Beckles and Verene Shepherd (Kingston, Jamaica: Ian Randle Publishers, 1991), 173–182; Jeffrey P. Koplan, "Slave Mortality in Nineteenth-Century Grenada," *Social Science History* 7 (1983): 311–320; K. O. Laurence, "The Development of Medical Services in British Guiana and Trinidad 1841–1873," *The Jamaica Historical Review* 4 (1964): 59–67; C. H. Senior, "Asiatic Cholera in Jamaica (1850–1855)," *Jamaica Journal* 26 (1997): 25–42; Richard Sheridan, "Mortality and the Medical Treatment of Slaves in the British West Indies," in *Caribbean Slave Society and Economy*, 197–208.
23. David Geggus, "Yellow Fever in the 1790s: The British Army in Occupied St. Domingue," *Medical History* 23 (1979): 38–58; Karol K. Weaver, *Medical Revolutionaries: The Enslaved Healers of Eighteenth-Century Saint Domingue* (Urbana-Champaign: University of Illinois Press, 2006).
24. Nancy Leys Stepan, "The Interplay Between Socio-Economic Factors and Medical Science: Yellow Fever Research, Cuba, and the United States," *Social Studies of Science* 8 (1978): 397–423; François Delaporte, *The History of Yellow Fever: An Essay on the Birth of Tropical Medicine* (Cambridge, MA: MIT Press, 1991); José López Sánchez, *Carlos Finlay: His Life and Work* (Havana, Cuba: Editorial José Martí, 1999); S. A. Anayán, "Contribución de los científicos cubanos al estudio de la epidemiología y cuadro clínico de la fiebre amarilla [Contribution of Cuban Scientists to the Study of the Epidemiology and Clinical Description of Yellow Fever]," in *Ensayos Científicos. Escritos en Homenaje a Tomás Romay* (La Habana, Cuba: Academia de Ciencias de Cuba, Museo Histórico de las Ciencias Médicas "Dr. Carlos J. Finlay," 1968), 493–508; Juan A. del Regato, "Carlos Juan Finlay (1833–1915)," *Journal of Public Health Policy* 22 (2001): 98–104. Important modern exceptions to this passionate debate, which has reached an impasse, are the following works exploring other dimensions in the rich universe of Cuban medical history: Pedro Pruna Goodgall, *La Real Academia de Ciencias de la Habana, 1861–1898* (Madrid: CeSIC, 2002); Enrique Beldarraín Chaple, *Los médicos y los inicios de la antropología en Cuba* (La Habana, Cuba: Fundación Fer-

nando Ortíz, 2006), 27–28; Reinaldo Funes Monzote, *El Asociacionismo científico en Cuba, 1868–1898* (Madrid: CeSIC, 2004); and Adrián López Denis, "Melancholia, Slavery, and Racial Pathology in Eighteenth-Century Cuba," *Science in Context* 18, no. 2 (2005): 179–199. A fine historiographical overview, now in need of updating, is Gregorio Delgado García, "Los Estudios de la Historia de la Medicina en Cuba," *Cuadernos de la Historia de la Salud* 66 (1983); and an intriguing overview is Ross Danielson, *Cuban Medicine* (New Brunswick, NJ: Transaction Press, 1979).

25. David Arnold, *Colonizing the Body: State Medicine and Epidemic Disease in Nineteenth-Century India* (Berkeley: University of California Press, 1993).

26. See also Karol Weaver, "She Crushed the Child's Fragile Scull: Disease, Infanticide, and Enslaved Women in Eighteenth-Century Saint-Domingue," *French Colonial History* 5 (2004): 93–109.

27. Considering the proportion of men who entered lunatic asylums as a result of suffering from neurosyphilis (or general paralysis of the insane), these two institutions could be seen as arising, in part, from similar problems of contested social behaviour and sexuality.

28. On this subject, see Philippa Levine, "'A Multitude of Unchaste Women': Prostitution in the British Empire," *Journal of Women's History* 15, no. 4 (2004): 159–163; and also Levine, *Prostitution, Race, and Politics: Policing Venereal Disease in the British Empire* (New York: Routledge, 2003).

29. For a discussion on the role of medicine in the construction of identity in the colonial environment, see Mary Sutphen and Bridie Andrews, eds., introduction to *Medicine and Colonial Identity* (London: Routledge, 2003).

30. See Marcos Cueto, ed., *Missionaries of Science*; Rita Pemberton, "A Different Intervention: The International Health Commission/Board, Health, Sanitation in the British Caribbean, 1914–1930," eds. Juanita De Barros and Sean Stilwell, Colonialism and Health in the Tropics, special issue, *Caribbean Quarterly* 49, no. 4 (2003): 87–103; John Farley, *To Cast Out Disease: A History of the International Health Division of the Rockefeller Foundation (1913–1951)* (New York: Oxford University Press, 2004); Anne-Emanuelle Birn, "Revolution, the Scatological Way: The Rockefeller Foundation's Hookworm Campaign in 1920s Mexico," in *Disease in the History of Modern Latin America: From Malaria to Aids*, ed. Diego Armus (Durham, NC: Duke University Press 2003), 158–182; and Birn, *Marriage of Convenience: Rockefeller International Health and Revolutionary Mexico* (Rochester: University of Rochester Press, 2006). See also Steven Palmer, "Central American Encounters with Rockefeller Public Health, 1914–1921," in *Close Encounters of Empire: Writing the Cultural History of U.S.-Latin American Relations*, ed. Gilbert Joseph, Catherine Legrand, and Ricardo Salvatore (Durham: North Carolina Press, 1998), 311–332; and Steven Palmer, "'O Demônio que se transformou em vermes': a tradução da saúde pública no Caribe Britânico, 1914–1920," *Historia, Ciencia, Saude: Manguinhos* 13, no. 3 (2006): 571–589.

31. There is an interesting parallel (and contemporaneous) debate about the alleged 'immunity' of black Africans and African Americans to suicide and mental illness. See chapters by Parle and Fearnley in John Weaver and David Wright, eds., *Suicide in the Modern Western World: Historical Perspectives* (Toronto: University of Toronto, 2008).

32. Esteban Mira Caballos, "Sanidad e Instituciones Hospitalarias en Las Antillas (1492–1550) [Health and Sanitary Institutions in the Antilles, 1492–1550]," *Asclepio* [Spain] 46 (1994): 181–196.

33. For a sample of the international literature on the history of madness, see Roy Porter and David Wright, eds., *The Confinement of the Insane: International Perspectives, 1800–1965* (Cambridge: Cambridge University Press, 2003).

34. On this subject, see Enrique Beldarraín Chaple, "Cambio y revolución: El surgimiento del sistema nacional único de salud en Cuba, 1959–1970," *Dynamis* [Spain] 25 (2005): 257–278; and Beldarraín Chaple, "La salud pública en Cuba y su experiencia internacional (1959–2005), *História, Ciências, Saúde: Manguinhos* [Brazil] 13, no. 3 (2006): 709–716.

1 "For the benefit of the planters and the benefit of Mankind"

The Struggle to Control Midwives and Obstetrics on the Island of St Croix in the Danish West Indies, 1803–1848·

Niklas Thode Jensen

As in most pre-emancipation Caribbean sugar colonies, the enslaved population in the Danish West Indies (now the US Virgin Islands) never managed to reproduce their numbers. The most important reason for the demographic decline was a staggering child mortality rate. When the Danish government abolished the slave trade in 1803, this problem could no longer be ignored because the external sources of new enslaved workers were cut off. Consequently, after the British occupation during the Napoleonic Wars (1807–1815), the Danish administration on the main island of St Croix tried to improve and expand the system of trained and authorized midwives that already existed. In this way, the administration hoped to be able to reduce the mortality among the enslaved children "for the benefit of the planters and the benefit of Mankind".[1]

In this chapter, I will examine the construction of this unique system of midwives on St Croix between the abolition of the slave trade in 1803 and the emancipation of the enslaved in the Danish West Indies in 1848. The system was based on the metropolitan Danish system of midwives trained and authorized by the government, yet it developed into a singular colonial hybrid with government-sanctioned training and authorization of enslaved women as plantation midwives. No other Caribbean colony seems to have had a similar system at that time. The examination will reveal the multiple clashes of power and culture involved in the attempt to construct the system. On one level, it sparked a struggle to gain control over births and obstetric practices among the Danish administration, the planters of mainly British stock, and the enslaved Afro-Caribbean mothers. Here, European and African cultures of midwifery and perceptions of knowledge and superstition collided. On another level, Danish and British administrative cultures of midwifery and medicine opposed each other. On yet a third level, considerations of economy intersected with attempts at humanitarian reform.

The central argument of this chapter is that in early nineteenth-century Crucian society, midwifery—and, by extension, medicine—constituted a contested field. Neither the colonial administration, nor the planters, nor the enslaved workers had complete control of practices and perceptions. Instead, the field of midwifery and medicine was the scene of a continual negotiation of power among the three parties. For instance, constant compromises had to be reached to address the regard for the plantation economy, the survival of the newborn, and the views of the enslaved.

In the historiographic perspective, this approach is new in the study of medicine in enslaved populations. Previously, the field has been dominated by demographic, social, and medical scientific approaches represented by eminent scholars like Berry Higman, Kenneth Kiple, Richard Sheridan, Richard H. Steckel, and Todd Savitt. However, these approaches have recently been expanded by Sharla Fett, in her book, *Working Cures: Healing, Health, and Power on Southern Slave Plantations*.[2] Taking my inspiration from her, I have moved the focus to the Caribbean and, at the same time, tried to fine-tune Fett's perception of "medicine as an art of resistance" into an argument for midwifery and medicine as a space of not just outright resistance, but the always unsettled negotiations of power between free and enslaved.[3]

THE DEMOGRAPHY OF THE ENSLAVED AND THE ISSUE OF CHILD- AND MATERNAL CARE

During the last three decades, a substantial amount of international scholarly research has investigated the demography of the enslaved populations in the Caribbean. This has led to a consensus that, prior to emancipation, the enslaved populations of most sugar-producing Caribbean colonies (and neighbouring sugar-producing areas) rarely managed to reproduce their numbers. The reason was high mortality connected to the rigours of sugar production, and especially to high child mortality.[4] The problem of negative demographic development was well known to planters and officials across the Caribbean from the latter half of the eighteenth century and accentuated by the abolition of the slave trade by Britain in 1807. Contemporaries discussed and tried out various measures to alleviate the problem, and as child mortality accounted for a substantial part of the excess mortality, many measures focused on child- and maternal care.

In a comparative Caribbean perspective, attempts to deal with issues of child- and maternal care were initiated on two levels: by private planters and/or by colonial governments. In the British West Indies, the private initiative seems to have dominated. Plantation doctors called for better treatment of the mothers, including improvement of maternity wards and better education of midwives, whom they generally accused of being incompetent and negligent.[5] This perception of the role of midwives vis-à-vis doctors is in line with the attitude in Great Britain, the United States, and other British colonies in the eighteenth and early nineteenth centuries, when midwives were gradually expelled from their domain by doctors who acted as man-midwives.[6] In some colonies—for instance, on Barbados—the doctors seem to have taken over the role as midwives on the plantations completely.[7] Planters also tried to increase fertility by rewarding, with gifts of money or goods, enslaved mothers who managed to keep their children alive. Other measures included reducing the workload for pregnant women and women with babies, and supplying them with special medical services, while at the same time limiting the period of breastfeeding with the aim of facilitating a new pregnancy.[8] In contrast, government initiatives appear to have been very few. Maternity wards did become statutory in Jamaica in the 1790s, but this does not seem to have had much impact on the actual number of such wards on the island.[9]

In the French West Indian colonies of Guadeloupe and Martinique, the development was somewhat different. This was possibly because of the colonial power's tradition, dating back to the eighteenth century, of maintaining a hierarchical system of state trained, authorized, and funded midwives; a "continental" tradition shared by countries like Denmark, Sweden, and the Netherlands.[10] In the French West Indies, development in the beginning of the nineteenth century was characterized by attempts to establish government training and authorization of midwives. However, these initiatives were haphazard and rarely managed to reach beyond the major cities. Significantly, it was often local doctors and surgeons who managed to block new initiatives on economic and professional grounds. It was not until the middle of the nineteenth century that the islands saw the establishment of public, stable, long-term, free, professional education and licensing of midwives. Accordingly, during the first half of the nineteenth century, the large majority of midwives in the French West Indies were still trained in the traditional fashion, and the new obstetric skills remained with the surgeons and doctors in the cities.[11]

THE DEMOGRAPHIC PROBLEM ON ST CROIX

The common pattern of a declining enslaved population manifested itself on the main sugar-producing island of St Croix in the Danish West Indies. The population regime during the years 1780 to 1804 was a one percent decline per year.[12] This negative trend continued steadily after the Danish government abolished the slave trade in 1803. By 1846, the enslaved population of the island had been reduced to 70 percent of the 1804 level, from 22,076 to 15,310 individuals. Even discounting manumissions (the formal emancipation of individuals form slavery), the demographic decline was somewhere between 1.0 and 0.5 percent a year.[13]

The reason for the negative demographic trend on St Croix was thus not manumissions, but rather a deficit of the rate of fertility to mortality. Mortality among enslaved workers on the sugar plantations was high throughout the entire period of 1803 to 1848, and the number of births never rose above the number of deaths. In 1804, the annual mortality was approximately 38 per 1,000 enslaved workers, and in 1846, it had risen to approximately 44 per 1,000 enslaved. The main cause of the elevated mortality level was a substantial child mortality rate. Up to 40 percent of all deaths were children under the age of five years, and approximately 25 percent of all deaths among children under the age of one year occurred during the first two weeks of life, which amounts to 10–15 percent of all deaths.[14]

The fertility of the enslaved population on St Croix is difficult to calculate because of a lack of data. However, the fertility does seem to have been rising slightly throughout the period from fewer than 30 births per 1,000 enslaved individuals per year in 1804 to approximately 34 births per 1,000 enslaved in 1846. In comparison, the fertility in Denmark at the same time was 30–32 births per 1,000 inhabitants. Thus, the fertility among the enslaved was not as low as claimed by many contemporaries.[15] In conclusion, the main reason for the negative demographic trend in the enslaved population of St Croix was not low fertility but rather a staggering child mortality rate.

THE SYSTEM OF MIDWIFERY IN THE DANISH WEST INDIES

In the period of 1803 to 1848, the Danish administration on the island of St Croix set out to expand and develop the system of midwives. The aim was to improve the care of the labouring enslaved women and their newborns. In theory, the system was designed like a pyramid. The top was made up of two royally appointed and state-employed midwives, one stationed in each of the towns of Christiansted and Frederiksted. This arrangement had existed since 1768, when the first two midwives received licenses as royal midwives.[16] In the hierarchy of the Danish West Indian colonial health system, the royal midwives were under of the supervision and control of the royal *landfysikus* (the royal physician). They were always trained at *Den Kongelige Fødsels- og Plejestiftelse* (the Royal Birth and Nursing Foundation) in Copenhagen and of Danish extraction. Their licenses were exact copies of midwives licenses in Denmark and thus the obligations listed in them were the same. First of all, the midwives were required to serve all the women on St Croix—the poor for free, and the wealthy at a fixed moderate rate. The enslaved were not mentioned in the licence, which is only natural, as the license was based on conditions in Denmark. However, the two royal midwives were obviously not able to serve the thousands of enslaved women on St Croix and, accordingly, the following obligation in the licence becomes of interest: " . . . to assign to themselves [i.e., the royal midwives] such local subjects whom they might find suitable and willing and whom, when in time they become sufficiently capable to pass the examination by the landfysikus, may also be allowed to practise as midwives. . . ".[17] In other words, the royal midwives were instructed to employ local women and train them in midwifery, and if the apprentices passed the examination by the landfysikus, they were allowed to work as midwives. However, apparently the royal midwives did not observe this obligation in the years prior to 1803. In that year, landfysikus Johan Mathias Frederik Keutsch (1775–1815[18]) wrote in the first medical report from the Danish West Indies that in the countryside of St Croix—i.e., on the plantations—births were only attended by old, untrained, enslaved women. To alleviate this condition, Keutsch suggested that the royal midwives, and possibly the landfysikus too, undertook the task of training six to eight enslaved women as plantation midwives.[19] Two years later, the prominent St Croix planter, Peter Lotharius Oxholm (1753–1827[20]), expanded on this view by claiming that it was these old, untrained, enslaved midwives who were responsible for the high mortality among the newborn enslaved children. According to Oxholm, the untrained plantation midwives did not do any harm in "natural births" (births without complications), but in difficult cases, they did not call the plantation doctor or a trained midwife fast enough. Furthermore, Oxholm added, the plantation midwives often tried to get the baby out by force, which caused the death of the child.[21]

The call for training of enslaved plantation midwives does not seem to have been acted upon until after the second British occupation ending in 1815 and the issuance of *Instruks for Stifts- og Landphysici* (Instructions for Physicians of Dioceses and Lands) on 4 March 1818. These instructions required that " . . . in places where no examined midwife is to be found . . ."—i.e., on the plantations—the landfysikus had to see to it that untrained midwives obtained the necessary guidance.[22] During the 1820s, the royal midwives began to apprentice young enslaved women from the plantations of St Croix.[23] The planters funded the training, and afterward, the apprentices returned to the plantations and took over as plantation midwives. The duration of the apprenticeship seems to have been two to three years, during which time the apprentice assisted the royal midwife in her daily work.[24] At the end of the apprenticeship, the royal midwife received a fee[25] and the apprentice was examined by the landfysikus and another authorized local doctor.[26] If she passed the exam, the apprentice was licensed as a plantation midwife. These trained and licensed plantation midwives came to form an intermediate stratum in the hierarchy of midwives.

Still, not all plantations got a formally trained and authorized plantation midwife—quite the contrary, in fact. In the medical reports from the 1820s and onwards, the doctors in private practice commented in unison that nearly all plantations had an enslaved woman who assisted as midwife, but that only a few of them had received formal training with royal midwives or doctors.[27] Thus, these plantation midwives without training remained the third, lowest, but numerically largest, stratum in the hierarchy of midwives.

From the years prior to 1848 there exists no precise information on how many plantation midwives there were on St Croix or what kind of training they had received. However, a register from 1852 shows that

in the western jurisdiction of Frederiksted (comprising town and plantations), there were twenty-five midwives, four of whom were trained by a
royal midwife or doctor.[28] A comparable register from 1864 shows that in
the central district of the island (Kingshill), there were eight plantations
with midwives trained and examined by royal midwives and licensed doctors, twenty-nine plantations with midwives without formal training, and
thirty-eight plantations with no midwife at all. Finally, a third register
from the same year shows that in the eastern town of Christiansted, there
were four midwives examined by doctors, and in the country district of
Christiansted, there were a total of eleven plantation midwives, none of
whom was formally trained.[29] Based on this evidence, it is clear that, in
the years following emancipation, only about one-fifth of all plantation
midwives in the three districts of St Croix had received formal training
or been examined. As previously mentioned, the medical reports from the
doctors in private practice do not give reason to believe that the situation
was any better before the emancipation.

In 1826, the interim landfysikus, Poul Elias Wintmöhl Schlegel (1784–
1849[30]), noted in his medical report that the planters were less inclined
than before to apprentice their bondswomen to the royal midwives. In
Schlegel's opinion, legislation would not have any effect but he called
for the state-owned or so-called 'royal' plantations (about 10 percent of
all plantations on St Croix) to make a good example by sending their
enslaved midwives for training.[31] To what extent the private leasers of
the royal plantations followed this example is not clear, yet it is certain
that some of the royal plantations had an enslaved woman registered
as a "midwife".[32] Thus, she was not just an ordinary "sick nurse", who
could be found at any plantation hospital. However, only a few of the
midwives on the royal plantations were formally trained.[33]

Many reasons can be suggested for the decreasing number of apprentices with the royal midwives. However, in view of the fact that in
the period of 1820 to 1848, the plantations on St Croix suffered from
increasing economic strain due to bad harvests, falling prices of sugar,
and lack of manpower, the planters had strong economic motives to keep
all hands on the plantation and save the fee of having a royal midwife.
Yet, the planters' expenses from having one enslaved woman trained and
examined were negligible compared to what they spent each year on doctors bills, the plantation hospital, and other health-related expenses.[34]
Naturally, it was cheaper in the short run to neglect the training of a
midwife and carry on the tradition of relying on the experience of old
enslaved women—especially since no law forbade it. Another contributing cause might have been problems making the enslaved women accept
the European birth practices introduced by the trained midwives. Later,
we will see that these practices of European obstetric science opposed
the enslaved women's traditional notions of taboos and rites of passage
during labour.

On plantations that did not have a midwife at all, there were several ways to acquire one. If the plantation was situated near one of the towns, the royal midwife could be called in. A cheaper alternative was to fetch one of the free coloured women in town, who seem to have pursued midwifery as a side business.[35] A third possibility was to rent or borrow a midwife from a neighbouring plantation in the same way that planters rented or borrowed enslaved men trained in various trades.[36] In the very few instances when this rented plantation midwife was trained, she often conducted midwifery on several plantations in the neighbourhood.[37] The use of external midwives is revealed in account books from several plantations. It is not possible to discern if the midwives in question were royal midwives or plantation midwives from the neighbouring plantations, but the latter case is the most likely. Only very rarely do the accounts show a doctor functioning as "accoucheur" (man-midwife) among the enslaved.[38]

Concerning the royal plantations, it is curious that the government body in charge of them, the *Likvidationskommissionen* (the Liquidation Commission), did not heed Schlegel's call to make a good example of them by stipulating a demand for training and examination of plantation midwives in the lease contract. In fact, the reproductive field is absolutely absent in the lease contracts and regulations in spite of the administration's interest in the field in these years. Other approaches in the reproductive field that the Likvidationskommissionen might have tried in order to improve the fertility and the survival of the newborn was, for instance, to reward the mothers by reducing their workload or by giving them gifts of money. In the last years of the 1820s, one lieutenant Brady described the use of this reward system on private plantations on St Croix:

> At births and deaths, the families in which they occur generally receive about ten pounds of sugar and two gallons of rum. At [Estate Mannings Bay] and upon some other estates, lying-in women receive two bottles of Madeira wine, and other comforts.[39]

It is not clear how common it was to reward enslaved mothers, but it does not seem to have been practiced on the royal plantations.

THE DANISH MODEL

Based on the previous section it is evident that the local colonial administration's attempts to structure the system of midwifery in the Danish West Indies were modeled on the system in Denmark. In the period of 1803 to 1848, the metropolitan Danish system of midwifery developed into a finely meshed and efficient system, which covered all of Denmark and had significant impact on the lowering of neonatal mortality. The system was based on the Midwife Ordinance of 21 November 1810, which applied to the kingdom of Denmark (and to the kingdom of Norway until its independence from Denmark in 1814) but not to the Danish West Indies. Following this ordinance, Denmark was subdivided into midwife districts, with one royal midwife in each district. In 1850, there were 686 such districts in Denmark outside Copenhagen.[40] All state-employed royal midwives were trained at the Royal Birth and Nursing Foundation in Copenhagen, but if no trained midwife were to be found in a district, a local woman could be trained and authorized by the local landfysikus. This midwife was then put in charge of midwifery in the district while another local woman was sent to Copenhagen for training. If a labouring woman chose to use an unauthorized midwife, she still had to pay a fixed salary to the royal midwife in the district. Finally, in cases of difficult labour, the state midwife was obliged to call for the landfysikus.[41] Accordingly, the formal and traditional role of Danish doctors was to supervise the midwives, not to act as man-midwives.[42] On St Croix, one can recognize the hierarchy of the Danish system in the division between the Danish-trained, state-employed royal midwives; the locally trained and licensed plantation midwives (enslaved women); and the untrained plantation midwives (enslaved women). But in contrast to the situation in Denmark—where the trained, state-employed midwives seem to have gradually replaced the untrained midwives by the first half of the nineteenth century[43]—the situation on St Croix does not seem to have changed after 1826. Neither the number of Danish trained and state–employed midwives on the island, nor the number of locally trained and licensed plantation midwives, seem to have increased.

MIDWIVES, DOCTORS, AND ADMINISTRATION: CONFLICTS OF KNOWLEDGE, TRAINING, AND ECONOMY

In spite of their privileged position, the royal midwives did not have a legally sanctioned monopoly on midwifery. This created problems from the very beginning, as is visible from the fact that the royal midwives accused the enslaved, unauthorized plantation midwives and free coloured midwives of stealing their customers.[44] As an example, the royal midwives Madam Biørn (in Christiansted) and Madam Clark (in Frederiksted) complained in 1815 to the local government that Afro-Caribbean women conducted midwifery without authorization.[45] The government rejected the complaint and declared in an ordinance of 9 December 1815 that, since it was impossible for the two royal midwives to conduct all births on the island, other authorized midwives were permitted to set up businesses on the island and subject themselves to licensing for practice.[46] The authorized midwives referred to by the government were probably midwives that might arrive from Denmark, but to Danish midwives, only the positions as royal midwives were economically attractive. In 1820, the government reminded the doctors of their duty to supervise all midwives[47] and to report if their behaviour gave reason for complaint.[48] Finally, in 1821, the government stressed that midwives were only allowed to practice if they had passed examination by the landfysikus or another local authorized doctor.[49] These regulations seem to have been aimed primarily at the unexamined free coloured midwives who, however, did not change their behaviour. They practiced in the towns and were thus the closest competitors in the royal midwives' primary market. Despite the government's attempts, the problems continued. In 1835, a new complaint was filed by the royal midwife in Christiansted concerning unauthorized persons practicing midwifery.[50] In 1837, landfysikus Schlegel proposed a new procedure to control the practice of the plantation midwives. His idea was to put the plantation doctors in charge of issuing written certificates documenting the practical skills of plantation midwives and who had been responsible for their training. If the certificate was recommending, the landfysikus could issue an authorization to practice on plantations other than the one where the midwife was living.[51] However, the proposal was not approved.

As is evident from the above discussion of the system of midwifery in the Danish West Indies, the problem was not the issue of finding a midwife, but the knowledge she had, or rather, did not have. Most of the doctors did not entertain the slightest confidence in the skills of the plantation midwives and described them as generally ignorant of obstetrics because only few of them had received formal training.[52] In 1829, for instance, the interim landfysikus, William Stephen Jacobs (1779–1843[53]), made a powerful expression of this attitude in his medical report:

> . . . The state of midwifery on estates is miserable, very few having been instructed. I frequently attend with the Danish midwifes in difficult and tedious cases, and I have the same fault to find with them all, which is, that they are always in a hurry, and anxious to have the business terminated, and are too desirous of having instruments used, when only a little patience is necessary.[54]

In addition to this alleged ignorance, the plantation midwives kept stubbornly to their own traditional knowledge and practice, and they were unwilling to listen to the exhortations of the plantation doctors.[55] The doctors' critique was not, however, founded only on strictly professional concerns. Many of them were themselves "accoucheurs" with the wealthy Euro-Caribbean citizens in accordance with British traditions.[56] In other words, there were aspects of professional and economic competition between the doctors and the entire group of midwives. By contrast, the relationship between doctors and midwives in Denmark was much better. This was because legislation and tradition separated the domains of doctors and midwives, and the state controlled the professional skills of both groups. Because there were many more midwives than doctors in the Danish countryside, and because the midwives enjoyed the trust of the locals, the doctors were forced to maintain a good relationship with the midwives.[57]

To counter the dangerous situations that might occur due to their lack of training, the plantation midwives were instructed to call for the plantation doctor, another accoucheur (doctor), or the royal midwife in the event of problems during labour.[58] This was in accordance with the abovementioned instructions for physicians of Dioceses and Lands in Denmark, which demanded that all midwives seek the help of a doctor if a difficult labour arose.[59] However, calling the doctor was generally the last resort to prevent mother and child from dying. The special means that only the doctor had at his disposal was, first, his knowledge of how to turn the baby manually. Second, he had a range of instruments, which the midwives were not allowed to use, such as instruments for delivery by forceps, surgical removal of the child through the birth passage and, as a last resort, caesarean section.[60] The first known incidence of caesarean section on St Croix was performed by landfysikus Schlegel on an enslaved woman named Sophia in 1821.[61] Third, the doctor had at his disposal pharmaceuticals like *Secale cornutum*, which causes uterine contractions.[62] The labouring enslaved women were aware of the effect of *Secale* and asked for the drug if they felt the labour took too long.[63]

As previously mentioned, the idea of lowering neonatal mortality through improvements in the standard of the plantation midwives had existed since it was proposed by Keutsch and Oxholm at the beginning of the nineteenth century. Since then, the administration had tried to 'raise the standard' by having apprentices trained in the art of midwifery. However, the success was limited. It was not until 1832 that the administration turned the idea into a real plan for action. On 4 February of that year, Governor General Peter von Scholten (1784–1854) sent a memorandum to landfysikus Schlegel which contained a draft for a new ordinance employing ten new examined midwives on St Croix. Von Scholten explained the reason for the draft in this way:

> I will only point to one reason for this decrease [in the enslaved population], which we have been taught from experience, namely the death of the Negro children in the first 9 days after birth. The reason for this seems to be the bad midwives who, with only a few exceptions, are employed at the plantations . . . [64]

Accordingly, the purpose of the draft was to stop the decrease in the enslaved population by lowering the neonatal and infant mortality rates. The task of the new examined midwives was to strengthen the supervision of the labouring women on the plantations and to increase the knowledge of obstetrics through educating the plantation midwives and enslaved women. Because the government was not able to pay a salary substantial enough to attract midwives from Denmark, von Scholten wanted to select ten Afro-Caribbean women, presumably free coloured women, and send them for a 1-year internship at the Royal Birth and Nursing Foundation in Copenhagen. After their exam, the ten midwives were to return to their new positions in the Cruzian countryside.[65] Von Scholten's draft shows that, at this time, if not earlier, the administration was aware of the potential importance of educated midwives. The draft also demonstrates that the administration was not focusing on the long-standing and popular Euro-Caribbean presumption that it was the promiscuity and self-inflicted venereal diseases of the enslaved that caused the decrease in the population.

However, nothing came of von Scholten's draft. An analysis of the apprentices at the Royal Birth and Nursing Foundation in Copenhagen shows that, in the period of 1806 to 1848, only one woman from the Danish West Indies was admitted, and she was of Danish extraction.[66] The main reason why the draft was not made into an ordinance seems to have been that it was economically inconvenient at the time. According to a memorandum from landfysikus Schlegel dated 1837, the plantation owners were unable to pay the additional tax on each slave, which was the economic basis of von Scholten's draft. Furthermore, Schlegel pointed out, because of the emancipation of the enslaved in the British West Indies in 1834, the enslaved population in the Danish West Indies would also have to be emancipated within the foreseeable future. As it was unlikely that the ex-enslaved would be able to afford to pay for the services of trained midwives, and thus maintain a new elaborate system of midwives, Schlegel advised against the idea. In addition to these economic arguments, Schlegel also stated a number of other reasons in support of the existing, time-honoured system of plantation midwives. First, he claimed that cases of difficult labour were rare on St Croix due to the warm climate; when they occurred, all the plantations had a doctor on contract who could be called in. Second, Schlegel claimed that tetanus among newborns was not as common as it had been previously, and that this was due to the fact that the system of midwifery was working quite well. Finally, he noted that the plantation midwives had the confidence of the enslaved women, which the royal midwives did not.[67] Thus, he hinted that midwives trained in European obstetrics might not be accepted by the enslaved women. In conclusion, Schlegel was of the opinion that, even if the system of midwifery was not perfect, it was adequate.

About ten years later, in 1846, the thought of improving the training of midwives re-emerged. This time it was the doctor of the garrison in Frederiksted, Rasmus Pedersen Worm (1786–1863[68]), who used his annual medical report to complain about the ignorance of the plantation midwives. He claimed that he was often called out to cases of labouring women, which any trained midwife would have been able to handle on her own. Therefore, and "for the benefit of the planters and the benefit of Mankind", he called for more trained midwives on the island.[69]

Based on the statements by von Scholten, Keutsch, Worm, Schlegel, and Jacobs, a picture emerges of three conflicting views among doctors and the administration as to how the system of midwifery was to be structured. Von Scholten, as a representative of the administration, and Keutsch and Worm as representatives of both administration and state doctors, were all in favour of the 'Danish' model—the training of midwives to take care of births on the plantations. Schlegel, who as landfysikus was both a doctor and member of the administration, positioned himself in a pragmatic middle, inasmuch as he found the existing system to be time-honoured and difficult to change due to the weak economy. Finally, the substitute landfysikus Jacobs expressed the opinion of the majority of the doctors on the island, namely that the plantation midwives were incompetent. Training or improvement was not an issue at all. Seen on the basis of the national affiliation, which Jacobs himself and the majority of the doctors on St Croix had to the Anglo-Saxon world (Britain, its colonies, and the United States), and the disdain with which doctors in this world regarded midwives at the time, it is no wonder that many of the doctors shared this view. Jacobs' temporary position as landfysikus did not change his opinion of midwives. It is no greater wonder that von Scholten and the doctors trained in Denmark and employed by the administration showed the same attitude as the medical establishment in Denmark, namely that midwives ought to be trained. More interesting is landfysikus Schlegel's middling position. As the premier officer in the medical hierarchy of the colonial administration, and as a doctor trained in Denmark, one would have expected him to support the 'Danish' model. However, he chose a pragmatic line. As mentioned earlier, the reason was primarily the economy, yet it may also have been a matter of responsibility. As landfysikus, Schlegel was himself responsible for the proper functioning of the midwifery system.

In the end, the administration shelved the question of improving the system of midwifery. The reason for this reticence following the draft of 1832 may be found—if we are to believe Schlegel's account—in the events that took place in the year 1834. This was the year of emancipation in the British West Indies, and the administration in the Danish West Indies could no longer harbour any doubt that something similar would take place in the Danish islands sooner or later. The only question was how long the emancipation could be postponed before the enslaved revolted. The administration needed time to study the British example and to see what happened afterwards so as to be better prepared for emancipation and to minimize the economic damages.[70] In this situation, it was not opportune, as Schlegel remarked in 1837, to experiment with costly improvements to the system of midwives, which in all probability could not be maintained after emancipation. This was especially the case since the economy of the plantations was ailing. However, Schlegel's suggestions for almost cost-free improvements of the existing system do not seem to have been heeded either.[71]

THE STRUGGLE OVER BIRTHS:
ENSLAVED 'SUPERSTITION' VERSUS DOCTORAL 'SCIENCE'

Descriptions of practices surrounding births and midwifery among the enslaved population on St Croix are rare. However, in the first medical report from the Danish West Indies, dated 1803, some of the doctors on the island described the 'superstition' in the reproductive field, which they claimed existed among the enslaved.[72] As mentioned earlier, child mortality among the enslaved, including neonatal and infant mortality, was staggering, and through the entire period doctors consistently pointed to lockjaw (*tetanus neonatorum, trismus nascentium*) as the most important cause.[73] In the medical report of 1803, Drs William Stedman (1764–1844[74]) and Hugh Morris Lang (1779–1864[75]) listed three possible causes for "nine day lock jaw", i.e., deaths among newborns caused by tetanus in the first nine days after birth: retention of meconium (child's first stools), wrong treatment of the umbilical cord, and polluted air. According to Stedman and Lang, the first factor was immaterial because all plantation midwives gave the newborn an enema of castor oil. The second factor was far more serious because of the 'superstition' connected to the umbilical cord. Stedman and Lang claimed that, normally, the plantation midwives did not examine the umbilical cord until the seventh or eighth day after birth, which was the reason why the cord generally became infected and caused nine-day lockjaw. To this can be added landfysikus J.M.F. Keutsch's description from the same medical report:

> . . . the Negroes' nasty habit of binding the umbilicus with a thick and long string, wrapping it in a large piece of coarse linen and afterwards binding one maybe two coarse umbilicus-cloths around the child's abdomen as tight as possible, must absolutely cause the umbilicus to become squeezed, the tissue irritated and inflamed. . . [76]

Landfysikus Keutsch considered this treatment of the umbilical cord to be wrong, and the sole reason for the tetanus deaths. Since it was not possible to treat tetanus effectively, he asserted that one should try to prevent tetanus by bathing the child every day and gently dressing the umbilicus. However, it was even more important to try to educate the enslaved midwives. Only through them could the treatment of the children be improved.

To Stedman and Lang, the third factor was also connected to the 'superstition' of the enslaved. They explained that:

> . . . it is a common practice among Negroes not to allow the smallest particle of free air to be admitted into the chamber of a lying-in woman for 4 or 5 days after delivery . . . That impure air is one of the most frequent causes of this complaint we are led to believe from many circumstances.[77]

To remove the impure air (miasma), Stedman and Lang recommended that all planters build a special airy maternity ward where the children could be bathed in cold water every day. These procedures had been tested with great success on one of the plantations where they attended as plantation doctors.[78]

The occurrence of such maternity wards on the plantations seems to have become more common during the 1820s and 1830s. When new plantation hospitals were constructed, a maternity ward was often added. However, it cannot be said that this was a general trend.[79] This description of the situation is supported by the previously mentioned lieutenant Brady, who in the late 1820s, described how births on some plantations took place in maternity wards and on others in the house of the labouring woman.[80] Whether labouring women also gave birth in plantation hospitals without maternity wards is not certain, but in any case, the labouring women do not seem to have spent their maternity leave before and after the birth there. It appears that after the birth they were relieved from work for 3–6 weeks, during which time they stayed in their own houses.[81]

Despite the new maternity wards and the good intentions of the doctors, it seems to have been difficult to make the enslaved women change their ways and use the new facilities. In the previously mentioned article by Oxholm from 1805, he explains that when the planters forced the enslaved women to abandon the tightly sealed slave houses or huts, they became "dissatisfied"[82], and only slowly did they change their habits.[83] This resistance on the part of the enslaved women is especially interesting because the reactions of the enslaved to the government or private health initiatives concerning them are rarely visible in the existing source material. The enslaved women's dissatisfaction with their removal from the closed houses or huts is understandable in light of how the enslaved understood the newborn child. In his book, *Various Remarks Collected on and about the Island of St. Croix in America* (1788), Dr Johan Christian Schmidt (1728–1807) explained that the enslaved were afraid their newborn would be stolen or eaten by witches. If a witch had the opportunity to look into the eyes of the child during the first eight days after birth, she could steal its breath and thus kill it.[84] This was possibly the reason why the house or hut had to be locked tight for the first nine days after birth. Another explanation with similar features comes from twentieth-century West Africa (the Akan tribe of Ghana, amongst others), which was the ancestral home of many enslaved in the Danish West Indies. Here, the newborn was perceived as belonging to the spirit world for eight to nine days after birth and thus as ritually non-existent. Not until nine days had passed were the newborns counted among humans, and if the child died before then, it had never existed.[85] In other words, there seem to have been perceptions of childbirth both in West Africa and among the slaves on St Croix in the period just prior to the period 1803–48, which included a tabooed rite of passage lasting about nine days. The previous quotation from Stedman and Lang shows that a similar perception still existed in the period from 1803 to

1848. The clash between this magico-religious perception of birth and the newborn child on one side and the physiological European perception of the diseases of the newborn and the treatment of nine-day lockjaw on the other were inevitable.

Judging from the evidence above, it appears to have been necessary for the planters, at least initially, to force the enslaved women to use the maternity wards. By depositing the women in the ward, they achieved two goals: to remove the labouring women from the village of the enslaved, where 'superstition' allegedly ruled with destructive force; and to obtain the conditions and facilities for treatment demanded by the doctors. In addition, it became easier for doctors and managers to monitor and control both the pregnant and labouring enslaved women and the suspicious activities of the plantation midwives. On this basis, it is possible to view enslaved births as a field in which a conflict between an Afro-Caribbean and a European perception and practice of health played out. As mentioned earlier, this conflict was not confined exclusively to the maternity wards, but also took place between the European doctors and royal midwives on one side, and the suspicious unexamined midwives in alliance with the labouring women on the other. Judging from the slowly increasing number of maternity wards on the plantations, it would appear plausible that the victor in this struggle was the doctors, and by extension, European medical science. However, as the unexamined plantation midwife was still in charge of the majority of births among the enslaved, it is not evident that the practices surrounding births became European because some enslaved women were removed to maternity wards.

From this perspective, it is possible to perceive the resistance of the enslaved women to the European conception and practice of birth as a part of a negotiation of power in which none of the parties were in charge, but all engaged in a continuous process of compromises and changes. The planter and the plantation doctor could decide the location of the birth, but the content—the practice—was far more difficult to control. Ideally, it required the plantation doctor to be in charge of the birth itself, and for this to happen, he had to transcend the taboos of the enslaved surrounding confinement. If relocation of labouring women to the well-ventilated maternity ward could create "dissatisfaction", it is beyond doubt that the doctor's takeover of the birth itself could create a high degree of "dissatisfaction", not just among the labouring women, but also among the entire enslaved population at the plantation. Notwithstanding the planters' economic calculations in relation to the doctor's salary, the risk of unrest may have been a significant reason why the plantation doctors did not take over the domain of the plantation midwives. The number of doctors on St Croix was in fact large enough to make this scenario possible; nonetheless, it did not happen.[86] To avoid making the enslaved population even more uncooperative and sabotaging, it was in the interest of the manager to send for the doctor only when there was no other alternative to both mother and child dying. In other words, a compromise had to be established between the regard for the economy of the plantation, the survival of the newborn, and the views of the enslaved.

Such a compromise could have been personified by the trained and examined plantation midwife. As she was both an enslaved woman who was known by the locals, and trained in European obstetrics, she could potentially mediate the tensions between the norms of the doctors and the planter on one side and those of the enslaved on the other surrounding births.[87] However, as previously mentioned there were very few of these trained plantation midwives. This might have been due to the economic strategy of the planters or due to the fact that not even the trained plantation midwives had an easy job being accepted by their enslaved sisters.

CONCLUSION

The system of midwives on St Croix is central to answering the question of what the Danish colonial administration did to maintain and improve the health of the enslaved population. In the period from 1803 to 1848, the administration tried to expand and improve the hierarchical system of midwifery in the Danish West Indies in an effort to lower child mortality. The model for both the design and the improvements was the successful system of midwives in Denmark. However, the efforts of the colonial administration were not successful, presumably because they were not supported by legislation. Training and examination of plantation midwives seem to have been ruled out in the economic strategies of the planters, possibly due to problems with the integration of the European birth practices of the trained midwives into the cultural norms of the enslaved. Governor General Peter von Scholten's proposal to train district midwives foundered on a bad financial situation in the 1830s and on the foreseeable emancipation of the enslaved. Accordingly, it was not because the administration failed to see the possible advantages in an efficient system of midwifery. Von Scholten's draft shows that the colonial administration was aware of the connection between child mortality and the negative development in the enslaved population. Thus, the importance of this field was not neglected because of the common perception that the declining population was due to the promiscuity of the enslaved.

Because the administration's initiatives foundered, the untrained plantation midwives remained in charge of large parts of the system of midwifery. Among the untrained midwives, the doctors, and the royal midwives there existed several related conflicts of interest: an economic competition, a professional antagonism, and a related cultural opposition. The doctors' critique of the plantation midwives' lacking abilities was not just a sign of professional egotism and jealousy, but also of the cultural antagonisms between the doctors and the Danish royal midwives on one hand and, the Afro-Caribbean plantation midwives on the other. Between the royal midwives and the plantation midwives, the cultural antagonisms expressed themselves in the enslaved women's lack of confidence in the former and confidence in the latter. The plantation midwife was part of the same Afro-Caribbean culture as the labouring women and she knew the traditional practices and the English–Creole language. Conversely, the royal midwives were both culturally and linguistically foreign in the world of the enslaved. Accordingly, the enslaved women's trust in their conduct of something as intimate as births almost inevitably had to be low.

The enslaved women's distrust of the royal midwives was met with a similar professional and cultural distrust by the doctors. They criticized the birth practices of the enslaved as being rife with harmful superstition, which produced increased child mortality and thus had a negative effect on the important development of the enslaved population. The doctors wanted the births of the enslaved to be subject to European medical practices and thus under the supervision of the doctors themselves. To achieve this, the enslaved women in labour were moved to special maternity wards. The existence of such wards in some plantation hospitals may indicate that the doctors were successful in this conflict between the two perceptions of health over the control of the place of birth. However, the birth itself was generally conducted by uneducated plantation midwives. The reason for this was not just economic considerations, but also the "dissatisfaction" in the enslaved population which might result from the doctor taking over the domain of birth.

In conclusion, this case study of midwives and midwifery on the island of St Croix sheds new light on the continuous negotiation of power between the three parties in Danish West Indian society: the administration, the planters, and the enslaved. These negotiations reveal that the reproductive health of the enslaved was not just influenced by considerations of economy and humanitarian reform, but involved strategies of power and control.

NOTES

* This chapter is a translated and edited version of a chapter in the author's PhD thesis titled, *"For the Health of the Enslaved. Disease, Health and the Effects of the Health Policy of the Colonial Administration of the Danish West Indies, 1803–1848 Among Plantation Slaves on St. Croix"*. The PhD was funded by the Danish Government Council of the Humanities (*Forskningsrådet for Kultur and Kommunikation*) and approved by the Department of History at the University of Copenhagen in October 2006.

1. Board of Health (BH), Medical reports (Med. rep.), Danish West Indies (DWI), no. 1252,1846, Danish National Archive (DNA). Original text in Danish.

2. Sharla Fett, *Working Cures: Healing, Health, and Power on Southern Slave Plantations* (Chapel Hill: University of North Carolina Press, 2002), 1–12.

3. Ibid., x.

4. For instance, Barry W. Higman, *Slave Populations of the British Caribbean, 1807–1834* (Baltimore, MD: Johns Hopkins University Press, 1984), 72–76, 307–311, 324–329, 374–375; Geneviève Leti, *Santé et société esclavagiste à la Martinique, 1802–1848* (Paris: L'Harmattan, 1998), 7–9, 23–30; Alex van Stipriaan, *Surinaams Contrast, Roofbouw en overleven in een Caraïbische plantagekolonie, 1750–1863* (Leiden, Netherlands: Koninklijk Instituut voor taal-, land- en volkenkunde, 1993), 316–318; Michael Tadman, "The Demographic Cost of Sugar: Debate on Slave Societies and Natural Increase in the Americas," *The American Historical Review* 105, no. 5 (2000): 1534–1575.

5. Barbara Bush, *Slave Women in Caribbean Society, 1650–1838* (London: James Curry Ltd, 1990), 135; Richard Sheridan, *Doctors and Slaves. A Medical and Demographic History of Slavery in the British West Indies, 1680–1834* (Cambridge: Cambridge University Press, 1985), 230; David Collins, *Practical Rules for the Management and Medical Treatment of Negro Slaves in the Sugar Colonies* (London, Vernor, Hood and Sharp 1811; New York: Books for Libraries Press, 1971;), 137–138. Citations are to the 1971 edition.

6. Harriet Deacon, "Midwives and Medical Men in the Cape Colony before 1860," *Journal of African History* 39 (1998): 271–292, 272–274.

7. Higman, *Slave Populations*, 262.

8. Ibid., 349.

9. Ibid., 352.

10. Irvine Loudon, *Death in Childbirth. An International Study of Maternal Care and Maternal Mortality, 1800–1950* (Oxford: Clarendon Press, 1992), 398–427.

11. Marie-Antoinette Menier, "Hommes sages contre sages-femmes à la Guadeloupe (1829–1842)," *Bulletin de la Societé d'Historie de la Guadeloupe* 87–90 (1991): 3–31, 4–5, 12, 23, 26–27; Leti, *Santé et société*, 84–87.

12. Svend E. Green-Pedersen, "Slave Demography in the Danish West Indies and the Abolition of the Danish Slave Trade," in *The Abolition of the Atlantic Slave Trade. Origins and Effects in Europe, Africa, and the Americas*, eds. David Eltis and James Walvin (Madison: University of Wisconsin Press, 1981), 234–235, 238–239.

13. Jesper Bering Asmussen, "Slavedemografi. St. Croix' Landdistrikter, 1803–1848" (master's thesis, University of Aarhus, 1983), 35–36. Asmussen's unpublished results correspond to results published by Hans Christian Johansen, yet they are more precise because Asmussen is only dealing with St. Croix. See Hans Christian Johansen, "Slave Demography of the Danish West Indian Islands," *The Scandinavian Economic History Review* 29 (1981): 1–20.

14. Asmussen, "Slavedemografi," 53, 58–59, 61.

15. Ibid., 66–67, 69.

16. West Indian Local Archives (WILA), box no. 3.40, Register of instructions, 1723–1784, DNA.

17. WILA, box no. 3.40, DNA. Original text in Danish.

18. Kristian Carøe, *Den Danske lægestand, 1479–1900.* (Copenhagen: Gyldendal, 1977), III: 107; V: 80.

19. Danish Chancellery (DC), Common Department, Commission concerning an ordinance about the medical police 1803–1814, Incoming cases, negotiations and correspondence, box no. G125C, DNA (hereafter called DC, box no. G125C, DNA).

20. Carl Frederik Bricka, *Dansk biografisk Lexikon.* (Copenhagen: Gyldendalske Boghandels Forlag, 1887–1905), 12: 507–508.

21. Peter Lotharius Oxholm, *Nogle Anmærkninger over en Afhandling om Negerhandelens Ophævelse udi Maanedsskriftet Minerva af Februarii 1805* (Copenhagen, n.p. 1806), 27.

22. Jacob Henrie Schou, *Chronologisk Register over de Kongelige forordninger og Aabne Breve, samt andre trykte anordninger, som fra Aar 1670 af ere udkomne, tiligemed et nøiagtigt udtog af de endnu gieldende, for saavidt samme i Almindelighed angaae Undersaatterne i Danmark og Norge, forsyndet med et alphabetisk Register* (Copenhagen, n.p. 1823), section XVIII, 38. Original text in Danish.
23. BH, Med. rep., DWI, 1826, DNA.
24. BH, Med. rep., DWI, 1837, DNA.
25. WILA, box no. 10.2.1., 31 May 1837, DNA. The direction of the state debt and the sinking fund, archive no. 423, DNA (hereafter DSD, DNA). Estate Longford, 1828, box no. 1129
26. BH, Med. rep., DWI, 1826, 1844, DNA.
27. BH, Med. rep., DWI, 1825, 1826, 1828, 1829, 1830, 1834, 1835, 1836, 1837, 1838, 1844, 1846, DNA.
28. Records of the Government of the Virgin Islands, the former Danish West Indies, 1672–1917, entry 82, box 220, Record Group (RG) 55, National Archives and Records Administration (NARA) (hereafter RG55, NARA).
29. Entry 82, box 319, RG55, NARA.
30. Carøe, *Den Danske lægestand*, III: 180; Ibid., V: 92.
31. BH, Med. rep., DWI, 1826, DNA.
32. WILA, box no. 46.21, Estate Retreat, 1839, DNA. WILA, box no. 46.21, Estate Work & Rest, 1833, DNA. WILA, box no. 46.17.45, Estate Longford, 1843, 1846, DNA. WILA, box no. 46.17.32, Estate Hermon Hill, 1835, DNA. Entry 1109, box 2435, Estate Jolly Hill, 1840, RG55, NARA. BH, Med. rep., DWI, 1826, DNA; appendix to the medical report by landfysikus Schlegel.
33. DSD, box no. 1129, Estate Longford, 1828, DNA. WILA, box no. 46.17.32, Estate Hermon Hill, 1835, DNA.
34. DSD, box no. 1129, Accounts for 1828, DNA.
35. BH, Med. rep., DWI, 1839, 1842, 1846, DNA.
36. BH, Med. rep., DWI, 1825, 1826, DNA.
37. BH, Med. rep., DWI, 1844, DNA.
38. Entry 1109, box 2438, Estate Mount Victory, 1828, RG55, NARA.
39. Arnold R. Highfield, ed., *Observations Upon the State of Negro Slavery in the Island of Santa Cruz. The Principal of the Danish West India Colonies With Miscellaneous Remarks Upon Subjects Relating to the West India Question and a Notice of Santa Cruz* (London: Simpkin & Marshall & Longman Reid & Co., 1829; Christiansted St. Croix: Antilles Press, 1996), 13. Citations are to the 1996 edition.
40. Anne Løkke, "Did Midwives Matter? 1787–1845," in *Pathways of the Past. Essays in Honour of Sølvi Sogner*, ed. Hilde Sandvik, Kari Telste, Gunnar Thorvaldsen (Oslo: Novus Forlag, 2002), 71–72.
41. Christian Poulsen Nørbom Petersen, *Den Danske Medicinal-Lovgivning eller samling af de forordninger, placater, kongelige rescripter og resolutioner, reglementer, instruxer, fundatser, collegialbreve og andre offentlige aktstykker, som vedkomme læger, apothekere og gjordemødre i Danmark*. 3 vols. (Copenhagen: J. H. Schubothe, 1833), 1: 81–89.
42. Nick Nyland, *De praktiserende læger i Danmark, 1800–1910. Træk af det historiske grundlag for almen medicin* (Odense: University of Southern Denmark, 2000), 247.
43. Løkke, "Did Midwives Matter?" 61–66.
44. WILA, box no. 3.30, Pro Memoria by midwife A.C. Lindefield in Christiansted, 1786, DNA.
45. WILA, box no. 2.2.1, DNA; WILA, box no. 2.16.5, DNA.

46. WILA, box no. 2.1.6, p. 634.
47. WILA, box no. 3.18.1, 1820: document no. 59.
48. WILA, box no. 10.2.1, 26 October 1821.
49. WILA, box no. 3.18.1, 1821: document no. 15.
50. WILA, box no. 10.2.1, 23 January 1835.
51. WILA, box no. 10.2.1, 31 May 1837.
52. BH, Med. rep., DWI, 1825, 1828, DNA.
53. Carøe, *Den Danske lægestand*, III: 98; Ibid., V: 79.
54. BH, Med. rep., DWI, 1829, DNA. Original text in English.
55. BH, Med. rep., DWI, 1834, DNA.
56. WILA, box no. 10.2.1., Draft from landfysikus Schlegel, 31 May 1837, DNA.
57. Nyland, *De praktiserende læger*, 247–249.
58. BH, Med. rep., DWI, 1834, 1836, 1838, DNA.
59. Schou, *Chronologisk Register*, section XVIII, 38.
60. BH, Med. rep., DWI, 1832, 1834, 1842, 1843, DNA.
61. Poul Schlegel, "Beskrivelse af en Sectio Cæsarea foretaget paa negerinden Sophia paa St. Croix i Christiansstæds Bye d. 6te Febr. 1821,"*Bibliothek for Læger* 3 (1823): 140–149.
62. *Secale cornutum* is also called ergot (fungus in rye) and contains ergotamine, a powerful toxin that causes muscle contractions.
63. BH, Med. rep., DWI, 1842, DNA.
64. WILA, box no. 10.2.1., DNA. Original text in Danish.
65. WILA, box no. 10.2.1., DNA.
66. The Royal Birth and Nursing Foundation. Copybook of matron's instructions and a protocol on apprentices, 1806–1838, no. 186, DNA.
67. WILA, box no. 10.2.1, Draft from landfysikus Schlegel, 31 May 1837, DNA.
68. Carøe, *Den Danske lægestand*, III: 233; Ibid., V: 100.
69. BH, Med. rep., DWI, 1846, DNA. Original text in Danish.
70. Jens Vibæk, "Dansk Vestindien, 1755–1848. Vestindiens storhedstid," in *Vore gamle tropekolonier,* ed. Johannes Brøndsted (Copenhagen: Fremad, 1966), 2: 271–273.
71. WILA, box no. 10.2.1, Draft from landfysikus Schlegel, 31 May 1837, DNA.
72. DC, Med. rep., box. no. G125C, 1804, DNA.
73. BH, Med. rep., DWI, 1830, 1831, 1838, 1846, DNA.
74. Carøe, *Den Danske lægestand*, III: 195–196; Ibid., V: 44.
75. Ibid., III: 117; Ibid., V: 82.
76. DC, Med. rep., box. no. G125C, Landfysikus JMF Keutsch, 1804, DNA. Original text in Danish.
77. Ibid., Drs. Stedman and Lang, 1804, DNA. Original text in English.
78. Ibid.
79. WILA, box nos. 3.81.690, 46.17.5, 46.17.6, 46.17.15, 46.17.30, 46.17.32, 46.17.33, 46.17.44, 46.17.45, 46.17.53, 46.17.54, 46.17.72, 46.20, 46.21. DNA; DSD, box no. 1113, DNA.
80. Highfield, *Observations*, 24.
81. For instance, WILA, box nos. 45.17.55, 45.17.5., DNA.
82. The Danish word is "misfornøjet", which translates to "displeased" or "dissatisfied".
83. Oxholm, *Nogle Anmærkninger*, 27.
84. Johan Christian Schmidt, *Various Remarks Collected on and about the Island of St. Croix in America* (St. Croix Christiansted: The Virgin Islands Humanities Council, 1998. Originally published in Copenhagen, 1788), 29.
85. Bush, *Slave Women*, 146.

86. Approximately 600 births per year divided among 15 doctors equals about 40 births per doctor per year. In addition, the royal midwives took care of births.
87. A similar mediating function between local practise and authorized obstetrics can be seen among midwives in Denmark. See Anne Løkke, *Døden i Barndommen. Spædbørnsdødelighed og moderniseringsprocesser i Danmark 1800 til 1920* (Copenhagen: Gyldendal, 1998), 309–310.

2 "Any elderly, sensible, prudent woman"
The Practice and Practitioners of Midwifery during Slavery in the British Caribbean

Tara A. Inniss

Little is known about the practice and practitioners of midwifery in the British Caribbean during the time of slavery. As in Europe, physicians were not usually called to attend women giving birth in plantation society unless there were complications. When either the mother or the infant appeared to be in distress, it was often too late to send for a physician located on another estate or in town. Women who were experienced in delivering babies assisted parturient women. Sometimes called midwives or nurses, these women resided either on the plantation or on neighbouring estates. In other instances, particularly in urban areas, the midwives attending enslaved women were white or free coloured women who resided near plantations or households. When summoned, they traveled to attend the delivery. Once the child was delivered safely, they were paid a fee.

This chapter will look at the practice, competition, and professionalization in midwifery during the slave period in the British Caribbean. The practice of midwifery in the British Caribbean was a contested space with gender, race, free/enslaved status, and cultural beliefs dividing practitioners (both physicians and midwives) and the patients they attended. Although midwives held intimate knowledge of women's bodies and pregnancy, their knowledge and practices were often marginalized by physicians who viewed them as both incompetent health practitioners and unworthy competitors in the health marketplace. However, there was an accepted place for trained and untrained female midwives in plantation society established by both custom and need, and their services continued to be called upon in the majority of births in the free and enslaved populations.

Midwifery was one of the few skilled occupations dominated by women, and consequently, free and enslaved midwives competed for these potentially lucrative positions on estates. Estates often shifted between the services of free white or coloured midwives and the enslaved women living on the premises. Both groups were rewarded for their services, but remuneration differed greatly, with enslaved women receiving much less in compensation than their free counterparts. However, it is important to note that midwifery, as a profession dominated by free and enslaved women, offered fewer financial rewards than did skilled professions monopolized by men.

However, health work performed by women was undervalued in another respect: their skills were denigrated and their work was condemned by physicians and elite patients. Black midwifery practices were racialized. Nevertheless, enslaved women relied on their care and knowledge which involved a ritualized space of health and healing based on African-derived beliefs and practices. Little is known about the way in which this space was constructed, but data collected from research on African-American midwifery and practices reported in twentieth-century Trinidad can be used to examine some of the cultural beliefs and rituals that may have informed black midwifery practice in the early nineteenth-century British Caribbean. Understanding the practice and practitioners of midwifery during slavery helps to situate the health work of women within the history of medicine and health provision in the colonial British Caribbean.

The limited references to midwifery in the British Caribbean historical record provide some information on the socioeconomic, cultural, or ethnic backgrounds of midwives, but it is necessary to draw on sources for the early colonial period, as well as other geographical areas to supplement this information. The history of African-American midwifery is well developed, and the analysis of midwives from the United States as intermediaries in childbirth can help advance our understanding of the importance of midwifery practice in the lives of enslaved persons in the British Caribbean.[1] Moreover, research on midwifery in early twentieth-century Toco, Trinidad, also lends insight into the practices and beliefs of midwives in a rural community and how they may have been related to the folk knowledge handed down over generations since slavery.[2]

Maternal and infant health have recently become important avenues of historical inquiry, especially among medical historians in the United Kingdom, Europe, and the United States. Irvine Loudon is pre-eminent among these historians. He documents the factors leading to fluctuations in the maternal death rate for over a century and a half in several regions throughout the world. Although he does not specifically refer to birthing practices in the colonial Caribbean, his study does provide exhaustive information on the practice of 'traditional' midwifery and man-midwifery in England in the late eighteenth and early nineteenth centuries. He also discusses the training in English and Scottish medical schools, which British Caribbean physicians likely received. His work also reveals the attitudes physicians held toward women and their health complaints in the early nineteenth century.[3]

Medical treatises and slave management manuals are useful for any discussion of practices used by planters to ensure the health of the enslaved. Sometimes written by physicians, such publications instructed planters and plantation managers on the successful management of sugar plantations.[4] These sources are valuable for their insights into maternal and infant health during the slave period, when many planters were concerned about the high mortality rates of slaves. Although several of these sources were not published specifically in reference to Barbados or the period in question, planters, plantation personnel, and physicians consulted them throughout the Caribbean and for much of the slave period.

MIDWIFERY PRACTICE, COMPETITION, AND PROFESSIONALIZATION

Observations on midwifery practice have been reported since the mid seventeenth century. Richard Ligon reported that husbands called on a neighbour to attend to enslaved women during childbirth. According to Ligon, the neighbour "gives little help to her delivery, but when the child is born (which she calls her Pickaninny) she helps to make a little fire near her feet."[5] By the nineteenth century, when most planters recognized that greater attention had to be paid to parturient mothers, most large estates employed a midwife or nurse, or at least consulted one. A distinction was made between "a proper Midwife" who was called upon to deliver the infant and a nurse who would look after the new mother during her confinement.[6] On some estates, this may have been the same woman, but this reference indicates that contemporaries distinguished a professional midwife from a nurse. Nonetheless, it was recommended that every estate should have a midwife and/or a woman to provide post-natal care for mother and infant.[7]

It is not clear what qualifications were needed to be designated a midwife or nurse in plantation society. According to David Collins, a planter and physician practicing in St Vincent:

> Any elderly, sensible, prudent woman who has borne children, may easily be instructed in the art of delivering others. A few lessons from any gentlemen of the faculty or even from one of her own sex, will qualify her sufficiently for your purpose; the principal part of what she has to learn being, not to attempt too much, and to demand other assistance, when the presentation of the child is not according to nature.[8]

No standard existed for the selection of midwives or nurses, who, in Collins' opinion, only provided support and coaching to pregnant women. Moreover, midwives largely respected the professional boundaries physicians placed upon midwifery and called upon their assistance in emergencies.[9]

Gendered notions of whose professional expertise was greater in difficult deliveries come across in the writings of several physicians in the region. It was generally accepted that skilled women could attend most deliveries, but that in complicated labours, "men of science must be early resorted to."[10] As in general health-care provision, where physicians vied for control of the health marketplace with quacks, enslaved doctors, and doctresses, the practice of midwifery was a contested space.

Physicians were invested financially and psychologically in the perpetuation of slavery. Many depended on estates for their regular income, and several young physicians traveled to the region in order to make money and establish themselves as both physicians and landowners. Such opportunities for lucrative practice and land ownership could never have presented themselves for physicians in England or the rest of Europe at the time. Therefore, physicians were critical of local practitioners, including midwives, who cut into their profits. They perceived their medical knowledge and the training they received as superior to what was offered locally. They criticized black men and women who provided inexpensive health care. If black and white women could do the work of obstetrics, then what position did the white male physician hold in the general provision of health care? Collins and his contemporaries believed that their knowledge helped preserve maternal and infant life, especially if there were complications in delivery.

'Men of science', however, may not have been adequately trained in midwifery practices or the expanding specialization of obstetrics. Maria Lucia Mott questions the assertion that formally trained physicians practicing in colonial Brazil were better qualified in delivering children than midwives due to their limited exposure to obstetrics training.[11] A significant proportion of degree-holding physicians practicing in the British Caribbean were graduates of Scottish medical schools, where students (unlike their English counterparts) were required to study midwifery in addition to anatomy, pharmacy, and surgery. However, little is known about how widely their knowledge was put into practice, especially in light of the competition posed by female midwives practicing in the region.[12] Some physicians had instruments that were used in abnormal or prolonged deliveries. Collins, for example, insisted that physicians attending enslaved populations should have at least one pair of obstetrical forceps.[13] They also could administer opiates such as laudanum or opium to mothers in pain. Enslaved or free midwives did not have access to such instruments or medications.

A physician could live a fair distance from an estate, particularly in rural districts. Consequently, it was unlikely that he could be summoned to, and arrive at, an emergency in a timely manner. Mother and child could die or, at least, be gravely injured before the physician arrived. Moreover, the methods of physicians could cause more harm if they were able to arrive in time to make a difference. During difficult deliveries, Hans Sloane, an English physician practising in Jamaica in the early eighteenth century, administered courses of bleeding to his pregnant patients, which further depleted them.[14] In the nineteenth century, physician–*accoucheur* practice still involved several techniques that often placed both mother and child in harm's way. Unsterilized forceps could leave both mother and child susceptible to bacterial infection. In fact, any instrument that was used on a patient was not likely to be sterilized. Forceps deliveries were complicated, and many physicians who had them in their possession may have been unable to deliver the child without some significant damage to the infant or mother. Additionally, physicians did not wash their hands when performing vaginal examinations.[15] It is unclear whether the health of mother or infant was any further improved with the presence of a physician during difficult births. Collins observed that deaths in childbed were "not very great in warm climates", but there is little empirical evidence to substantiate his assertion.[16] Nevertheless, physicians used their perceived medical authority to challenge female midwifery practice.

Planters also sought to regularize the services offered to and by midwives. In spite of the evidence which suggests that parturient enslaved women preferred the presence of female family members and enslaved midwives to physicians, several physicians practicing in the region recommended the establishment of separate lying-in facilities in estate hospitals. M.G. Lewis, a Jamaican planter, mentioned his visits to the 'lying-in apartment' on his estate, where a physician also made daily visits. Such facilities helped managers and physicians monitor the progress of ante- and post-partum women and their infants, especially when they feared the incompetence of midwives. Another Jamaican observer strongly recommended the establishment of separate lying-in facilities supervised by "properly instructed midwives." He witnessed "many women educated as midwives at considerable expence [sic]" and observed that "children [were] better taken care of than formerly." There is no mention of who instructed the midwives or whether they were enslaved or free.[17]

Many enslaved women, however, were delivered at home in the company of "a woman, generally one of their own relations or friends."[18] Attendance of informally trained female relations was customary when an externally contracted or estate midwife could not be found. Old Doll, an elderly slave on Newton Plantation in Barbados, for example, acted as midwife to her niece, Mary Thomas, when she delivered her son. However, when the child died, Sampson Wood, the manager, blamed Old Doll and Mary Thomas for the child's death.[19] Enslaved midwives were easy targets for blame should the child succumb to illness or sudden death in the first days of life.

When capable enslaved midwives could not be found, owners or managers often contracted white or free coloured women with midwifery skills. On Newton Plantation, a white woman was contracted to take the place of the elderly enslaved midwife when she became enfeebled and unable to perform her duties. Higman suggests:

> White sick nurses and midwives were generally drawn from the estate tenantry but were generally used only when skilled slave women could not be found to perform these functions.[20]

Newton estate records reveal that in the late eighteenth and early nineteenth centuries, three white women—Mary Evelyn, Ann Crichlow, and Frances Gibson—were contracted at different stages as midwives to the estate.[21] Gibson was replaced as midwife by a slave belonging to Newton in 1818, who was paid substantially less than she was.[22] Plantation midwifery was one of the many knowledge-based skills that owners and managers could extract from their labour force without laying out tremendous expenditure.

Midwives were judged on their past successes of delivering healthy babies to healthy mothers. Their reputation as cautious facilitators of labour, rather than hasty interventionists, won the patronage of women, planters, and physicians. One difficult case that could not be managed, or a succession of failures to bring about the safe delivery of child and mother, could signal a loss of confidence in a midwife's abilities, and, in slave society, a loss of economic and social status.

There has been no significant research done on the economic and social status of free or enslaved midwives in the Caribbean. However, Deacon's study on urban Cape Colony midwives suggests that many remained in an impoverished state. Unlike some of the other economic activities enslaved and free women engaged in, such as marketing and prostitution, midwifery provided an unstable income.[23] Whereas enslaved women could depend on the support of the estate, the uncertain nature of midwifery kept many free women impoverished. Employable 'elderly' women participated in the profession, but as elderly—and frequently single—women, their economic status in society was much lower than that of their younger married counterparts.[24] Mrs. Bynoe, for example, was a white midwife residing in the Garrison in 1805 whom several persons described as "a very poor Woman who acts in the Character of Midwife and is frequently from home." The only slave she could afford to buy was reportedly lame and in ill health.[25] Aging free women working in the capacity of midwives found it difficult to survive without the support of husbands or family members. In Antigua, a woman named Mary, who in 1815 was reportedly 100 years old, was described as "a good midwife." Her son contributed to her support for many years when she could no longer support herself. She received 1 shilling 6 pence per week from a charitable organization until she died.[26]

Both enslaved and free midwives received monetary payments for their attendance of enslaved women. Enslaved midwives were one of the few enslaved, female-dominated occupational groups in plantation society to receive cash payments from estate managers. It was customary for members of male-dominated occupational groups, such as masons, carpenters, and boilers, to receive cash payments. However, as Higman suggests, unlike their male counterparts, enslaved midwives were given small cash payments for safely delivering women as an incentive to increase fertility and the standard of care mothers and newborns received.[27] In addition to small sums of money, enslaved midwives were also given non-monetary consideration for their work. It is unclear, however, to what extent enslaved midwives received cash payments exclusively for the unique service they offered. At Newton, Frances Gibson, who was designated as 'sick nurse', was paid £15 per annum, and in 1815, she received £9 for twelve women she delivered.[28] When an enslaved woman took over midwifery duties in 1818, she was given 6 shillings 3 pence per delivery and conceivably no annual salary.[29] The disparity in income levels for the two racial groups was quite large.[30]

In spite of their training and the faith that planters and managers placed in them, enslaved midwives, like many midwives in Europe at the time, were often stereotyped as incompetent.[31] Their informal training made them vulnerable to physicians, planters, and managers who often blamed them for high infant mortality rates. Edward Long, a late eighteenth-century Jamaican planter, wrote that "many children are annually destroyed, as well as their mothers, by the unskillfulness and absurd management of Negroe midwives."[32] Untrained midwives in Europe were stigmatized in similar ways, but in the colonial Caribbean, the practice of midwifery was both racialized and denigrated. Little comparative research has been done on the practice of colonial and imperial midwifery. Harriet Deacon, however, describes how black midwives in Cape Colony were the focus of such stereotypes:

> This provided an opportunity for a neat combination of the European image of the 'untrained' midwife as a dirty, drunk and gossipy old woman, refusing doctors' aid, protecting immoral mothers and procuring abortions, and the colonial image of the Khosian and slave woman as a dirty, lazy primitive, inebriated and immoral 'creature.'[33]

In the colonial Caribbean, black midwifery was perceived in similar ways. Planters and managers could use 'incompetent' enslaved midwives as scapegoats for the poor conditions into which many infants were born.

Few descriptions exist in documentary sources of black midwifery. However, one of the nurses or midwives who was present at the delivery of Governor Nugent's first son in Jamaica was an old black nurse named Nurse Flora. Lady Nugent said little about general midwifery practices in the colonial Caribbean, but she shared her observations. Nurse Flora's presence at the birth of the Nugent's child was tolerated, but was not welcomed. She

> brought a cargo of herbs, and wished to try various charms, to expedite the birth of the child . . . I was really in a fright, for fear she would try some experiments on me. But the maids took all her herbs from her, and made her remove all the smoking apparatus she had prepared for my benefit.

Nurse Flora was an experienced midwife who regaled Nugent with her "many stories of pinching and tying women to the bedpost." Nurse Flora's presence was more of an amusement to Nugent and the other white women who attended her labour. After the delivery, she was forced to keep her distance from Nugent by the "English maids." Nugent wrote that she did not want the old nurse to "pinch, or suffocate me to death with her charms."[34] This is a contrived description of black midwifery in the Caribbean, but it demonstrates that black midwives probably used African-derived midwifery practices to ensure the comfort of the mother and the health of the newborn. Nurse Flora's prolonged and dutiful attendance of Nugent was comparable to the amount of time that nurses spent with enslaved mothers, especially on estates where nurses or midwives stayed with mothers during the lying-in period. However, Nugent did not appreciate Nurse Flora's presence or knowledge. She dismissed Nurse Flora's brand of midwifery as incompetent and bizarre.

From the time women reported their pregnancies, midwives, such as Nurse Flora, were consulted. Holding intimate knowledge of women's pregnant bodies, midwives anticipated due dates by charting the phases of the moon since conception.[35] They coached women throughout their pregnancies, monitoring both their physical and spiritual health. They were also charged with making baby clothes and tending to the health needs of pregnant women.[36]

Research on childbirth practices in the twentieth-century African diaspora indicates the readiness with which women looked to midwives or other women in the community for health and spiritual advice. Scholars exploring African-American midwifery practices emphasize their importance. Zeina Omisola Jones points out that African-American midwives were involved in "mothering the mother."[37] Jacinta Gertrude Fraser argues that they held "ritual and physiological knowledge of women's bodies."[38] Such beliefs are reflected in historical and contemporary reports of the African-derived beliefs and customs that surrounded childbirth and postnatal care. These are essential to the reconstruction of the cultural context of midwifery practice, particularly in the absence of documentation for the British Caribbean during the slave period. The midwife was instrumental in imparting and reproducing this knowledge. She paid attention to the "rituals and observances necessary for the successful reintegration and re-entry of both mother and baby into society."[39] In some twentieth-century sources, it is evident how enduring these beliefs and customs were. It was believed, for example, that negative thoughts of pregnant women could result in the physical deformity or mental retardation of the infants born to them.[40] Pregnancy made women and their unborn children susceptible to spirits and the malice of others in the community.[41] Midwives were believed to help mediate these dangers during pregnancy. Protective measures were taken by pregnant women and their midwives before and after childbirth to guarantee the spiritual well being of the child, family, and the community.

Plantation personnel, midwives, and other women monitored women for complications in pregnancy, which signaled more than physical distress for mother and infant. Melville J. Herskovits and Frances Herskovits reported that during prolonged pregnancies or deliveries in Toco, Trinidad in 1939, midwives believed that the baby was "tied up" inside the mother and that, "'Somebody is doing things to keep it from being born'". Similarly, breech births "are held in great mistrust". The dangerous presentation was believed to be the Devil coming "to kill the mother". The circumstances of the child's birth, if born breeched, were kept a close secret to the family since other families would not allow their children to marry children born in this way.[42] In normal presentations, black midwives in Toco preferred their patients to squat over a cloth-covered, large wooden tray that was placed, rather than lying down. The mother was kept active during labour until she was fully dilated, and "[t]hen the midwife rub[bed] the vaginal passage and abdomen with 'sweet, good oil'."[43] However, if there were no complications, the correct disposal of the afterbirth was more important than the actual delivery of the child.[44]

Immediately after birth, midwives usually administered herbs and drinks to "clean out" the mother, or expel the placenta and afterbirth. In Toco, the midwife would pound wild coffee otherwise known as *malame*, boil it, and give it to new mothers in large quantities to "'bring out all the bruised blood'". The midwife was also responsible for massaging or "beating" the new mother's belly.[45] A wide piece of cloth was also bound around the mother's abdomen to help contract the womb.[46]

All of the physical remnants of the birth had to be carefully treated and disposed of. Improper disposal of the umbilical cord or the afterbirth could inhibit the mother's healing or signal developmental problems for the child later in life. Jamaican midwives reported that the umbilical cord could not be dropped "on the floor because then the child will be unable to control its urine".[47] When the umbilical cord was cut in Toco, "the scissors, of the ordinary type, are put beneath the place of the baby's head is to lie, and left there for nine days, when the mother and child first emerge from the house".[48] The Herskovits' informant also reported, "on the ninth day the umbilicus is given to an older relative who dig a hole for it and plant a coconut, banana or plantain tree over it" for the benefit of the child once it grows older. It is called the child's 'navel-string tree'". If someone damaged the tree, the child must receive monetary compensation.[49] The afterbirth also needed protection from disturbances. Herskovits and Herskovits wrote that this ritual was done to prevent post-partum pain in the mother. It was placed in a calabash and put on a bed of buck-buck or 'fig' (banana) leaves with salt and rum or bay rum, and buried. A fire was lighted over it, and kept burning for nine days; if this fire went out, it was rekindled.[50]

The nine-day seclusion of mother and child has been recorded in the slave period. Lewis reported that one of his nurses on his estate in Jamaica reported, "Oh, massa, till nine days over, we have *no hope* of them."[51] During this time, newborns were not seen as fully part of the human world, and much superstition surrounded the child's spiritual and physical health. Caution was taken during the nine days before the child and mother could be introduced to the rest of the community. During the seclusion in Toco, the mother's diet was watched carefully. She was given soft foods and plenty of "cooling teas". She was also prevented from doing any heavy work during this period.[52] Family and community members celebrated when mother and child were brought out of their nine-day seclusion. In Trinidad, Herskovits and Herskovits witnessed family members asking the ancestors to bless the child. Community members also brought gifts for the benefit of the child and the family.[53] Beckwith reports that in Jamaica, baths were prepared for infants on the ninth day, into which family members would throw coins for luck.[54]

In the slave period, physicians suggested that women should receive cautious care and attention after the successful delivery of their infants. Collins recommended that they should receive extra blankets to keep warm. He also suggested that the quarters where post-partum women rested should remain quiet. Women were also designated a nurse to attend to them and their newborns.[55] The midwives who attended women during delivery likely continued daily visits, especially to monitor the healing of the newborn's navel. Other women in the family or community also played immediate post-partum supervisory roles, guiding new mothers in the care and maintenance of newborns.[56] The black midwife was seen as not only an authority in the physical health of the child and mother, but also as an authority in the spiritual health of the newborn's family and the wider community. She supervised the physical act of childbirth through cautious facilitation, and by preventing dangers to their spiritual well being; she mediated the sacred world of womens' and infants' health.

CONCLUSION

The health work of women as midwives is relevant to any discussion of health-care provision in the colonial Caribbean. During slavery, health care was inscribed with enduring gender and racial hierarchies that continued to dominate the medical landscape well into the twentieth century. Western European formal medical training and practice clashed with African-derived, apprentice-based midwifery practice to create a competitive health-care marketplace in slave society to which both free and enslaved women had access. Although other health-care professionals often maligned their profession, midwives provided a vital service to mothers and their newborns. They dutifully attended parturient women and ensured that newborns were brought safely into the world. Midwives helped women through difficult pregnancies and assisted medical professionals. Although midwives were important, their careers were unstable. Professional rivalries and income disparities existed between free and enslaved midwives. Physicians seemingly outranked them in the wider arena of health-care provision and often dismissed them.

NOTES

1. Zeina Omisola Jones, "Knowledge Systems in Conflict: The Regulation of African American Midwifery," *Nursing History Review* 12 (2004); Gertrude Jacinta Fraser, *African American Midwifery in the South: Dialogues of Birth, Race and Memory* (Boston: Harvard University Press, 1998).
2. Melville J. Herskovits and Frances Herskovits, *Trinidad Village* (New York: Alfred A. Knopf, 1947).
3. Irvine Loudon, *Death in Childbirth: An International Study of Maternal Care and Maternal Mortality 1800–1950* (Oxford: Clarendon Press, 1992).
4. Richard B. Sheridan, *Doctors and Slaves: A Medical and Demographic History of Slavery in the British West Indies, 1680–1834* (Cambridge: Cambridge University Press, 1985); Thomas Dancer, *The Medical Assistant; or Jamaica Practice of Physic: Designed Chiefly for the Use of Families and Plantations* (Kingston, Jamaica: Alex, Aikman, 1801); William Sells, *Remarks on the Condition of the Slaves in the Island of Jamaica* (London: J.M. Richardson, Cornhill and Ridgways, 1823).
5. Richard A. Ligon, *A True & Exact History of the Island of Barbadoes* [1657] (London: Frank Cass, 1998), 47–48.
6. "The Treatment of Negroes in Barbados in 1786 and in 1823," *Journal of the Barbados Museum and Historical Society* 11, no. 1 (1934): 29.
7. David Collins, *Practical Rules for the Management and Medical Treatment of Negro Slaves in the Sugar Colonies* [1803] (London: Vernor, Hood, and Sharp, 1971), 159.
8. Ibid.
9. "Quaker Records 'at a Meeting of the Midwives in Barbadoes 1677'," *Journal of the Barbados Museum and Historical Society* 24, no. 3 (1957).
10. Collins, *Practical Rules*, 159.
11. Maria Lucia Mott, "Midwifery and the Construction of an Image in Nineteenth-Century Brazil," *Nursing History Review* 11 (2003): 40.
12. Loudon, *Death in Childbirth*, 192–193; W. J. Bell, "North American and West Indian Graduates of Glasgow and Aberdeen to 1800," *Journal of History of Medicine* 20 (1965): 411–415.
13. Collins, *Practical Rules*, 400.
14. Hans Sloane, *A Voyage to the Islands Madera, Barbados, Nieves, S. Christophers and Jamaica: With the Natural History . . . Of the Last of Those Islands; to Which Is Prefix'd an Introduction, Wherein Is an Account of the Inhabitants, Air, Waters, Diseases, Trade, Etc.* 3 vols. (London: British Museum, 1707–1725), cxxxi, cxl, cxlvii.
15. Loudon, *Death in Childbirth*, 186.
16. Collins, *Practical Rules*, 164.
17. Sells, *Remarks on the Condition of the Slaves in the Island of Jamaica*, 18.
18. Quoted in Barry Higman, *Slave Populations of the Caribbean, 1807–1834* (Barbados: The University of the West Indies Press, 1984), 352.
19. Karl Watson, *A Kind of Right to Be Idle: Old Doll Matriarch of Newton Plantation* (Bridgetown: University of the West Indies and the Barbados Museum and Historical Society, 2000), 124.
20. Higman, *Slave Populations of the Caribbean*, 263.
21. Jerome S. Handler and Frederick W. Lange, *Plantation Slavery in Barbados: An Archaeological and Historical Investigation* (Cambridge, MA: Harvard UP, 1999), 100; Higman, *Slave Populations of the Caribbean, 1807–1834*, 263.
22. Higman, *Slave Populations of the Caribbean, 1807–1834*, 263.
23. See Welch for discussion on economic activities of women in Bridgetown. Pedro Welch and Richard Goodridge, *"Red" and Black over White: Free-Coloured*

Women in Pre-Emancipation Barbados (Bridgetown, Barbados: Carib Research and Publications, 2000), 56–57.

24. Harriet Deacon, "Midwives and Medical Men in the Cape Colony before 1860," *Journal of African History* 39 (1998): 280.

25. Depositions: Mrs. Bynce's Treatment of Her Slave. 14 Nov. 1805, Seaforth Muniments GD 46/17/80 f. 93, National Archives of Scotland, Edinburgh.

26. Association for the relief of Distressed Negroes &c. in Antigua, "Third Report of the Association for the Relief of Distressed Negroes, &C. In Antigua: Particularly among the Discarded Negroes" (London: Association for the Relief of Distressed Negroes, &c. in Antigua, 1815).

27. Higman, *Slave Populations of the Caribbean*, 263.

28. Robert Haynes, "Abstract of Newton Plantation in Barbados, 1 Jan. to 31 Dec. 1815", Newton Estate Papers, MS 523/166, University of London, London, England.

29. Higman, *Slave Populations of the Caribbean* 263.

30. Research on Cape Colony's enslaved midwifery suggests, "Most midwives of slave origin were poor: midwifery practice may have been one way of earning money while enslaved, but it was not lucrative". Deacon, "Midwives and Medical Men in the Cape Colony before 1860," 280.

31. Ibid., 272.

32. Edward Long, *The History of Jamaica: Or, General Survey of the Antient and Modern State of That Island: With Reflections on Its Situation, Settlements, Inhabitants, Climate, Productions, Commerce, Laws, and Government*. vol. 1 (London: T. Lowndes, 1774), 436.

33. Deacon, "Midwives and Medical Men in the Cape Colony before 1860," 275.

34. Frank Cundall, ed., *Lady Nugent's Journal: Jamaica One Hundred Years Ago* (London: Adam and Charles Black, 1907), 164.

35. Fraser, *African American Midwifery in the South*, 214–215.

36. Copy of Plantation Journal for the Estate of Peter T. Brooke Esq called 'Langfords' Mar. 1832, Brooke of Mere [Antigua] Muniments Box VIII/6/1021, U of Manchester Library, Manchester.

37. Jones, "Knowledge Systems in Conflict," 167.

38. Fraser, *African American Midwifery in the South*, 217; Jones, "Knowledge Systems in Conflict," 167.

39. Jones, "Knowledge Systems in Conflict," 167.

40. Fraser, *African American Midwifery in the South*, 219.

41. Ibid., 221.

42. Herskovits and Herskovits, *Trinidad Village*, 114–115. In these cases, midwives administered various concoctions to stimulate labour. Midwives took cobwebs from the ceiling, boiled them, and gave the concoction to the mother to drink. "Then baby born. Must born, even if lion tie him. Before the drink is finished, is born".

43. Ibid., 113.

44. Fraser, *African American Midwifery in the South*, 226.

45. Herskovits and Herskovits, *Trinidad Village*, 114.

46. M.G. Smith, *Kinship and Community in Carriacou* (New Haven, CT: Yale University Press, 1962), 88.

47. Martha Warren Beckwith, *Black Roadways: A Study of Jamaican Folk Life* (New York: Negro University Press, 1969), 55.

48. Herskovits and Herskovits, *Trinidad Village*, 113. Incidentally, Ibo midwives place sharp objects that are used to cut the umbilical cord under the beds of labouring women to cut the labour and post-partum pains. See "The Cauling Midwife: A Historical Journey of Midwifery through the Hands of Mid-

wives of African Descent," *Birth in the Tradition* 9 May (2004). <http://www.birthinthetradition.com/1.0bitt_hist.html.

49. Beckwith, *Black Roadways*, 55.
50. Herskovits and Herskovits, *Trinidad Village*, 113–114.
51. M. G. Lewis, *Journal of a West India Proprietor, Kept During a Residence in the Island of Jamaica*, 2 vols. (London: John Murray, 1834), 97.
52. Beckwith, *Black Roadways*, 57; Herskovits and Herskovits, *Trinidad Village*, 117.
53. Herskovits and Herskovits, *Trinidad Village*, 118.
54. Beckwith, *Black Roadways*, 57.
55. Collins, *Practical Rules*, 159–160.
56. Fraser, *African American Midwifery in the South*, 234.

3 From the Plantation to the Academy

Slavery and the Production of Cuban Medicine in the Nineteenth Century

Steven Palmer

In 1839, the surgeon Ambrosio Moreno removed a tumour from an infant just born into slavery on a plantation in the province of Havana and discovered that the growth contained bones and teeth.[1] He donated the medical curiosity to the Anatomy Cabinet of the San Ambrosio Hospital's School of Practical Anatomy, whose director was the hospital's Chief Surgeon, Nicolás Gutiérrez. Moreno also wrote up his finding as a clinical note for a Havana medical journal, *El Reportorio Médico-Habanero*, a paper founded by Gutiérrez, and edited by one of his medical faculty colleagues.[2] These transactions trace an important circuit in Cuba's extraordinary nineteenth-century medical universe, one that connected plantation medicine with the academic and commercial pinnacles of the art, science, and business of healing. The schooled and licensed medical practitioner engaged in a lucrative practice on the sugar plantations of the hinterland, maintaining the corporeal machinery of the *ingenio* (sugar mill complex), and simultaneously gaining clinical and surgical experience while generating clinical material that could provide useful native content to the development of medical institutions and professional exchanges in the capital. In the process, the practitioner enhanced his own stature within the metropolitan scientific community in a way that might open up professional and commercial possibilities in the capital following a stint in the countryside.

When Moreno's specimen was put on display, Havana had one of the densest populations of titled medical practitioners in the world. As Cuba became the world's richest centre of sugar production in the century between 1770 and 1870, Havana and its sugar-producing hinterland emerged as a medical metropolis. No other place in the Americas came close to Cuba in the quantity and educational background of its licensed medical practitioners, and the large numbers of highly qualified physicians and surgeons in rural areas was a phenomenon unique in Latin America at this time. The capital city boasted a thriving university medical school that attracted *criollo* and peninsular youth from around the island.[3] They were joined by a numerous and diverse immigration of doctors and surgeons from Spain, France, and Great Britain. Together, these galens made up the core market for a series of medical periodicals that circulated in the city, and justified the growth of hospital, professional, and scientific institutions. This medical splendour was a product, above all else, of the great wealth and expansion of Cuba's slave-based plantation economy at a time when the price of slave bodies was rising.

Doctors were a crucial part of the social relations of production in this slave system. They tried to preserve its labouring bodies and organize sanitary practices on plantations with increasingly large complements of slaves. At the same time, physicians and surgeons found clinical material in this great mass of subordinate and stressed bodies. They conducted surgical, therapeutic, and medicinal trials on them, and published the results in medical periodicals in Havana and beyond. Slave sickness and health were raw material for the production of a professional and academic universe whose magnificence and political importance were enshrined in 1861 when Nicolás Gutiérrez finally realized his dream of calling to order the first session of the Royal Academy of Medical, Physical, and Natural Sciences of Havana, an august body of learned men of the island, made up overwhelmingly of criollo physicians and surgeons.[4] We should keep in mind that medical practitioners on the plantation may also have saved lives, and intervened to keep overseers and owners from sending slaves who could not physically endure labour back to work. Some doctors were proponents of abolition, and some participated in the attenuated Cuban war of liberation (the Ten Years' War of 1868–1878) that, despite falling short of its objective, did edge the colonial state toward ending slavery. For the purposes of this chapter, however, I would like to set aside the possible humanitarian and healing activities of Cuban doctors. The slave plantation complex of Havana and its environs during the first four-fifths of the nineteenth century was an infernal agro-industrial system that ran on a labour system characterized by suffering, violence, torture, and premature death; physicians and surgeons were important components in its reproduction. This is the murky ethical bargain—one practitioners were aware of, though in terms peculiar to the era—that lay beneath Havana's nineteenth-century medical brilliance: medicine was an integral part of the slave-based sugar production process itself, and the injuries and infirmities of slaves, in turn, provided raw material for the production of Cuban medicine.

This Spanish Caribbean story echoes one told some twenty years ago by Richard Sheridan in his important study of doctors and slaves in the British Caribbean.[5] It differs in time period, with the bulk of Sheridan's cases coming from the eighteenth century—prior to the termination of the slave trade—while my evidence comes largely from the nineteenth century—after the end of the legal trade. There are crucial differences in the nature of academic and plantation medicine in the two settings and time periods, and more importantly, in the market demand for medical treatment of slaves, which was greater following the end of the slave trade. Nevertheless, Sheridan documents a similar dynamic, whereby planters and physicians in the British Caribbean sugar colonies applied the rational discourse of medicine in an effort to maximize slave production. *Doctors and Slaves* also portrays a comparably learned stratum of elite practitioners composing medical treatises, for the most part, on the management of slave health and sickness and on questions of medicine in the tropics.

There is another important difference, however, between the eighteenth-century British Caribbean medical circuitry described by Sheridan, and the nineteenth-century Cuban one explored here. In the British West Indies, the relatively thick medical universe of white doctors would wither away with the end of slavery, and its relationship to subsequent colonial medical institutions in the nineteenth and twentieth centuries— let alone its relationship to medical life during the independence era—is unclear and discontinuous. The Cuban nexus of plantation and academic medicine, on the other hand, was at the heart of the development of criollo medical institutions and leaders that would play an important role in anti-colonial, and then national, civil and political society. Though rarely explicitly opposed to Spanish colonial rule, or (until the very final years of the struggle) supportive of the Cuban wars of liberation (1868–1878, 1895–1898), the powerful and illustrious community of criollo medical men headquartered in Havana wrote themselves into national destiny. They did so by creating a native scientific edifice of some distinction in the midst of a Spanish scientific milieu that, if undergoing a period of dynamic renewal in the metropolis, had a poor expression in its Cuban colony. The Medical Faculty of the University of Havana and the Royal Academy of Sciences of Havana would become pillars of nineteenth-century criollo civil society.[6]

Each of these institutions insured themselves a place in the nationalist pantheon. The medical school became an important patriotic symbol, by association, with the eight criollo medical students (the Martyrs of 1871) who were executed by Spanish firing squad during the first Cuban war of liberation after being accused of desecrating the gravestone of a leading advocate of Spanish colonial rule. The relatively minor nature of the incident that provoked such draconian punishment underlines how closely Spaniards had come to associate medical studies with the articulation of criollo interests. The Academy of Sciences earned its place in the patriotic lexicon by association with its most famous member, Carlos Finlay, the Cuban star in the firmament of medical history. Finlay proposed in 1881 that yellow fever was a mosquito-borne disease; though his views were long dismissed, most of the particulars of his hypothesis, and the accuracy of much of his experimentation, were later demonstrated in Havana by Walter Reed's team of US military doctors, assisted by a number of Cuban physicians (including Finlay himself).[7] As a result, Cuban medical historiography, which can be considered well developed in some areas, has not been inclined to delve into the slave plantation associations of a criollo medical society that animates nationalist discourse to the present day.[8]

"A LUXURIOUS CARRIAGE": THE MEDICAL
UNIVERSE OF HAVANA AND ITS ENVIRONS

Adrián López Denis has written with great insight on the sudden appearance of a sophisticated and sometimes highly original medical discourse in late eighteenth-century Havana. From 1790 to 1805, the *Papel Periódico de la Havana* [sic], one of the first Cuban newspapers, had a positive impact on the development of local medicine, with over half of its scientific articles devoted to medical issues. In 1797, a half-dozen scientific titles appeared on themes ranging from botany, bee-keeping, and sugar engineering to the utility of chemistry, a defense of surgery, and a dissertation on yellow fever by the towering medical figure from this era, Tomás Romay.[9] López Denis focuses on the eccentric work, also begun in 1797, of a relatively unschooled and non-elite doctor, Francisco Barrera y Domingo's *Reflexiones Histórico Físico Naturales Médico Quirúrgicas*. Barrera was a Spaniard who had trained at a provincial hospital in Zaragoza. Hired as a surgeon by the Spanish Royal Navy, he established permanent residency in Havana in the early 1780s. Though of humble origin, and without a doctorate, he was an avid reader of medical literature and natural history, and he used his clinical knowledge of slave pathologies to present slavery as itself pathogenic. His *Reflexiones* contained a radical critique of eighteenth-century thoughts on race, and a particular rejection of ideas about the inherent barbarism of Negroes.[10]

Already by the end of the eighteenth century, then, Havana was a notable point of medical convergence in the Americas and the Atlantic world, and the city would consolidate its medical prowess and originality. The aggressive embrace of Enlightenment industrial discourse and practice by Cuba's criollo plantocracy, famously discussed by Manuel Moreno Fraginals, provided a generally conducive environment for the rapid development of a medical school at the University of Havana, the adoption of contemporary practices, such as anatomy and clinical pathology, and the promotion of surgery. At the same time, the sugar boom of the first half of the nineteenth century greatly increased the demand for slave bodies in Cuba at precisely the time that the English abolished the slave trade. Though planters continued to circumvent this by engaging in a dynamic contraband trade across the Atlantic that, by and large, satisfied their demand, the price of slave bodies tended to rise over the century, and it is likely that they were more prone to contracting diseases as plantation labour forces grew in size.[11] In this context, planters increasingly paid for medical attention, perhaps in some cases as an expression of the modernizing spirit of criollo slavocrat intellectuals like Francisco de Arango y Parreño (who was centrally involved in promoting medical reforms like the creation of the Midwives Academy at the women's Hospital de Paula in 1828).[12] In the retrospective words of the eminent nineteenth-century criollo ophthalmologist, Juan Santos

Fernández, who grew up in one of the great plantation zones in Matanzas in the 1850s: slaves were cared for because they came to cost from 500 to 1000 pesos each, "as a result of which medicine improved because they looked for the best doctor to attend them."[13] This begs the question of just what it was that planters thought physicians might do to improve the health of slaves—an important point that, given the limited effective offerings of medicine and surgery at this time, remains a crucial area for further research.

It is clear, however, that the market in slave medical care was good— good enough to attract many a foreign practitioner to the island. Medical immigration was assisted by Cuba's role as the initial landing place in the New World, and the island would become more attractive as a Spanish-American destination after 1810, when the wars of independence disrupted traffic and destroyed the economies in the rest of Spain's American colonies. The economic stagnation and political instability that followed independence and plagued the new Spanish-American republics through the 1850s provided further reasons for emigrant practitioners to cluster in Cuba, with its booming sugar economy and expansive medical marketplace. With the end of slavery in the British Caribbean in the 1830s, Cuba would also inherit some of the neighbouring islands' doctors. For example, Carlos Finlay's father, Edward, left Port of Spain, Trinidad, for Cuba in 1831 as part of this migration away from the dying slave systems of adjacent British islands, and would quickly leave Havana and go to the plantation zone of Puerto Príncipe. Then, after another brief stint in Havana, he would become the physician–proprietor of coffee estates using substantial complements of slave labour in Guanímar.[14]

The booming sugar economy and the rising value of healthy slaves also made medical schooling unusually appealing to criollo youth, even those from prosperous planter backgrounds. In other parts of Spanish America, medical enrolments languished for much of the nineteenth century as elite youth shunned the arduous and protracted training process, not to mention the dubious economic payoff and social stature (medical studies were easily a distant fourth place to law school, the military academy, and the seminary as an academic pursuit of oligarchy).[15] In Cuba, on the contrary, medical school enrolments were brisk, with a graduating cohort of 49 in 1850, and the numbers studying medicine rising precipitously from 93 in 1857 to 204 in 1864, when they represented over one-third of university students before dropping back to the low hundreds during the Ten Years' War of 1868–1878. Still, the famous first-year cohort of 1871, eight of whose members were sent to the wall, was a surprising fifty-two in number—this during the dire years of the war. Compare these figures to Chile, where four criollos finally graduated from the university's medical program in 1842 after ten years of study; or Peru, where only 10 of 142 students enrolled in the University of San Marcos in 1854 were studying medicine.[16]

Many of these criollo graduates set off in short order on a peculiar journey of apprenticeship. As Juan Santos Fernández put it, looking back on this golden era:

> they went to the ingenio hospitals because they knew that they offered abundant clinical material and good remuneration, and within a few years those who were active and studious came back to the capital with a fortune and no small experience, but having lived a rude life which was only tolerable during one's youth.[17]

Already in the late 1790s, Barrera y Domingo would observe that, in his seventeen years practicing medicine in Cuba, he had seen a great number of doctors engaged in this journey of apprenticeship, and had "to confess that, at the cost of grave damages to the poor negroes, although without hurting their consciences, some physicians and surgeons have become relatively skilled in their profession." He thought very little of the quality of most of the doctors he had come across, however, insisting that even among the licensed, there were many illiterates, and many more ignorant. Of course, he did not classify himself among this group, though he, too, was the product of just such a journey of apprenticeship: "I have put into practice, in this great city of Havana, my tried method of curing developed in a great many houses of the large ingenios, where I have saved thousands of miserable negro slaves with the almost miraculous cures I have affected."[18] The French physician, Henri Dumont, who worked on the plantations of Cuba in the 1860s, called this circuit a "tournée."

The pattern was common enough that it became a trope of Cuban *costumbrismo* (a short fiction genre of nineteenth-century Latin America that portrayed social types). In José María Cárdenas y Rodríguez's 1845 satire, "A Country Doctor", the narrator, one Tumbavivos (roughly, "entomber of the living") recalls his days, fresh from receiving his Licenciate in medicine, when he set out for a country practice. He soon strikes a deal with the "fat and healthy" owner of the ingenio Concurso, don Próspero Débito, "who needed a *facultativo* [titled doctor] for his property." As part of the bargain, the young galen receives his salary, food supplies, and "a maid at my disposition who was at the same time a washerwoman, cook, seamstress, and anything else I wanted." He is also given dispensation to "come to terms" on nearby farms, and to "attend on whoever called for me." Although the story does not cover the nitty-gritty of practicing medicine on slaves, the doctor's successful fooling of the country folk into thinking he has cured their self-limiting conditions with classic medical hocus pocus allows him to conclude:

> I spent six years in the countryside, at the end of which and with the good reputation I had acquired, and most of all with a nice bit of metal,

I was able to come back and establish myself in the city where, as everyone knows, I am one of the most famous *facultativos*.[19]

Of course, not all planters or (in the case of the many absentee owners) estate administrators were willing to pay the steep price of the schooled and titled practitioner—or the potentially steeper price of making his slaves available for further schooling the newly minted doctor. Honorato Bernard de Chateausalins, a doctor with long experience caring for "thousands of slaves" between 1820 and 1850 in the region of Madruga, wrote a best-selling medical manual for the use of planters. Chateausalins noted that most of the healing on fincas was provided by "low-rank surgeons and leading barbers"—the lowest category of titled surgeon with little formal schooling. But the book was written against the same "tournée" that Fernandez described, which was precisely the norm:

> a young European, recently arrived from Spain, France, England and so on, retires to the countryside, makes his first experiments on the negro slaves and lacking the experience necessary to repair the direct modifications that the climate brings to the nature of a disease, its causes, symptoms, cures, medicinal doses, and so on, practices medicine on the beaches of Havana or Veracruz the same way he would in Madrid, Paris, or London; he commits an infinite number of errors until the experience of many years is overcome, but at the expense of the hacendados; the extraordinary mortality rates that can be seen are a result of their inexperience.

The itinerant French curer registered the dislike of many planters for the orthodox medical approaches of schooled practitioners in including in his second edition, written in 1854, a homeopathic section "for those Señores Hacendados who want to cure their slaves by this method." He also reported the widespread lay practice of planters or administrators ministering to slaves using copies of Buchan's *Domestic Medicine* in translation or other similar medical manuals.[20]

While more solid evidence on the nature and economy of this medical apprenticeship would be nice, a basic pattern emerges clearly from the descriptions, commentaries, and biographical data: the standard medical bargain in Cuba saw foreign and criollo practitioners establish their credentials, their clinical skill and surgical technique, their therapeutic repertoire, and their capital through an apprenticeship journey around a plantation circuit, or through residency on particular plantations, with the majority of them establishing themselves in a larger urban centre after its completion. Some of these doctors, of course, settled in the rural areas, some as plantation owners themselves. The Trinidad visionary, Justo Germán Cantero, was one such planter who developed therapeutic mineral baths on his ingenio San Isidro to manage the health of slaves. Though solid research has not been done on this subject, it is not unusual to find planters with medical credentials, and it may be that, by the early nineteenth century, perhaps also due to the increasing value of slave bodies, planter sons were encouraged to pursue medicine as a practical education.

Juan Santos Fernández is one example of the male offspring of wealthy planters whose medical education was encouraged by his family, though circumstance, inclination, and changes in the sugar industry would lead him away from running the family ingenios. The following anecdote suggests that some of the riches available to plantation doctors came from treating the owners rather than the slaves, but it is worth noting that part of what inspired Fernández to go into medicine was the great impression made on him as a boy by the local doctor who had attended his mother during a serious illness. The dashing young doctor in his mid-twenties had arrived at the ingenio in his "luxurious coach", drawn by "three perfectly bridled horses." When the doctor's treatment yielded happy results, Fernández heard that his grandfather had sent the physician 100 ounces of gold, "of the kind that used to circulate with the head of Carlos III, equivalent to 1,700 pesos, and for her part my mom gave him a splendid mount" worth 60 ounces of gold.[21] Indeed, some doctors or surgeons appear to have made enough capital from their practice and other adventures to finance entry into the increasingly expensive world of slave-based sugar production. One who may fit this bill is José Leopoldo Yarini y Klupffel, the subject of another intriguing study by López Denis. Originally from Italy, Yarini came to Cuba with a Spanish passport in the context of the Napoleonic wars, toiled in the rural interior for some years as a school teacher, and was then able to pay his way through medical school at the University of Havana. Only a few years after receiving his title as a Latin Surgeon in 1811 and snagging a surgeon's post in the Spanish garrison in Matanzas, he appears as a prosperous plantation owner in this dynamic sugar frontier.[22]

CONNECTING PLANTATION AND SCIENTIFIC MEDICINE

Cuba was characterized throughout the nineteenth century by a super-abundance of licensed medical practitioners. Compared to other parts of the Americas, the numbers are staggering. In his political essay on Cuba, published in 1825, Humboldt calculated 61 "patrician physicians", 333 surgeons, and 100 druggists in Havana alone.[23] One standard medical history puts the number of practitioners of all kinds in the whole island at about 600 in 1833 (in Jamaica in the same year, on the eve of abolition, the number was 200, and it would drop precipitously soon after).[24] Good records can be obtained from some of the *Guías de forasteros* (an annual directory of colonial Cuba), published for most years in the nineteenth century. The 1842 guide provides a full registry of accredited medical practitioners in Cuba at a time of economic buoyancy and at the peak of the Cuban slave plantation's "classic period"—a time after the Haitian revolution when Cuba inherited the mantle of the world's pre-eminent sugar producer by developing industrial production methods that used large contingents of slave labourers. In and around Havana alone, there were 433 practitioners "offering services" in 1842 (and this does not include those on the regulating body, the Royal Governing Board of Medicine and Surgery, or Spanish military medical officers). What immediately stands out beyond the sheer numbers is that, for the time, this was a relatively educated and titled bunch. More than one-sixth (seventy-three) of these were actual Doctors in Medicine (graduates of a lengthy, arduous, expensive, and multi-tiered university medical training program, followed by public examination). Almost half (190) were Doctors or Licenciates in medicine and/or surgery—that is, they were graduates from university programs and titled by the royal licensing board. *Romancista* surgeons, some schooled, but most empirics and apprentices, and phlebotomists, all of them licensed after undergoing examination by the authorities, and among them a number with the status of mulatto and black, accounted for about one-third of the practitioners.[25]

Table 3.1 Titled Medical Practitioners Resident in Havana and Environs, 1842.

Professors of medicine and surgery	Doctors	51
	Licenciates	28
Professors of medicine	Doctors	6
	Licenciates	16
Latin surgeons	Doctors	12
	Licenciates	87
Romancista surgeons	Doctors	1
	Bachelors	3
	Priests	2
	Dones	52
Phlebotomists	Masters	88
Dentists		10
Midwives	White	6
	Mulata and black	9
Miscellaneous		17
Facultativos resident on haciendas and country estates	Doctors	3
	Licenciates	25
	Romancistas	17
Total listed in Guia		433

Source: *Guía de forasteros en la siempre fiel isla de Cuba para el año de 1842* (Habana: Imprenta del Gobierno y de la Real Sociedad Patriótica por Su Majestad, 1842), 266–276.

The guide registered 291 practitioners in the rest of Cuba, with the largest concentrations in Puerto Príncipe (34), Matanzas (22), Cienfuegos (13), Ciudad de Cuba (17), and Guanabacoa and Guines (8 each)—all important centres of Cuban sugar production at the time.[26] There were at least 37 doctors and 100 Licenciates—that is, almost half of the medical men of these provincial towns and their environs were titled physicians or surgeons, which is an extraordinary ratio for secondary and semi-rural areas of Latin America at this time.[27] It is also worth mentioning, given the healing roles often played by pharmacists, that there were a total of 267 Doctors and Licenciates in Pharmacy in Cuba in 1842—over half of them outside Havana (and with the largest extra-metropolitan concentrations in Matanzas and Puerto Principe, the leading sugar regions).[28] As Santos Fernández put it, citing as an example Juan Francisco Calcagno y Monti, a physician originally from Turin who, in 1820, set himself up in Güines (at the time undergoing a boom in sugar production), "in those bygone days one found doctors of great learning in the countryside."[29]

The doctors of plantation and metropolitan medical institutions were complemented at the elite level by the garrison medicine of the Spanish military. In the first half of the nineteenth century, there was significant overlap between garrison doctors and the rest, since many of the military posts were filled by local surgeons (this would change after 1854, when a new law was passed that prohibited all but Spanish military doctors from holding positions in the garrison hospitals).[30] Also titled and learned were a middle stratum of coloured phlebotomists, dentists, and midwives. Under an old Spanish law, only those who could demonstrate "purity of blood"— that is, clear European ancestry—could receive a title of surgeon or physician. Though this restriction was breaking down elsewhere in the new Latin-American republics, it was still very much applied in Cuba: José de la Encarnación Valencia, who sat on the Protomedicato as an examiner of phlebotomists and who ran a barber shop in Havana, had his application for a surgeon's license rejected on these grounds in the 1830s. Eleven of the twenty-six phlebotomists (barber–surgeons) listed in the *Guía de forasteros* in 1834 were "of color", as were fourteen of the seventeen midwives certified by the Protomedicato in 1828. (Typical of Latin America, Cuba's professionals lamented that no criollo women would train at the new school of midwifery after its creation in 1824 because of the association of even the learned heights of the trade with coloured status—though six of fifteen listed in Havana in 1842 were *doñas*.)[31]

Titled practitioners with some African descent also formed part of the circuit connecting plantation medicine to the learned world. They seem to have been primarily an urban phenomenon, which means they would have had limited contact with the plantation world (though they would certainly have practiced on the slaves in the retinue of Havana's patrimonial families). It is entirely possible that these titled phlebotomists or dentists also undertook tooth-pulling and minor surgical tours of the hinterland. Carlos

Blackley, a black dental surgeon originally from Charleston, and with a title obtained in London, ran a large practice in Havana with a number of junior dental practitioners for twenty-five years. It is entirely possible that he himself was a slave owner, and that some of the junior practitioners were his slaves; and it is easy to imagine him mounting the odd expedition through plantation zones as part of his business. Elite coloured practitioners were not yet, however, part of the formal network of medical knowledge–creation, and the precariousness of their position is illustrated by the fact that Blackley was finally ruined when he was accused of involvement in the 1844 conspiracy of "the Ladder" (alleged by the authorities to have been a planned uprising with involvement by many free people of colour and intended to reproduce the Haitian revolution in Cuba).[32]

Between this urban constellation and the plantation infirmary was a great assortment of popular healers, as well as the traveling homeopath, medicine man, foreign mountebank, and exotic country healers. Yarini describes the palaver that occurred in Guamacaro, Matanzas, during the cholera epidemic of 1833, when the bogus ministrations to stricken slaves of a British quack, Dr Mackie, were upstaged by the successful treatment of two slaves by a "wandering country Doctor, a Chinese curandero who was a native of the Philippine islands." Though the reference is notable in that this predated the arrival in Cuba of indentured Chinese labourers who brought Chinese medical practices with them, Yarini provides no details on the curandero's treatment.[33] Beneath the ingenio hospital was a complex world of reconstituted African healing practices and beliefs. Since the clandestine slave trade continued to thrive in Cuba up to the mid-century, there was a continuous influx of African medicine into the slave barracks. And between the *médico de ingenio* and the slave patient, there might be at least one nurse or infirmary attendant. Though we know virtually nothing about them, some would have played key mediating roles between doctor and patient, and translated for those slaves who had no Spanish. Working in the mid-1860s in the area around Wajay, the French physician anthropologist, Henri Dumont, compiled a glossary of fifty-seven medical terms and phrases in lucumí (the Yoruba language as spoken in Cuba), with the help of a Cuban surgeon who had worked on the clandestine middle passage and on a number of plantations. Dumont's work must have had its origins in the bilingual knowledge of infirmary attendants.[34]

Other evidence, however, underlines the fact that plantation doctors did not always work with infirmary attendants or have the ability to communicate linguistically with their patients. In his manual for planters, the experienced Chateausalins offered an elaborate glossary of body semiotics for the diagnosing of slave illnesses, something that assumed the average ingenio would have little, if any, medical intermediary between planter or mayordomo and slave.[35] In other parts of the Caribbean, information gleaned from infirmary curers, especially about medical botany, was rendered into early treatises on medicine in the tropics. Some recent studies, particularly

Julyan Peard's work on the Brazilian Tropicalista school of medicine, have shown that tropical medicine was not only a colonial discourse emerging from Western Europe in tandem with late nineteenth-century imperial conquests, but was also an autochthonous Latin American medical discourse that was in dialogue with European expertise from at least the mid-nineteenth century.[36] It would be nice to think that a further step might be taken by historians of medicine to find the patterns and methods that made African medical knowledge an active and constant source informing the emergence of tropical medicine. For now, we can only signal the existence of these overlapping healers and medical systems in the sugar hinterland, and note the interchange that must have taken place.

THE SLAVE CLINIC

The great size of the island's titled practitioners was sustained even as the Cuban sugar industry suffered some damage from the first war of liberation. The productivity of slave labour remained high until the period of abolition in the late 1880s, and planter commitment to using slave labour remained constant. However, estates also began to use other types of labour, including large complements of indentured workers and wage labourers, with as-yet-undetermined effects on the economy of plantation medicine.[37] The 1862 census registered 537 physicians and surgeons in the island, 220 of them in Havana.[38] Even in the bleak days of the Ten Years' War, in 1872, with notable migration of professionals out of Cuba, there were still over 150 Doctors and Licentiates in Medicine and Surgery listed in the *Guía de forasteros* for the city of Havana, and some 250 in the rest of the island. Again, this was a large figure for Latin America, and the qualitative indicators were also unusually high. The overall level of schooling had risen, medicine and surgery were now amalgamated disciplines for all practitioners, and barber–surgeons and phlebotomists were no longer listed.[39] Moreover, there is a likelihood that the profession had "nativized" itself, with the large cohorts graduating from the University of Havana in the 1840s and 1850s, slowly making up the core of the established community, and supplemented by criollos like Juan Santos Fernández and Carlos Finlay, who had done their medical schooling or specialist training abroad and had returned to take up practice in increasing numbers as the war drew to a close.

This consistently large, titled community of practitioners with a significant criollo presence was both the source and the audience of the medical and scientific institutions that flowered in the mid-nineteenth century. More work is needed to determine the role of slave doctors and the needs of plantation medicine in the initial period of Cuban medical enlightenment in the late eighteenth and early nineteenth centuries, though the general context is clear enough, and figures like Barrera y Domingo suggest the links were much stronger than has been represented up to now. A second period of great medical dynamism ran from the late 1830s until the founding of the Real

Academia de las Ciencias de la Habana in 1861. The two leading figures of this era, Nicolás Gutiérrez and Julio Jacinto Le Riverend—the first a criollo; the second a naturalized French immigrant—are themselves examples of the way that plantation medicine fed academic, scientific, and indeed professional and "national" medicine.[40] From the mid-1820s onward, Gutiérrez, a surgeon, was an important member of the Havana medical elite. Eventually occupying a chair in the Faculty of Medicine and Surgery at the University of Havana, he actively promoted the development of anatomo-clinical medicine. Le Riverend also enjoyed a number of faculty positions at the university medical school, including holding the position of Chair in Anatomy and Surgery in the 1850s. In 1861, he and Gutiérrez would become members of the Royal Academy of Sciences of Havana, and Gutiérrez would become its first president, their life's dream of founding such an academy finally come true.

The creation of the Academy of Sciences capped two decades of active and continuous medical publishing in Havana, with Gutiérrez and Le Riverend taking an author credit on a number of medical textbooks and on manuals intended for public consumption.[41] Both also played leading roles in the creation of a medical press in Havana from 1840 through the 1850s: in 1840, Gutiérrez was director of *Medicina y Cirujía*, which metamorphosed into the *Reportorio Médico-Habanero*, and he later became a regular contributor to Le Riverend's *El Observador Habanero: periódico de medicina y de cirujía práctica* (1844–1848) and in the 1850s, to his *Revista Médica de la Habana* (1854–1857). By some measures, these medical periodicals, and others of the period, were short-lived, and they tended to merge into one another and share the same small core of promoters and editors, with Gutiérrez and especially Le Riverend often at the helm (see Table 3.2.). At the same time, over the course of two decades, Cuba was rarely without a medical journal that appeared on at least a monthly basis (and might, as in the case of the *Repertorio Económico de Medicina* of the 1850s, sustain a weekly edition over an extended period).

Table 3.2 Medical Periodicals Published in Havana, 1840–1860.

Medicina y Cirugía/Reportorio Médico-Habanero	1840–1843
El Boletín Científico	1843–?
El Observador Habanero: periódico de medicina y de cirujía práctica	1844–1848
Reportorio Económico de Medicina, Cirujía y Ciencias Naturales	1847
Repertorio Económico de Medicina, Farmacia, y Ciencias Naturales	1850–1851
La Emulación Médica	1854–1860
Revista Médica de la Habana	1854–1857
Revista Médica de la Isla de Cuba	1858
El Eco de París [published in Paris by Cubans]	1858–1859

Le Riverend and Gutíerrez had both completed apprenticeship stints on the sugar plantations of Cuba. Le Riverend spent some years in the 1820s, after arriving in the country from France, working as a "médico de ingenio," including a residency on a large complex owned by the first Conde de Peñalver, among the very richest members of the plantocracy.[42] Gutiérrez had a brief apprenticeship on the plantations after receiving his Bachelor of Medicine from the University of Havana, and prior to his enrolment in the doctorate. Although this dimension of their experience has been essentially left out of the existing accounts of the rise of Cuban medicine in the nineteenth century, the medicine practiced on slaves by schooled and titled practitioners was central to the institutional and discursive medical complex that they wove over these decades. Slaves were used for clinical analysis; medical, surgical, and pharmacological experimentation; and dissection and autopsy. They were also used as sources of therapeutic and medicinal knowledge. In all cases, the results became raw material for a developing criollo scientific literature that legitimized institutions, built prestige, and founded a Cuban criollo medical sensibility.

The history of autopsy and dissection in Cuba has not been written, but there are indications that, as occurred in the American South, slave bodies, and black bodies in general, were more likely to be opened up after death, either to confirm clinical assessment or to serve as medical school cadavers.[43] In the 1820s, during his stay on the island, Alexander von Humboldt was duly impressed by the Museum and School of Anatomy, and noted that in the general hospital, "those who enter are the old, the incurable, and the negros who have few months to live and who the plantation owners wish to get rid of to avoid having to care for them."[44] These aging and infirm slaves, literally dispossessed, were the wretches whose cadavers fed Havana's amphitheatres of anatomo-clinical knowledge. One "Rare Case of Autopsy" written up for the *Reportorio Económico de Medicina* in November 1850 by the medical student, Braulio Saez, expressed the nature of this process in its blunt prose: "A black having died in the Medical salon of the San Juan de Dios charity hospital . . . the cadaver was transferred to the amphitheater and, having proceeded to the opening of the cranium, we observed . . .".[45] Similarly, when a "parda desgraciada" (roughly, "miserable mixed-race woman") by the name of Gamboa raised suspicions in the clinical salon of Havana's charity hospital for women, the Hospital de Paula, due to her masculine character and refusal to allow nurses to undress her for bathing or urinating, there was no question what would happen to her when she expired: "in the presence of the honoured teacher, Dr. Fernando González del Valle and a group of studious youth, the autopsy went ahead" in order to explore the possibility that she was that much sought-after medical freak, the hermaphrodite.[46]

Physicians conducted experiments on slaves as a matter of course. As he described it in *El Observador Habanero*, Licenciado José María Montalvo was called in 1843 to attend to Alejandro, a slave on a hacienda in Wajay who was suffering from tetanus. Interested in "proving with whatever facts were at my disposal the efficacy of tobacco preparations in the cure of tetanus," Montalvo began a series of experiments with green tobacco leaves. His article described the results of the experiments not only on Alejandro, but also on six other slaves in the area.[47] Montalvo did not say whether the owner was informed of the experiment. Evidence that findings published in the papers of the day were tried out on slaves comes from an 1844 submission to *El Observador Habanero* from Dr Joaquín María Quintana of Guanajay as part of this same debate over local botanical applications for tetanus. Having read Nicolás Gutiérrez's article on the use of the guaco plant to cure tetanus, he "proposed to try out the plant in isolation at the earliest opportunity in order to assure myself of its efficiency." Soon after, he was called to Travesura, a coffee plantation owned by the *Alcalde mayor* and his brother, to treat a 12-year-old, Cuban-born slave, Germán, who had "presented himself in the infirmary." Diagnosing tetanus, he tried out his recipe of a cup of infused fresh guaco leaves every two hours, and reported happy results.[48] In some cases, the physician might even purchase the slave in order to conduct an experiment and, in the case of successful outcomes, subsequently profit through the use or sale of the body once it was returned to health. Le Riverend recalled one such instance from his own past in the pages of *El Observador Habanero*. He had been sent for by the owner of a slave suffering from seizures, and diagnosed it as epilepsy. "After telling his owner . . . of the slight hope that I had of curing this illness, he proposed to sell him to me for cheap, and after he passed into my ownership I subjected the negro to [a] cure." Le Riverend documents the experimental therapy he employed, and concludes with the news that "since the year 1840 when he was sold to don Serafín Echeverría he has not had another episode."[49]

An interesting example of medical research on slaves is Justino Valdés Castro's *Memoria sobre lactancia*, winner of a literary prize in 1849, and published some years later in the *Revista Médica de la Habana*. Citing Le Riverend's own *Memoria sobre la leche* as an authoritative precursor, Valdés Castro presents a medical treatise on how to choose a wet nurse from among slave women. Here, careful physiological analysis of the advantages of breast and nipple shapes among certain African ethnicities, and the types of contagious diseases to look for, are combined with an anthropological analysis of temperament. In the end, *congas* (a designation used for several peoples from Central Africa) are determined to make the best wet nurses, though an individual phrenological exam and careful examination of the mouth for yaws are recommended prior to making a decision. Valdés Castro, evidently a self-styled reformer, nicely expresses the contorted moral calculus faced by the medical counsellor to slaveholders. He writes that:

> separating her children from her loving breast, to divert food that nature gave to them, to nourish others that do not belong to her; this, if you like, is *inhuman* [emphasis in original]. She is a mother, and

cannot look with indifference upon this change, one that might well be the cause of the death of the child that she truly loves.

The doctor proposes that the humane resolution to this moral dilemma is to grant the wet nurse her freedom "as payment for the maternal love that has been robbed from her" (though presumably only after she has proven her worth with the adoptive infant and suffered the death of her own).[50]

It is true that few of these examples come from the world of field labour on the plantation. This point remains for further study; the absence of clinical and experimental notes concerning slaves subjected to brutal punishment, or victims of industrial accidents, may have had more to do with the rules of public discourse and decorum. We can glimpse such a horrific world, however, in the pages of Henri Dumont's *Antropología y patología comparadas de los negros exclavos*, written in 1876. The work, considered a classic of early Cuban anthropology, was based on data compiled in 1865–1866 while Dumont was on a "tournée" around plantations in the interior of the island. The author was careful to note, however, that much of the data was given to him by a Dr Moreno (actually don Fernando Moreno, a romancista surgeon listed as resident of Havana in 1842), a practitioner he had met on the ingenio of Guanabacoa who had been the surgeon aboard the good ship Minerva when she made no less than eight contraband slaving trips to Africa between 1818 and 1820. Moreno had given him accounts of these voyages and "a large number of notes and observations on the negros he had assisted on the different ingenios of Cuba."[51] The work of Dumont, then, which should also be understood as a contribution to notions of distinct racial pathologies that were part of the developing discourse of tropical medicine, shows nicely how the medical knowledge accumulated by the plantation doctor—both elite (and in the case of Dumont, foreign) and ordinary surgeon—expressed itself at the level of formal scientific discourse in the metropolis.[52] Toward the end of his work, Dumont explores the common and disabling curvature of the leg and breakdown of the knee joint common to adult slaves in Cuba, and explains it as a result of the normal practice of forcing slave children to lift and carry excessively, indeed cripplingly, heavy loads from the age of six onward. Having diagnosed the problem, Dumont proposes a remedy that indicates in disturbing fashion the object of medical attention on the plantation: rather than proposing the elimination of the crippling practices of slave child labour, the handy Frenchman designs a leg brace that will allow slaves to maintain productivity as the condition develops.[53]

CONTINUITIES

Starting again in the 1870s, Cuba's criollo physicians and surgeons began to elaborate a complex institutional nexus on the foundations of the

Royal Academy of Sciences, and lived another glorious moment of scientific study, debate, and invention. A medical press established itself more firmly, clinical societies were formed, bacteriological laboratories built, island-wide medical congresses held, and revolutionary papers given at home and abroad—the most famous being that of Carlos Finlay on the mosquito transmission of yellow fever, delivered to his Havana colleagues in the Academy (following an earlier presentation of the core ideas at an international health conference in Washington, D.C.). These medical institutions were among the most important in an expanding criollo civil society that renewed the pressure on Spanish colonial control, and pushed the envelope of reform and calls for autonomous government in the years prior to the second war of independence of 1895–1898. However, not even this latter massive disruption of normal professional life could hold the doctors down. By the time of the census undertaken during the US occupation, the medical community had more than rebounded and numbered about 500 doctors. If, as Reinaldo Funes has recently noted, citing a contemporary source, Havana had more physicians per capita than any other city in the world in 1899 (at 1:492, a strong claim), the institutions and the expectations that sustained this dense, *fin-de-siècle* community were not far removed from those that had emerged out of the medicine practiced on slaves.[54]

Of course, the nexus of plantation medicine and metropolitan medical science and professionalism unraveled as slavery withered in Cuba between 1868 and the final stage of emancipation in 1886.[55] Country doctors still tended to the brutalized and sick bodies of slaves, as Manuel Delfín describes acerbically in his recollections of time spent as a young district physician in the western province of Pinar del Río in the late 1870s and early 1880s. New medical procedures were required of them to skirt the laws regulating slave protection and emancipation. For one thing, excessive corporal punishment of slaves might now be prosecuted, and planters and overseers expected the doctor to cover up their crimes. The Ley Moret of 1870 emancipated all slaves over sixty years old and, as Delfín put it, "the owners fought tooth and nail to avoid liberating the sexagenarian slaves—as it was the doctor who resolved doubts about age . . . I recall a number of times I was threatened if I said that certain negros were sixty years old." Though Delfín maintains that he refused to participate in this kind of medical barbarism to the point of being jailed for refusing to follow orders, the implication is that the practice was common.[56] In any case, he was not long in heading back to Havana where, by 1887, he had established himself comfortably as part of the metropolitan medical elite. He may have been among the last to try this tournée. The good economic times and professional prospects for practitioners in rural areas were coming to an end. As an editorial in the *Abeja Médica* carped in 1893, "the rural doctor . . . is left to lament the loss of the *igualas* or contracts that he once established with the owners of slaves, and to lend those same services not to sick people gathered in one spot, but rather to those scattered all about; and with very little or no remuneration."[57]

Notably, until the bitter end, young medical scientists like Juan Santos Fernández availed themselves of the clinical and experimental opportunities offered by what remained of the slave plantation. Setting up shop as an eye specialist in Havana in 1875 after completing his medical studies in Europe, Fernández got his practice started by treating the eye problems of the slaves still owned by his extended family and other acquaintances of Matanzas. His grandfather's aging slave, the 70-year-old Félix, attributed his eye problems, according to Fernández's notes, "to a contusion produced by a whipping he received some time ago."[58] He also dabbled in plantation medicine himself. In 1879, he recorded somewhat sheepishly details of a "morena [colored woman] operated on in the countryside in the ingenio of Dr. [Gabriel] Casuso . . . one day when he invited me to visit the finca." The two doctors had botched the operation, in part, Fernández confessed in his notebook, because he was in a rush to return to Havana and they had improvised an operating chamber "all in too much of a hurry and without anesthesia."[59] Fernández spent much of his career compiling data on patients of African descent. He carefully recorded the race of all his patients, and if they were black, he noted the African ethnicity if it could be ascertained, to generate clinical data that he hoped would allow him to determine ophthalmic pathologies specific to the black race. Roughly simultaneous with the composition of Dumont's work, which won the Academy of Science prize in 1877, Fernández would be among the founders of the Anthropological Society of the Island of Cuba, along with four other medical doctors.[60] It is not coincidental that Fernández was the central player in the expansion of Cuban medical associationism in the late nineteenth century, founder of the island's bacteriological and anti-rabies-vaccine institute modeled on the Pasteurian method, editor of the country's most important medical newspaper, author of hundreds of scientific publications, and president of the Academy of Sciences from 1897 to 1899, and from 1901 to 1922. The symbiosis of criollo medicine and the slave plantation had laid strong roots that would continue to sustain the Cuban medical complex well after the abolition of slavery in the 1880s, and the War of Independence of 1895–1898.

The nineteenth-century Caribbean can be characterized as a "laboratory of modernity", López Denis reminds us, due to its contribution to the "development of imperial technologies that fueled successive waves of European expansion into the tropics."[61] Other appropriate metaphors might be "clinic of modernity" or "surgery of modernity"—at least as far as the domain of medicine is concerned. As eighteenth century turned to the nineteenth, and Cuba inherited the mantle of export agriculture juggernaut by perfecting the modern technology of slavery, medical practitioners clustered in unprecedented numbers to tend its wounds and ailments, fix up slave bodies for more work inside the machine, hone their skills, try out new remedies, and announce the results of their great slave clinic in the pages of a new medical press. Then, if they were lucky, they might march triumphant back to Havana and other metropolitan centres, riches in tow, to academic chairs, elite practice, and social prestige. The criollos among them, who might very well have come from the provincial plantocracy themselves, stood some chance of re-entering the world of sugar as doctor–planters; various foreign physicians and surgeons, perhaps arriving with some capital already, used their tours of the ingenios of the interior to augment their wealth and observe the system with an eye on amassing wealth, and perhaps even entering the industry as owners themselves. This chapter has sketched out the existence and rough shape of such a community of medical practitioners, and explored some of the ways that they served the slave-based sugar industry, and were in turn served by it. In doing so, I have proposed that medical practitioners were an integral part of the production of sugar using slave labour, and that this practice on slaves itself generated important capital and clinical material for the production of Cuban medicine.

NOTES

1. This chapter is the result of research carried out with a grant from the Social Sciences and Humanities Research Council of Canada. The author would like to thank Reinaldo Funes, José Antonio Piqueras, and Vicent Sanz for an invitation to present an early version of this chapter to a distinguished group of Cuban historians attending the seminar, "Cuba y la plantación esclavista. Economía, sociedad, política y medioambiente en la primera mitad del siglo XIX," Fundación Antonio Núñez Jiménez de la Naturaleza y el Hombre, La Habana, 7 and 8 December, 2005; and Adrián López Denis for lively and learned comments on an earlier draft. Special thanks to Rebecca Scott.
2. *El Reportorio Médico-Habanero* 1, no. 1 (1840): 3. On the Anatomy Museum, *Guía de forasteros en la siempre fiel isla de Cuba para el año de 1842* (Habana: Imprenta del Real Gobierno y Capitanía General y de la Real Sociedad Patriótica por S.M., 1842), 206–207.
3. The term *criollo*, quite distinct from the use of the term 'creole' in the English Caribbean, was a carefully constructed (and to some extent, formally policed) ethnic category for those born in Cuba, but who could claim clear and unadulterated European descent on both sides of the family. Though a *sine qua non* for elite status in Cuban society, criollos were still subject to policies of discrimination on the part of Spanish colonial authorities which kept them from many offices and privileges and which favoured peninsular Spaniards in a variety of ways.
4. Pedro M. Pruna Goodgall, "National Science in a Colonial Context: The Royal Academy of Sciences of Havana, 1861–1898," *Isis* 85, no. 5 (1994): 412–426; and Pruna Goodgall, *La Real Academia de Ciencias de la Habana, 1861–1898* (Madrid: Consejo Superior de Investigacion Científica, 2002).
5. Richard B. Sheridan, *Doctors and Slaves: A Medical and Demographic History of Slavery in the British West Indies, 1680–1834* (Cambridge: Cambridge University Press, 1985).
6. Pruna Goodgall, "National Science in a Colonial Context".

7. The definitive Cuban historiographical position on Carlos Finlay is that of José López Sánchez, *Carlos J. Finlay: His Life and Work* (Havana: Editorial José Martí, 1999). Summaries of work on the Student Martyrs of 1871 can be found in Jorge F. Le Roy y Gálvez, *Dos conferencias sobre el 27 de noviembre de 1871* (La Habana: Centro de Información Científica y Técnica, Universidad de la Habana, 1975); and Jorge F. Le Roy y Gálvez, *La inocencia de los estudiantes fusilados en 1871* (La Habana: Centro de Información Científica y Técnica, Universidad de la Habana, 1971). For a heretical, modern French take on Finlay, see François Delaporte, *The History of Yellow Fever: An Essay on the Birth of Tropical Medicine* (Cambridge, MA: MIT Press, 1991); his book can be considered, in part, a polemic against Nancy Stepan's widely read article, "The Interplay between Socioeconomic Factors and Medical Science: Yellow Fever Research, Cuba, and the United States," *Social Studies of Science* 8, no. 4 (1978): 397–423.

8. A historiographical overview is Gregorio Delgado García, "Los Estudios de la Historia de la Medicina en Cuba," *Cuadernos de la Historia de la Salud* 66 (1983). An intriguing attempt to break the mould and explore the social history of medicine in the nineteenth century, which ultimately founders on the rocks of ideological orthodoxy and macrohistorical overview without historiographical foundation, is Ross Danielson, *Cuban Medicine* (New Brunswick, NJ: Transaction Books, 1979). Two recent works of great quality that incorporate the historiography of the past quarter century are Pruna Goodgall, *La Real Academia de Ciencias*, and Reinaldo Funes Monzote, *Despertar del asociacionismo científico en Cuba, 1876–1920* (Havana: Centro Cultural Juan Marinello, 2004; Madrid: Consejo Superior de Investigacion Cientifica, 2003).

9. On the publications of 1797, a year the eminent historian of medicine, José López Sánchez, has called the year of "scientific eclosion" in Cuba, see Enrique Beldarraín Chaple, *Los médicos y los inicios de la antropología en Cuba* (La Habana: Fundación Fernando Ortíz, 2006), 27–28.

10. Adrián López Denis, "Melancholia, Slavery, and Racial Pathology in Eighteenth-Century Cuba," *Science in Context* 18, no. 2 (2005): 179–199.

11. On the increasing susceptibility to disease as plantation labour forces reached 200 and above, calculated for the British Caribbean, see Barry Higman, *Slave Populations of the British Caribbean, 1807–1834* (Baltimore, MD: John's Hopkins University Press, 1984), 332.

12. Manuel Moreno Fraginals, *Sugarmill: The Socioeconomic Complex of Sugar in Cuba, 1760–1860* (New York: Monthly Review, 1976); Jorge Le-Roy y Cassá, *Historia del Hospital San Francisco de Paula* (Habana: 1958), 385–397; and Le Roy y Cassá, *Apuntes para la historia de la obstetricia en Cuba* (Habana: Imprenta Ancha del Norte, 1908), 8–12. For a recent discussion of the free trade, but never free labour, modernizing liberal criollos, see José A. Piqueras, "El mundo reducido a una isla. La unión cubana a la metrópoli en un tiempo de tribulaciones," in *Las Antillas en la era de la revolución*, ed. Jose A. Piqueras (Madrid: Siglo XXI, 2005), 319–342.

13. Juan Santos Fernández, *Recuerdos de mi vida*, 2 vols. (La Habana: 1918–1920), I: 310. On Juan Santos Fernández, see Pruna Goodgall, *La Real Academia de Ciencias*, 140–144, and passim; Funes, *Despertar del asociacionismo*, passim; and Steven Palmer, "Juan Santos Fernández," in *Dictionary of Medical Biography*, ed. W. F. and Helen Bynum (Westport, CT: Greenwood Press, 2006). The prices of slaves fluctuated dramatically over the first two-thirds of the nineteenth century, but roughly doubled between 1820 and 1860, and could indeed reach as high as 1500 pesos; see Laird

Bergad, *Cuban Rural Society in the Nineteenth Century: The Social and Economic History of Monoculture in Matanzas* (Princeton, NJ: Princeton University Press, 1990), 67–85; and Laird Bergad, Fe Iglesias García, and María del Carmen Barcia, *The Cuban Slave Market, 1790–1880* (New York: Cambridge University Press, 1995), 47–51.

14. The data comes from López Sánchez, *Carlos J. Finlay*, 51–58, though the author in no way suggests that the father's geo-professional motivations were related to the market in slave medicine.

15. John Tate Lanning, *The Royal Protomedicato: The Regulation of the Medical Professions in the Spanish Empire* (Durham, N C: Duke University Press, 1985), 138–145.

16. The enrolment and graduation numbers are from José A. Martínez-Fortún y Foyo, *Historia de la medicina en Cuba* (Havana: Ministerio de Salud Pública, 1958), 54, 78, except for the data of 1871, which comes from Le Roy y Gálvez, *Dos conferencias*, 3. On the Latin American comparison, see Steven Palmer, *From Popular Medicine to Medical Populism: Doctors, Healers and Public Power in Costa Rica, 1800–1940* (Durham, NC: Duke University Press, 2003), 43–44.

17. Fernández, *Recuerdos de mi vida*, I: 310.

18. Francisco Barrera y Domingo, *Reflexiones histórico físico naturales médico quirúrgicas. Prácticos y especulativos entretenimientos acerca de la vida, usos, costumbres, alimentos, bestidos, color y enfermedades a que propenden los negros de Africa, venidos a las Américas* [1798] (La Habana: Ediciones C.R., 1953), 12.

19. José María Cárdenas y Rodríguez, "Un médico de campo," [1847] in *Costumbristas cubanos del siglo XIX*, ed. Salvador Bueno (Caracas, Venezuela: Biblioteca Ayacucho, 2006), 103–109.

20. Honorato Bernard de Chateausalins, *EL VADECUM de los hacendados cubanos, ó guía práctica para curar la mayor parte de las enfermedades. Obra adecuada á la zona torrida y muy útil para aliviar los males de los esclavos* (Habana: Imprenta de Manuel Solar, 1854), xvi, viii. For an extended discussion of this manual, see Beldarraín, *Los Medicos y los Inicios de la Antropología en Cuba*, 32–42.

21. Fernández, *Recuerdos de mi vida*, I: 69–70.

22. Adrián López Denis, "Sugar in the Times of Cholera," http://en.wikiversity.org/wiki/Sugar-in-the-times-of-cholera.

23. Alexander von Humboldt, *Ensayo político sobre la Isla de Cuba en 1825* (Paris: Casa de Jules Renouard, 1827), 157–158, fn. 1.

24. Martínez-Fortún y Foyo, *Historia de la medicina en Cuba*, 6; Sheridan, *Doctors and Slaves*, 46.

25. Pedro Deschamps Chapeaux, *El negro en la economía habanera del siglo XIX* (Habana: Unión de Escrituras y Artistas de Cuba, 1971), 135–137, 155, notes that eleven of twenty-six phlebotomists in 1837 were "de color", and that, though not able to gain title as practitioners due to their colour, phlebotomists "de color" did sit as examiners on the Protomedicato.

26. *Guía de forasteros . . . 1842*, 278–289.

27. Lanning, *Royal Protomedicato*, 138; and Palmer, *Popular Medicine*, 38–44.

28. *Guía de forasteros . . . 1842*, 289–301.

29. Fernández, *Recuerdos de mi vida*, 1, 312.

30. José María Massons, *Historia de la sanidad militar Española* 4 vols. (Barcelona: Ediciones Pomares-Corredor, 1994), II: 150–151.

31. Deschamps Chapeaux, *El negro en la economía habanera*, 153–165, 167–184.

32. Deschamps Chapeaux, *El negro en la economía habanera*, 158–162; on the "Escalera" uprising, see Louis A. Pérez, *Cuba: Between Reform and Revolution* (New York: Oxford University Press, 1992), 98–99.

33. José Leopoldo Yarini y Klupffel, "El cólera en Guamacaro", mss. Archivo del Museo Nacional de Historia de las Ciencias "Carlos J. Finlay", La Habana, n.p.; thanks to the generosity of Adrián López Denis for the text of this source. See his intriguing web project, "Sugar in the Times of Cholera," http://en.wikiversity.org/wiki/Sugar-in-the-times-of-cholera.

34. Beldarraín, *Los médicos y el inicio de la antropología*, 51–65.

35. For a detailed discussion of this section of the *Vadecum*, see Beldarraín, *Los médicos y el inicio de la Antropología*, 33.

36. Julyan G. Peard, *Race, Place, and Medicine: The Idea of the Tropics in Nineteenth-Century Brazilian Medicine* (Durham, NC: Duke University Press, 1999).

37. For a comprehensive analysis of this shift, see Imilcy Balboa Navarro, *Los brazos necesarios. Inmigración, colonización y trabajo libre en Cuba, 1878–1898* (Madrid: Biblioteca Historia Social, 2000); and Bergad, *Cuban Rural Society*, 245–287.

38. Martínez-Fortún y Foyo, *Historia de la medicina en Cuba*, 79. The census itself did not register professions in the city of Havana, and the author must have compiled the Havana figures from another source. Note also that the figures would no longer have included the lowest ranks of barber–surgeons and phlebotomists, who with the general amalgamation of medicine and surgery—which is reflected in the 1862 edition—were no longer able to receive titles from the authorities. See also *Noticias estadísticas de la Isla de Cuba en 1862* (Habana: Imprenta del Gobierno, Captanía Genera, y Real Hacienda por S. M., 1864), 11.

39. *Guía de forasteros . . . 1872*, 239–255.

40. Pruna Goodgall, "National Science in a Colonial Context," 412–426.

41. For example, Nicolás José Gutiérrez, *Curso de Anatomía al alcance de todos* (La Habana: [1848?]), n.p.; and Julio Jacinto Le Riverend, *Manual de higiene privada* (La Habana: Imprenta del Gobierno y Capitanía General, 1846); and Le Riverend, *Patología especial de la isla de Cuba o tratado práctico de las enfermedades observadas en dicha isla durante un período de treinta años* (Habana: Imprenta del Tiempo, 1858).

42. Julio Jacinto Le Riverend, *Lecciones sobre las enfermedades observadas en la Sala de Clínica de la Real Universidad de la Habana en el año escolar de 1858 y 1859. Fiebre amarilla.* (Habana: Imprenta del Tiempo, 1859), 47.

43. Todd L. Savitt, "The Use of Blacks for Medical Experimentation and Demonstration in the Old South," *The Journal of Southern History* 48, no. 3 (1982): 331–348; Sharla M. Fett, *Working Cures: Healing, Health, and Power on Southern Slave Plantations* (Chapel Hill: University of North Carolina Press, 2002), 142–168. In a personal communication, Pedro Pruna Goodgall has suggested to me that there was also a good supply of white bodies to be found among the Spanish troops struck down in great numbers each year, by yellow fever in particular.

44. Humboldt, *Ensayo politico*, 158.

45. "Caso Raro de Autopsia," *Repertorio Económico de Medicina, Farmacia, y Ciencias Naturales* 1, no. 9 (25 November 1850): 1.

46. M. Tagle, "La Parda Hermafrodita," *Revista Médica de la Habana* 10, no. 1 (1 September 1855): 152.

47. *El Observador Habanero; periódico de medicina y de cirujía práctica* 1, no. 2 (1844): 85.

48. *El Observador Habanero* 1, no. 5 (1844): 291.

49. *El Observador Habanero* 1, no. 1 (1844): 7.
50. *Revista Médica de la Habana* 1, no. 14 (1 January 1856): 218 and 209–229, passim. Le Riverend's findings on breastfeeding are reproduced in his *Manual de higiene privada*.
51. *Guía de forasteros . . . 1842*, 274.
52. Beldarraín Chaple, *Los médicos y los inicios de la antropología*, offers an extended discussion of Dumont's work.
53. Henri Dumont, *Antropología y patología comparadas de los negros esclavos* [1876] (Habana: n.p., 1922), 66.
54. Funes Monzote, *Despertar del asociacionismo científico en Cuba*, 41.
55. The classic work on the demise of Cuban slavery is Rebecca Scott, *Slave Emancipation in Cuba: The Transition to Free Labor, 1860–1899* (Princeton, NJ: Princeton University Press, 1985).
56. Manuel Delfín, *Treinta años de médico*, 27–34.
57. *La Abeja Médica. Revista de medicina, cirujía y ciencias auxiliaries* 2, no. 8 (August 1893): 2; thanks to Reinaldo Funes for this reference.
58. "Registro Clínico," libro 2, case 1370, Juan Santos Fernández Collection of Clinical and Surgical Notebooks, Archivo del Museo Nacional de Historia de las Ciencias "Carlos J. Finlay," La Habana. The name of the patient has been changed.
59. "Registro de Operaciones," libro 1, case 7808, Juan Santos Fernández Collection of Clinical and Surgical Notebooks, Archivo del Museo Nacional de Historia de las Ciencias "Carlos J. Finlay."
60. Funes, *Despertar del asociacionismo*, 77–83.
61. López Denis, "Melancholy, Slavery, and Racial Pathology," 180.

4 Race and the Authorization of Biomedicine in Yucatán, Mexico[1]

David Sowell

In January 1873, Dr Waldemaro G. Cantón addressed the *Sociedad Médico-Farmacéutica*, Yucatán's first professional medical association. Cantón praised the group for its organizational success, but urged his associates to move beyond the discussion of public hygiene and into the investigation of the "secrets" of Yucatán's vegetation. According to Cantón, *los naturales*—the indigenous Maya—knew the medical qualities of the natural world around them; white *médicos* did not.[2] The limited professional knowledge of the medicinal properties of the plants of interior Yucatán led the *gente rústica*—"ignorant commoners and country folk"—to turn to *curanderos*, "charlatans", and *yerbaleros* (herbalists) for relief from their afflictions.[3] In the minds of the emerging biomedical community, indigenous healers hindered the expansion of professional medicine, the authority of medical doctors, and, thereby, the advancement of civilization. The languages of race and medical systems permeated Cantón's address. His labeling of different types of healers as *charlatanes*, *curanderos*, *yerbaleros*, and *médicos* associated race with patterns of knowledge and distinct approaches to healing. To be a *médico* implied training at schools such as the *Escuela de Medicina de Yucatán*, where Cantón had received his education. By the mid-nineteenth century, it also implied that the healer was part of the emerging biomedical system. The vast majority of *médicos* were white. *Yerbaleros*, by contrast, referenced indigenous healers who utilized Mayan conceptions of diseases and healings. *Curanderos* were lay healers (most likely *mestizos*) who lacked professional training. Charlatans were those healers who practiced medicine without a license, or those who claimed abilities that they lacked. Cantón knew that the *gente rústica* overwhelmingly utilized the services of *yerbaleros*, *curanderos*, and charlatans. Cantón and other *médicos* thus faced serious competition as they sought to control medical practices in the region. Similar struggles to impose biomedical authority took place throughout the circum-Caribbean region and in most of Latin America.

The years after the founding of the *Sociedad Médico-Farmaceutica* saw biomedical practices emerge as the dominant medical system in Yucatán. Mayan healing patterns persisted, but as subordinates to biomedical approaches. The control of medical practices, patterns of knowing, and the authority to practice medicine sustained the power of biomedicine. Part of the biomedical system involved the professionalization of physicians into a medical corps with organizations designed to unify their members and to promulgate information through journals and other publications. The creation of a medical system also involved the development of educational institutions, hospitals, and organizations to coordinate public health practices. Activists in the creation of the biomedical system pursued political support for their project, including the authorization process that would define who could and who could not legally practice medicine.

This chapter traces the construction of biomedical authority in Yucatán. It is particularly attentive to the intersections of race and medicine. Four segments divide the narrative. The first locates Yucatán within the Caribbean region. The second explores the medical hierarchy of the colonial era, when *médicos*, clerics, and Spanish administrators created *curanderos* by defining what medical practices were legal for which races, along with the "proper" role of religious ritual in healing.[4] The third segment surveys the range of healers who operated in early twentieth-century Yucatán. The process of the authorization of biomedical physicians and the articulation of healing Otherness comprises the final segment. A brief conclusion summarizes how biomedical physicians in Yucatán used *curanderos*, *yerbaleros*, and other healers as a stepping-stone to their privileged status of authorized healers.

Yucatán does not fully adhere to the historic patterns of either the Caribbean or mainland Mexico. The development of sugar plantations and the importation of millions of enslaved African labourers dramatically altered the historical paths initiated by Spanish "discovery" and colonization of the region in the 1500s. Indigenous populations gave way to Europeans and Africans on most islands, laying the foundations for dominance of Africans and Europeans among contemporary populations. Sugar agriculture oriented the region's economy toward the exterior, principally Europe and the United States. Large numbers of indigenous people survived only in areas of the circum-Caribbean, especially Mayan peoples in Yucatán, lowland Guatemala, and what would become Belize. By contrast, dense indigenous populations sustained the Viceroyalty of New Spain, the largest colony in the Americas. The conquest of the polities of the central valley of Mexico led to the development of a rigid colonial structure in which the Spanish minority worked closely with indigenous elites to exploit the labour of hundreds of thousands of "commoners". Mixed-race *mestizos* quickly surpassed the numbers of Europeans in New Spain, though as late as 1800, the indigenous population outnumbered the combination of Spaniards and *mestizos* by a ten-to-one ratio. Colonial Mexico's economy relied upon the production of silver, large agricultural estates, and vast numbers of small producers; export agriculture played a minor economic role. Complex racial, economic, and political hierarchies characterized

Mexican society at the time of independence in 1821. Yucatán again differed from these patterns.

Yucatán is located within the "Upper Caribbean", a region traditionally dominated by the ports of Vera Cruz, New Orleans, and Havana. The region was united by trade routes, human migrations, disease transmission (especially yellow fever), and complex political relations—a microcosm of globalized connections.⁵ Yucatán historically refers to the entire peninsula, but the state analyzed in this chapter has been stripped of Campeche (1857) and Quinta Roo (1902). Racially, most Yucatec residents were either white or Mayan. Campeche hosted a significant population of African ancestry, but their numbers are quite small in contemporary Yucatán. Most residents were of Mayan descent. The Spanish conquest in the 1540s led to white minority rule, with authority flowing from the towns of Mérida, Valladolid, and Campeche. Small-scale agricultural operations dominated the region through the colonial period, with most indigenous communities remaining relatively intact in spite of repeated epidemics and Spanish pressures. Whites garnered tribute from Mayan communities governed by their own elite through the late 1700s. Many Mayas acculturated to white ways by moving to urban areas, whereas Mayan cultural patterns dominated the interior well into the twentieth century.

Yucatán shares several key features with the Caribbean. These include the ravages of epidemic disease, the development of an export economy, and the imposition of biomedicine upon earlier medical practices. Beginning with small pox in the late 1510s, waves of epidemic diseases swept through the region with devastating results. Typhus, influenza, the plague, and other diseases followed trading routes in and out of the region throughout the 1500s. Yellow fever became endemic to many Caribbean towns after its appearance in the 1640s. Cholera swept through the region several times over the course of the nineteenth century. Influenza followed in the 1910s. Each of these diseases afflicted Yucatán. Fortunately, the era of deadly epidemics appears to have passed, though HIV/AIDS might dampen that hopeful assessment. In their places, the epidemiological transition made distinct afflictions dominant; new diseases and illnesses became the primary concern of public health officials in the twentieth century.

Yucatán's export economy emerged in the mid-nineteenth century, making the regional economy more akin to its Caribbean neighbours. The binder twine produced from the leaves of the henequen plant became critical to the wheat industries of Canada and the United States. The profitability of the vast henequen plantations attracted considerable international investment after the 1870s, with the concurrent meddling in local affairs so common to the Caribbean. Thousands of local Maya, rebellious Yaqui peoples, and other imported labourers worked in conditions of near slavery to produce the "green gold" that made Yucatán Mexico's wealthiest state for many years. Yucatec elites used this wealth to modernize the state, including the creation of a system of public health and the construction of a 400-bed hospital in 1906. These facilities sustained efforts to make biomedicine dominant in the region.

The "racialization of healing" is deeply rooted in Mexican history. As Spaniards constructed a colonial apparatus, efforts to authorize their approach to medicine inadvertently led to the creation of *curanderos*, healers intimately linked to the Hispanic colonial process. Nahuan, Huastecan, Mayan, and other indigenous societies had deep-rooted medical traditions before their conquest by the Spaniards in the 1520s.[6] At least initially, Spaniards valued these indigenous healers, using the prestigious label of doctors (*médicos*) in describing them. The shortage of Spanish *médicos* in New Spain no doubt led the conquistadores to use the Nahua *tíctil* (healer) for medical relief, but so too did the efficacy of these healers in treating the fevers, wounds, and diseases suffered by the invaders. Spaniards valued indigenous healers until the 1550s.[7] Several factors coincided to redefine their perception of these healers. First, Spaniards came to think that the "basic physiological nature" of indigenous peoples differed fundamentally from their own. How else could one explain the horrendous effect of small pox, influenza, and typhus on natives? These "Old World" diseases certainly sickened Spaniards, but not with the catastrophic loss of life suffered by the indigene. If Nahua and other natives differed racially from the Spanish, then they surely required different healers and methods of medical treatment. As a result, Nahua Martín de la Cruz saw his status gradually shift from that of a doctor who might treat Spaniards—even the Viceroy— to a healer who should only treat his fellow natives.[8]

At the same time, Spaniards were institutionalizing their colonial apparatus, including those parts of it associated with medicine. Spaniards authorized their system of medicine through the establishment of educational and medical institutions, the *protomedicato*, and the Inquisition. In particular, the establishment of the *protomedicato* required that any healer would need authorization in order to practice medicine officially. The *protomedicato* had developed in fifteenth-century Spain with the responsibility of regulating the training of physicians and their examination and licensing, inspecting pharmacies, and punishing non-authorized healers.[9] In the 1530s, the *protomédico* authorized native healers, such as de la Cruz and Antón Hernández, as *médicos*, but later stipulated that they could only heal other Indians and only using "*their* kind of medicine". By 1553, newly authorized indigenous healers had lost their status as doctors and, from the Spanish perspective, became *amantecas* (craftsmen), a manual classification considerably below that of doctor.[10] This racialization of medicine paralleled the construction of a colonial edifice founded on racial categories that guaranteed Spanish supremacy in all institutions of power.

King Philip II named Francisco Hernández as *protomédico general* of the Indies in 1570. Philip charged Hernández with the establishment of a system for the regulation of medical practices in the region around Mexico City.[11] As *protomédico*, Hernández wrote quite passionately against indigenous healers, despite the fact that his magnum opus, *The Natural History of New Spain*, required extensive interaction and reliance upon those very practitioners. Hernández afforded them the status of empirics, in that "they neither study the nature of the illnesses and their differences", nor command the intricacies of humoural medicine.[12] He failed, however, to regulate the practice of medicine in the region, an obligation that would not be fulfilled until the establishment of a permanent *protomedicato* in 1646.[13] Hernández favoured knowledge gained from formal training in academic institutions, which explained his criticism of indigenous healers. "Proper" understandings of illness and healing were rooted in academic knowledge. Medical schools thereby constituted a second institution critical to the creation of *curanderos*. A complex set of requirements created several types of healers, ranging from the formally licensed *médicos*, to the academic surgeon (and his empirical counterpart), phlebotomists, apothecaries, and midwives. In theory, all healers would have to be examined and licensed by the *protomédico*, but in practice, most practitioners were unauthorized. Fully authorized healers usually attended only to the highest levels of Spanish society.[14]

The Tribunal of the Holy Cross, the third institution responsible for the creation of *curanderos*, began its formal duties in New Spain in 1571. Previously, bishops had focused their inquisitorial authority against "witches", a category that quite likely included a few healers. King Philip II determined that natives would remain under the jurisdiction of the bishops and not subject to the Holy Tribunal. Nevertheless, from the beginning of the seventeenth century until the end of the colonial period, natives were among the scores of people examined by the Inquisition. The obvious native ancestry led to the dismissal of charges against several prisoners; others faced trial.[15] Healers faced the Inquisition not because of their healing methodology per se, but rather because their practices included activities not sanctioned by the Church. Noemí Quezada identifies four patterns of punishable activities. First, the therapeutic activities of some *curanderos* included an appeal to, and the support of, supernatural beings. Second, some healers used hallucinogenic plants, such as peyote, to enter a trance through which they would establish contact with such beings. Third, others used "idols" or other images from the pre-conquest period in the process of curing. Finally, *curanderos'* use of divination in determining the illness and its treatment violated the Holy Tribunal's norms. The Holy Tribunal found only those *curanderos* who transgressed against Catholic religious norms guilty. Others were accepted as serving "a specific function by offering a solution to the health problems of most of New Spain through the use of an efficient traditional medicine".[16]

These efforts to authorize Spanish medical practices as dominant, and other approaches as illegal, created a space in which *curanderos* emerged. Just as *mestizos* reflected the mixture of indigenous and European peoples, so, too, did *curanderos* mix medical practices. Although law and official policy relegated *curanderos* to the treatment of only natives and *mestizos*, the shortage of *médicos* meant that they often treated Spaniards as well. During periods of medical emergencies, the *protomedicato* might extend short-term permits to *curanderos* to practice openly.[17] This tacit recognition of unauthorized *curanderos* revealed the inability of the colonial regime to create structures that could either regulate public health policies or eliminate undesirable medical practices.[18] Once created over the course of the sixteenth century, *curanderismo* coalesced around an amalgam of healing activities. *Curanderismo* defined as "traditional medicine" is a complex mix of knowledge and practices that intertwined elements of indigenous, African, and European medicine.[19] The authorization process established institutional and social spaces occupied by privileged *médicos*, spaces that biomedical physicians would occupy in the second authorization process.

Unlike many areas of the Caribbean region, neither force of arms nor disease eliminated the potency of Yucatán's Mayan inhabitants. To be sure, Spaniards asserted political, economic, and religious authority over the region, and fundamentally altered the social and cultural norms of Yucatán. Nevertheless, indigenous practices remained quite influential. Yucatán differed from most of the Caribbean in that African cultural norms had little influence in shaping medical practices (the area around Campeche being an important exception). Whites dominated cities such as Mérida, Valladolid, Progreso, and Campeche, along with the agricultural zones of northwest Yucatán that would produce henequen in the nineteenth century. Spanish descendents asserted only superficial control over most of the peninsula. Even this domination was profoundly shaken in 1848 as the uprising of the "Caste War" was barely suppressed by whites; by the 1870s, vast areas of the peninsula were still under the control of "barbarian" natives. In this context, Cantón's address not only called for the expansion of professional knowledge, it also constituted part of the ongoing white struggle against indigenous social and cultural power.

The efforts to authorize biomedicine took place within a dynamic period of Yucatec history. Wealth from henequen production transformed the capital city of Mérida over the course of Cantón's life.[20] By the early years of the twentieth century, the city boasted excellent rail connections to the port of Progreso, an aggressive program of urban modernization, and medical facilities comparable in quality to those of Mexico City. In this context, Cantón and other members of the biomedical community proudly launched an ambitious public health program in the 1890s. In time, they sought to limit the activities of healers who did not meet their own standards, whom they thought might retard the progress of the region, and who might compete with them for medical authority.

A wide variety of healers practiced their skills in Yucatán in the early twentieth century. The range of healers in urban and rural areas differed quite significantly. In the rural interior, many healers worked within the traditional medical system of the colonial period, practicing *curanderismo*, an amalgam of Spanish and Mayan medicine. Most adhered to more strictly Mayan practices, including the *yerbaleros* identified in the 1870s. By contrast, many urban *curanderos*, including biomedical doctors, homeopaths, and spiritists, utilized knowledge and approaches to healing developed in the nineteenth century. In this sense, biomedicine was a *new* approach to healing. Some urban healers mirrored their counterparts in the interior, although without immediate ties to rural agricultural or social settings. The vast majority of the titled doctors, medical facilities, and educational institutions were located in Mérida. From the city, biomedical physicians penetrated the interior to combat infectious disease or "unauthorized" healers.

Médicos were predominantly urban. Academic training and professional associations differentiated biomedical doctors from the majority of healers in the region. Most doctors studied at the *Escuela de Medicina de Yucatán*,[21] though others graduated from medical schools in Mexico City, France, Germany, Cuba, the United States, or elsewhere. These doctors formed various associations to promote their professional status, including the *Sociedad Médico-Farmacéutica* (1872), the *Sociedad Médica Yucateca* (1907), and the *Asociación Médica Mexicana* (1922). These organizations frequently led campaigns against *curanderos*. Initially, doctors used newspapers such as *La Emulación* as a forum for these efforts, but after 1891, they added the authority of the *Junta Superior de Sanidad* (Board of Health) to extend official recognition to titled doctors. By the 1920s, laws, professional associations, and the power of scientific knowledge combined in the struggle against *curanderos*, *yerbaleros*, and other non-titled healers.

The number of biomedical physicians and medical institutions expanded greatly in the generation after 1890. An estimated 90 authorized doctors worked in the state in 1895, a number that increased to over 250 by the mid-1920s. Although estimates vary, at least three out of four of these men worked in Mérida at the beginning of this period, a percentage that was unchanged by 1930. Most doctors were engaged in private practice and were not directly associated with either hospitals or public health agencies.[22] Physicians associated with hospitals, schools, and the Board of Health were in the minority, although they dominated public policy. In Mérida, doctors worked either in the Hospital O'Horan, the Ayala Asylum, or both. A small hospital in Valladolid offered free services to the poor, opening an institution of scientific medicine in the eastern portion of the state.[23]

At least two other types of healers practiced in Mérida. Biomedical practitioners labeled them as either *curanderos* or charlatans, often mixing the two terms in their public critiques, though they originated in quite distinct medical systems. *Curanderos* utilized Mayan and Spanish traditions that had long dominated the region. *Médicos* labeled as charlatans the homeopathic and spiritist healers, who, like biomedical physicians, utilized knowledge developed in the nineteenth century. Homeopathic doctors had been active in Mérida since the 1850s, with several of them holding positions at the School of Medicine and the Hospital O'Horan. Spiritists arrived in Mérida in the late 1860s.[24] Non-titled healers who drew upon biomedical knowledge might be labeled as charlatans.

Anthropologists have conducted extensive research on healing practices in Yucatán since the 1930s. The Carnegie Institution of Washington sponsored numerous scholars who produced a wealth of scholarship, including considerable information on traditional medicine in interior towns and villages.[25] Other scholars have conducted similar studies in the last generation.[26] Mayan healers dominated the interior. The villagers interviewed by Carnegie Institution scholars generally referred to healers by their Mayan names, rather than the Spanish terms used by Mérida's biomedical physicians. *H-men, dzadzac, pulyah, x-hiikab*, and *kaxbaac* dominated the countryside.[27] White *médicos* likely referred to them all as *curanderos*, a term by which Robert Redfield meant a healer who treated "illness with herbal and other medical or magical means".[28] This broad category might include the exclusively male category of *h-men*, who not only healed, but also performed ceremonies associated with the *milpa* and other agricultural activities.[29] *H-men* occupied a social status comparable to the urban *médico*.[30] *H-men* were *yerbaleros* to many whites, but Mayan villagers referred to herbalists as *dzadzac*. Both men and women might serve as herbalists (*yerbaleros/as*), though only women acted as midwives (*parteras*, or *x-hiikab*, "she who does massage"). Biomedical complaints often targeted *sobadoras*, literally translated as masseuse, a term that also included *parteras*.[31] A final healer reported by Redfield was the *pulyah*, one who worked with "black magic". This might be the *hechicero* (witch) cited in Inquisition trials.

Other healers operated in the interior. The most common healers were the rural inhabitants themselves who practiced household (*casera*) medicine, an eclectic blend of multiple medical practices. Healers with a smattering of scientific knowledge that doctors might label as charlatans also traveled from village to village.[32] Biomedical healers were not permanent members of most rural communities until the 1930s, though they were present on occasion. The most frequent penetration of the interior by *médicos* came with an outbreak of disease, such as the 1918–1919 influenza epidemic. Doctors and sanitary delegates associated with public health agencies visited more frequently after the development of revolutionary health programs in 1934.[33]

Biomedical physicians throughout the world have used licensure and professionalization as means to authorize their approach to healing. Sometimes this took the form of a demand for formal training; other times, physicians criticized the failure of "lay" healers to use scientific knowledge as the foundation to healing.[34] Through the process of professionalization, biomedical physicians created we/they divisions that categorized other healers as "inferior". In Yucatán, as it has been seen, racial ascription accompanied these inferior positions. Biomedical physicians also used craft associations, control of public agencies, publicity campaigns, and other tools to assert their professional status, which could be translated into demands for political authorization that excludes "them" from legally practicing medicine.

The *Sociedad Médico-Farmacéutica* (1872) represented the initial effort to unite members of Mérida's biomedical community. Although it numbered fewer than two dozen members, this professional association survived until the end of the century. The Medical-Pharmaceutical Society founded the newspaper *La Emulación* to support four professional goals: to stimulate the study of medical and pharmaceutical sciences; to foster scientific investigations; to combat "egotism" among medical professionals; and to "fight against *charlantanismo* and *empirismo*, whose pernicious influences are the origin of so many negative consequences that afflict humanity".[35] The *Sociedad Médico-Farmacéutica* advocated the development of public health institutions in Yucatán, at least partially to combat *curanderismo*. Cantón and other leaders noted that during periods of epidemic disease, such as during the cholera outbreak of the 1830s, political officials would create a Board of Health. It would then be disbanded after the crisis passed. Physicians associated with the Society argued in favour of a permanent Board with a much broader jurisdiction. The Society suggested that the lack of medical statistics hampered public health initiatives. For example, doctors had a very poor understanding of the cause of most deaths in the region, primarily because *curanderos*, *yerbaleros*, or charlatans treated most people without proper records. The Society therefore proposed that municipal leaders should require a medical certificate stating the cause of death before a person could be buried in municipal plots. This strategy, it was reasoned, would both improve the quality of medical statistics and reduce the number of non-certified doctors.[36]

Several types of healers drew the attention of the Society. "Indian" midwives so aggravated its members that the Society sought—unsuccessfully in the end—to create a program of obstetrics at the local hospital to train midwives.[37] *Médicos* also claimed that some nurses at the General Hospital with "partial" knowledge were administering medicine outside of the institution, a practice the Society labeled as charlatanism.[38] *Yerbaleros* posed a particularly difficult problem for biomedical physicians. Most herbalists operated in rural areas where "rustic people" favoured their services, in part because *yerbaleros* were members of the local community. Society physicians claimed that rural dwellers preferred to "die in their houses" than to seek out the services of "academics or professors of medicine".[39] Unfortunately, not only "rustics" sought out *yerbaleros*; many residents of the cities did as well. Only concerted action by members of the biomedical community could remedy the situation.[40]

A successor organization, the *Sociedad Médica Yucateca*, completed the labours of the *Sociedad Médico-Farmacéutica*. Its members created *La Revista Médica de Yucatán* in 1905, a paper that served as a long-term supporter of the professionalization of Mérida's biomedical community. The editors of the paper wrote that "in civilized nations there is a beautiful flow-ering of beneficial institutions [that exist] to offer the precious resources of science and of charity [to the] disadvantaged classes."[41] They purposely linked public health initiatives and professional standing. In assuming responsibility for public health, biomedical doctors insisted that only quali-fied, licensed healers should practice medicine. While that goal was ambi-tious and no doubt some years away, a first step would be to change the sanitary code so that anyone who died outside of the care of an authorized healer would have to undergo an autopsy, paid for by the victim's family.[42] Again, biomedical physicians saw death as a means of enhancing their medi-cal power over the Yucatec *pueblo*.

From the first issue of the paper, the city's medical corps expressed their confidence that their anti-*curandero*, anti-charlatan beliefs would soon be embedded in law and licensure requirements.[43] These steps were seen as necessary for the public good, as well as for the good of the profession. Dr Narciso Suoza Novelo later identified three types of healers that under-mined the fortunes of titled doctors. First, and not surprisingly, was the "plague of intruders called *curanderos*". Midwives who called themselves gynaecologists and patent medicine vendors were comparable dangers according to Suoza. Each, he said, claimed that they complemented the medical profession. Souza soundly rejected these claims. All types of heal-ers should be controlled by public agencies. In order to gain this power, Suoza urged that the Society seek "congressional protection of medical sci-ence through appropriate legislation".[44]

The Mexican government enacted a new Sanitary Code in 1891, a move that was promptly seconded in Yucatán. In that year, the *Sociedad Médico-Farmacéutica* realized its aspirations with the creation of a perma-nent *Junta Superior de Sanidad*.[45] Although its name would often change, the *Junta Superior de Sanidad* served as Yucatán's primary public health agency for the next fifty years. The body was divided into five divisions, which served as sanitary police; regulated public hygiene and prostitution;[46] oversaw public establishments, such as pharmacies, slaughterhouses, and restaurants; and conducted sanitary inspections. In addition, the Board of Health maintained epidemiological, mortuary, and vaccination statistics for the state, as well as conducted vaccination campaigns.[47] The region's first Sanitary Code fulfilled a second major objective of biomedical doc-tors, requiring all doctors to register with *Junta Superior de Sanidad*. The *Junta* would thereafter verify physicians' titles and would determine their competence by means of an examination. A second code strengthened these statues in 1911.[48]

The 1917 creation of the *Dirección General de Salubridad e Higiene* signaled a major expansion of public health activities and increased institu-tional power in the struggle against *curanderismo* and charlatans. Spokes-men for this new *Junta Superior de Sanidad* relied upon the rhetoric of scientific progress to support their activities. The *Junta* continued to inspect food, housing, and public facilities in Mérida, but in a far more systematic fashion. In addition, for the first time, it created a system of "sanitary delegates" who would live and operate in interior towns, where *curanderos* dominated healing practices. The sanitary delegates would be missionaries of science, seeking to convert into "tangible reality" the "natural right of progress".[49] Amplified legal authority aided the new body's efforts to regulate the practice of medicine in Yucatán. All titled surgeons, dentists, pharmacists, and doctors were required to register with *Dirección de Salubridad* to have their legal status confirmed. They would then have to pass an examination to verify their knowledge.[50] Within months of its founding, the *Junta* demonstrated its legal muscle when it fined Enrique Wanovichtz 500 pesos gold for repeated violations of the sanitary code's stipulation that a physician be titled and authorized in order to practice medicine.[51]

Homeopathic doctors proved far more problematic for physicians on the *Junta*. Followers of Samual Hahnemann asserted that they too practiced scientific medicine. They certainly had professional titles and formal academic training, some from the National School of Homeopathy in Mexico City, others from schools in the United States, Cuba, or Europe. Homeopathic doctors had practiced in Mérida since the 1850s. Some, such as Rafael Villamil, were leading physicians at the Hospital O'Horán and professors at the School of Medicine.[52] Dr Romualdo Manjarrez López thus faced a vexing task when Director Gil Rojas Aguilar asked him to recommend a policy for the Board of Health in dealing with homeopathic physicians. The administrative council of the homeopathic school in Mexico had asked Gil Rojas to request that Yucatán's state law be brought into agreement with the new federal constitution, thereby authorizing graduates of the school to practice legally in Mérida.[53] Manjarrez López recognized the sensitive nature of the issue, arguing that "social harmony" might permit the recognition of homeopaths. However, he insisted, the state government should not blindly authorize all titles from outside the state. Manjarrez López believed the National School of Homeopathy to be honourable, but its ideals and principles might be misguided, a coded critique of the homeopathic method. Still, it seemed "natural" that graduates of the school should be titled in Yucatán. The request was nonetheless denied, not on the grounds of belief systems—embedded in knowledge and education—but rather based on state versus federal authority. Manjarrez López reasoned that authorization needed to originate at the state, not federal, level. He recommended that homeopathic physicians be required to present their credentials to the Board of Health and, like graduates from other medical schools, undergo an examination to demonstrate their medical understanding.[54] Unspoken, of course, was the fact that homeopathic practices would not pass as appropriate knowledge in the eyes of the examining committee. Manjarrez López's jurisdictional logic thus avoided the underlying differences between the two medical beliefs, placing the legal system as the arbiter of "legitimate" medical practices.

Politicians, of course, dominated the legal system. Eduardo L. Menéndez argues that the labour and socialist organizations spawned by the Revolution were among the strongest advocates for public health programs sustained by scientific medicine. The "scientific medical solutions" envisioned by biomedical physicians were appropriated as constitutive elements of their own progressive ideology. Menéndez saw revolutionary support for public health most clearly in support of yellow fever campaigns, but also around questions of homeopathic medicine. [55] Homeopathic physicians gained partial legal status in 1922, when Socialist Governor Felipe Carrillo Puerto authorized the establishment of an *Escuela de Medicina Homeopática* in Mérida in opposition to the interests of biomedical physicians of the *Sociedad Médica Yucateca*. For several years, the Homeopathic School of Medicine was part of the *Universidad del Surreste*, a relationship that was abruptly severed in 1929 under a new administration. The *Escuela de Medicina Homeopática* operated through 1938, when it was ordered to close its doors.[56] It is clear that official favour determined whether homeopathic physicians were permitted to legally practice medicine.

Biomedical physicians also identified spiritists as charlatans. Officials of the *Junta Superior de Sanidad* informed the governor in 1922 that operators of the Spiritist Center, "*Luz y Unión*", were akin to "*hechiceros, brujos*, divinists, and *yerbaleros*" and were practicing sorcery, hypnotism, and other "absurd practices". In criticizing spiritists, biomedical physicians correlated their healing practices with those of indigenous healers, a characterization meant to belittle their social standing. Dr Miguel Castillo Torre and two police officers visited the Spiritist Center, speaking with both visitors and its director, Ignacio Góngora. Several patients reported that the medium prescribed and sold them various drugs. Director Góngora countered that he was hardly a charlatan, since he had been in business for over thirty years. Góngora told local officials that upon entering a trance, he sought out the protective advice of Francisco García A., a spirit "on the other side" who informed him of the person's illness and what medications were required.[57] Little seemingly came of this campaign, for ten years later, physicians complained that the spiritist facilities—"centers of barbarism"—still operated with the full knowledge of public authorities. Worse was the fact the local pharmacists readily filled the prescriptions from the centres. *La Revista Médica de Yucatán* lamented, "what a sad role that a professional might be mixed up in these affairs!"[58]

Midwives drew the same critiques as *curanderos*, homeopaths, and spiritists. Dr Carlos Cáseres noted progress in the regulation of physicians; no efforts were being made to monitor midwifery. While most midwives were "modest and moral" according to Cáseres, some practiced "the occult arts". Moreover, they gave injections and wrote prescriptions, which should be the sole prerogative of titled professionals. Worse, perhaps, for Cáseres was a recent congress of nurses and midwives in Mexico City. This gathering, he claimed, was a mix of the "logical and fantasy, the reasonable and absurd". The Revolution's spawning of self-regulating syndicates, Cáseres asserted, should be abandoned in favour of professional associations.[59]

Municipal authorities occasionally joined doctors in denouncing charlatans to the *Junta Superior de Sanidad*. Such was the case in 1927, when political boss Prudencia Pech from the village of Chicxulub claimed that Genaro Loría A. was presenting himself falsely as a doctor. Pech reported that Loría "is not a titled doctor", but that he did have sufficient knowledge to practice medicine in "necessary cases" and, anyway, he only charged fifty centavos a visit. The Board of Health ordered Pech to have Loría stop practicing until he could obtain the necessary permission from the Municipal Council.[60] In a similar case, the *curandero* Eduardo Peraza refused an order to cease practicing medicine, whereupon Governor Alvaro Torre Díaz ordered him arrested, and offered him the choice of a 100-peso fine or fifteen days in jail.[61]

Almost twenty years after he first called for a campaign against *curanderos*, Narciso Suoza Novelo joined Pedro Magaña Erosa to renew the struggle in 1931. In a speech before the third annual convention of Mexican medical societies, the pair outlined eight necessary steps to end the threat to their profession. The first step was to convince the public of the benefits of medical science, accompanied by an explanation of "the dangers that accompanied the empirical assistance of the sick". The public needed to rely upon science, rather than tradition. It was not enough, however, to explain the superiority of medical science; medical facilities should be established in rural towns and villages. Vaccinations, propaganda leaflets, and local conferences would help in the interior. In this task, local, state, and federal authorities, along with medical associations, needed to cooperate, a coordination that had been lacking prior to that time. With these two steps, a concerted campaign against non-registered charlatans could begin, demonstrating the "pseudo-scientific" nature of their practices. Pharmacists needed to be regulated much more closely, as did the drugs that they sold, especially to charlatans. Strong central authority and rigid enforcement of the law were the required final aspects of the campaign.[62]

The task of using medical knowledge to distinguish *médicos* from charlatans was challenging. Germán Pompeyo S. suggested that charlatans worked on the periphery of titled doctors, reaping the benefits of their labour. Unfortunately, medical science did not always attract the public's loyalty: "The doctor has knowledge, [but] silence and austerity accompanies science, which always searches for the severe truth offered as the beautiful product of investigation".[63] The implication in Pompeyo's analysis was that doctors needed to win the minds—and the hearts—of the public in order to strengthen the professional medical community. Pompeyo saw charlatans' appeals to passions as their strongest point, making "the most delicate fibres of the soul vibrate in the masses, which are fascinated by them to the point of craziness".[64]

Competition caused by the burgeoning number of physicians and the Depression increased complaints about *curanderos* and unauthorized practitioners. "*Curanderismo* is a true plague", concluded Dr Alejandro Cervera A. in 1933. Cervera identified six categories of charlatans, few of which would have been active in the nineteenth century. He argued that people associated with pharmacies or nurses practicing as doctors constituted an important category of charlatans. Both types, he concluded, had a little medical knowledge and often prescribed drugs without formal training. Vendors and hawkers of patent medicine, spiritists, and naturalists each occupied separate categories.[65] Another physician added three more categories: titled doctors who practiced outside their specialties, doctors who had lost their titles, and students who had not yet finished their education. Only university trained, biomedical physicians were "true" healers.[66]

Declining economic fortunes led the editors of *La Revista Médica de Yucatán* to ask if their subscribers thought a plethora of physicians existed in the region and, if so, how *curanderos* might contribute to the excess. Dr Alberto Berrón Guerrero, a leader in the *Sociedad Médica Yucateca*, blamed the medical community for many of its own problems. Yes, Berrón Guerrero opined, an excess of doctors existed, but *curanderos* were not at fault. Insofar as the vast majority of physicians resided in Mérida, physicians could help themselves by moving into the interior. Rural areas lacked adequate medical care, forcing peasants to seek out *curanderos*. This, for Berrón Guerrero, was expected, since "the bulk of the population is illiterate and believes in spiritists, in *yerbaleros* . . . in naturalists, in invisible doctors and in homeopaths".[67] However, until rural dwellers were educated, ending *curanderismo* was "anti-humanitarian" and "anti-patriotic". Better remedies for him included ending the economic crisis, limiting the number of foreign physicians and graduates from the local medical school, and creating rural clinics to increase the demand for specialists. He did call for the end of the practice of illegal medicine in Mérida, leaving more opportunities for titled physicians.[68] Dr Germán Pompeyo agreed that the creation of rural clinics that would deliver inexpensive care, offer physicians more jobs, and undermine the power of rural *curanderos*.[69]

Other physicians joined the conversation. Carlos Cáseres Pérez offered a somewhat different analysis than Berrón Guerrero. He agreed that the propensity to settle in Mérida was a major shortcoming in the region, but insisted that *curanderos* were part of the problem. Doctors should not seek to limit the number of graduates from the School of Medicine because scientific graduates were the best weapons against *curanderismo*. However, biomedical healers did need to communicate better and to demonstrate the superior health care created by scientific knowledge.[70] Ricardo Molina added that federal authorities had complicated the local situation by adding more and more requirements on titled physicians, while charlatans operated with impunity.[71] "Paradoxically, our system tends to favor those who operate outside the law, and to weigh heavily upon those who have chosen to obey it in keeping with the ideas that come with medical knowledge and the acquisition of medical titles."[72] Local authorities also deserved some blame, in that they accepted charlatans in the absence of licensed doctors. Rural areas, one editor wrote, required the "labour of a missionary" in order to demonstrate the value of a physician.[73]

Several years later, Dr Ciopriano Domínquez Rivero, from the interior town of Valladolid, offered a remarkably different analysis of rural medicine. Newly graduated physicians bound for a rural practice encountered three problems, in his opinion. A doctor first had to deal with the "ignorance of the pueblo", a problem stemming from the simple fact that doctors did not speak Mayan, nor most rural inhabitants Spanish. Doctors had to rely upon a translator, who was seldom trained in medicine and therefore unable to convey appropriate meanings of symptoms. As a result, misdiagnosis or poor prescriptions were common, resulting in a lack of trust for doctors among the Maya. Domínquez Rivero disagreed with those who claimed that widespread Spanish education was the answer. It made little sense to teach thousands of people Spanish: adding Mayan to curricula of medical schools would more conveniently solve the problem.[74]

Nor were traditional *curanderos* the only challenges to biomedical doctors. *Curanderos*, *yerbaleros*, and *hechiceros* had learned the "art of healing" not by knowledge, but by experience. Most dangerous, Domínquez Rivero argued, were the titled doctors who had abandoned their science while living in the interior and taken on the ways of empiricism. They had abandoned their scientific approach in favour of "instincts". Similarly, nurses, physician's aids, and pharmacists who claimed to know medicine, but who, in fact, had only partial knowledge, damaged the science of biomedicine and contributed to the lack of faith in its benefits. Rural officials, the third major problem in the region, assisted practitioners with partial knowledge. Officials seldom enforced the rules, took favours from charlatans, and contributed to the lack of respect for authority.[75] What then were the needs of rural medicine? Dedicated programs of rural health, with three years of Mayan language study required for doctors who would staff them. Rigid enforcement of existing laws was necessary, especially to deal with charlatans. Finally, public conferences on the benefits of scientific medicine could help to combat *curanderismo*.[76]

The influence of the Revolution on health care in Yucatán developed quite slowly. Not surprisingly, the creation of a federal, bureaucratic medical structure, replete with legal authorization and responsibilities, added another layer to the struggle against *curanderos* and helped further define the boundaries of charlatanism. Yucatec doctors, however, were far from pleased with all functions of the new federal entities. The revolutionary regime sought to control the production of all health care and the agents who delivered it.[77] These federal "intrusions" sparked local opposition. In 1927, for example, local physicians petitioned the Governor, protesting demands from the Sanitary Delegate of the federal *Departamento de*

Salubridad Pública that all local doctors register with the Department and that they report all cases of communicable diseases, in keeping with article 158 of the Federal Sanitary code.[78]

Local doctors argued that the proposal was unconstitutional, inimical to their relations with patients, and a boon to *curanderismo*. It was unconstitutional, the petition stipulated, because Articles 4, 14, and 16 of the constitution gave authorization powers to state authorities. If the Sanitary Delegate wanted the information, he could request it from the local *Junta Superior de Sanidad*, which already collected that type of data. The proposed registration would give rise to *curanderismo*, the petitioners argued, because it would damage the faith of patients in titled doctors, as well as force up prices. Patients would abandon titled doctors and seek out empirics, who had access to the same medicine but did not have to report to federal authorities.[79]

The syndicates spawned by the Revolution often took a leading role in linking local, state, and federal concerns. The *Asociación de Médicos y Profesionistas Conexos de Yucatán*[80] complained in late 1934 that "various judges and municipal authorities" were sponsoring *charlatanismo*. According to the Sanitary Code, the registry of deaths and burials were supposed to be the responsibilities of duly authorized physicians. Local politicians, they alleged, were allowing "non-authorized" persons to register deaths and burials for their personal gain and to the detriment of the profession. The Association asked that federal authorities halt such practices.[81] Within a month, a lawyer for the Judicial Service of the Federal Department informed the governor of Yucatán of the situation, asking him to take appropriate steps to comply with the rules of the Sanitary Code.[82]

In 1934, the revolutionary regime established a body for "*Servicios Médicos Ejidales*" that became quite active in the henequen zone.[83] The *Asociación de Médicos y Profesionistas Conexos de Yucatán* reported the next year that a henequen *hacendado* had informed them of the activities of *curandero*, Gregorio Cauich. Cauich, federal authorities were informed, "was a *curandero* dedicated to the illegal practice of medicine through witchcraft". Because Cauich was said to be in violation of federal and state Sanitary Codes, plus the Federal Work Law, the Federal Department of Public Health was asked to respond appropriately.[84] A flurry of correspondence brought together the Judicial Service of the Federal Department, its Sanitary Delegate, and the Governor of the State of Yucatán, the local *Junta Superior de Sanidad*, and municipal officials in Molas, where Cauich operated.[85]

Writing in the early 1940s, Drs José F. Díaz and Benjamín Gongora Triay proudly summarized the cooperative efforts of the federal and state governments to improve the public health of the region.[86] While evidence from the 1930s belies the harmony of state–federal relations, it is clear that an impressive institutional edifice had been constructed in the state. Led by the Hospital O'Horan, the Ayala Asylum, and the Children's Hospital (1940), social assistance was sustained by government authority and the Socialist Party. The Department of Sanitation and Beneficence (headed by the *Junta Superior de Sanidad*) managed state health programs. The Federal Sanitary Delegation included a laboratory, anti-yellow fever and anti-tuberculosis campaigns, various inspectors, and a growing administrative structure joined it. Rural schools begun in the 1930s and supported by the Socialist Party, became the backbone for a system of social security that developed after the 1940s. With the creation of the Ministry of Health and Assistance in 1943, the federal apparatus to guide medical policy was firmly in place.[87] Significantly, the institutions created by the state and federal governments rested on a scientific foundation.[88] So too did the academic and professional organizations that provided the physicians to these institutions and to the public. The many dimensions of Mexico's contemporary medical system were now in place, with full authorization powers sustained by state and federal political structures and a growing institutional edifice. At risk were indigenous healers, who were now illegal and faced the onslaught of both state and federal authority.

The twentieth-century authorization of biomedicine differed significantly from the authorization of Spanish medicine in the early colonial period. Absent from the second authorization was the church, in either its ideological influence or institutional contribution. The overtly racialized medical system of the colonial period, while now obscured, underpinned the medical discourse, expressed in the coded language of "progress" or "modernization". Whites led the civilizing mission of modernization; indigenous Mayans retarded progress. Still, while biomedical agents clearly linked *curanderismo* with Mayan and other indigenous peoples, most sectors of Yucatec society accepted *curanderismo*, just as they had in the colonial era.

The introduction of biomedicine into the Yucatán in the nineteenth century led to a reconceptualization of *curanderos*. After the 1850s, physicians associated with the emerging biomedical paradigm replaced the racial, religious, and social features that colonial *médicos* had used to distinguish *curanderos* from themselves with claims of scientific knowledge and professional conduct. They created professional communities that sought and achieved the exclusive privilege of practicing medicine, as well as the legal authority and power associated with state and federal institutions. In the descriptions of *curanderos* and charlatans, physicians revealed their sense of self, one that is visible throughout contemporary Mexico. These images of *curanderos* and charlatans help to illustrate the critical transition between the colonial and modern eras of Mexican medicine. At the dawn of the twenty-first century, many "biomedical representatives" continue to "dismiss village curers as quacks or superstitious charlatans". They allege "that the people who seek such cures are fools who are easily duped by charlatans in the guise of *curanderos*".[89] Although *curanderismo* is often effective and enjoys widespread popularity, it is deemed a "backward" approach to healing by agents of the government and biomedical institutions. People who seek the assistance of *curanderos* are relegated to an inferior social status, despite recent efforts to extend official support to the healing practices of *curanderos* and other traditional healers.[90]

NOTES

1. A preliminary version of this chapter was presented at the Juniata College Bookend Lecture Series and has been published in *Juniata Voices* 5 (2005). Parts used in that essay are reprinted with permission. The author acknowledges the helpful comments made at that forum and the readers of this significantly modified essay. The author gratefully acknowledges the editorial assistance of Emily Sowell in the preparation of this essay.
2. *La Emulación* (Mérida), January 1873.
3. *La Emulación*, November 1874.
4. For an overview of the Spanish medical system in New Spain, see Luz María Hernández and George M. Foster, "Curers and their Cures in Colonial New Spain and Guatemala: The Spanish Component," in *Mesoamerican Healers*, eds. Brad R. Huber and Alan R. Sandstrom (Austin: Texas University Press, 2001), 19–46.
5. José Ronzón, *Sanidad y modernización en los puertos del Alto Caribe, 1870–1915* (México, DF: Universidad Autónoma Metropolitana, 2004); Andrew Louis Knaut, "Disease and the Late Colonial Public Health Initiative in the Atlantic Ports of New Spain" (PhD diss., Duke University, 1994).
6. See, for example, Bernard R. Ortiz de Montellano, *Aztec Medicine, Health, and Nutrition* (New Brunswick, NJ: Rutgers University Press, 1990).
7. Carlos Viesca Treviño, "*Curanderismo* in Mexico and Guatemala: Its Historical Evolution from the Sixteenth to the Nineteenth Century," in *Mesoamerican Healers*, 47–49; Serge Gruzinski, *The Mestizo Mind: The Intellectual Dynamics of Colonization and Globalization*, trans. Deke Dusinberre (New York: Routledge, 2002), 47.
8. Viesca Treviño, "*Curanderismo* in Mexico and Guatemala," 49–50.
9. John Jay TePaske, "Regulation of Medical Practitioners in the Age of Francisco Hernández," in *Searching for the Secrets of Nature: The Life and Works of Dr. Francisco Hernández*, eds. Simon Varey, Rafael Chabrán, and Dora B. Weiner (Stanford, CA: Stanford University Press, 2000), 55–56. Many of the contributions of Hernández have recently been published in *Searching for the Secrets of Nature* and *The Mexican Treasury: The Writings of Dr. Francisco Hernández*, eds. Simon Varey, Rafael Chabrán, and Dora B. Weiner (Stanford, CA: Stanford University Press, 2000).
10. Viesca Treviño, "*Curanderismo* in Mexico and Guatemala," 50. Italics in the original.
11. TePaske, "Regulation of Medical Practitioners," 57–58.
12. Ibid., 55–56.
13. Ibid., 58.
14. Luz María Hernández Sáenz, *Learning to Heal: The Medical Profession in Colonial Mexico, 1767–1831* (New York: Peter Lang, 1997), 3–5.
15. Noemí Quezada, "The Inquisition's Repression of *Curanderos*," in *Cultural Encounters: The Impact of the Inquisition in Spain and the New World*, eds. Mary Elizabeth Perry and Anne J. Cruz (Berkeley: University of California Press, 1991), 39–41.
16. Ibid., 52–53.

17. Hernández Sáenz, *Learning to Heal*, 252–255.
18. Viesca Treviño, "Curanderismo in Mexico and Guatemala," 56.
19. X. Lozoya, "La medicina tradicional en México: Balance de una década y perspectivas," in *El futuro de la medicina tradicional en la atención a la salud de los paises latinoamericanos* (Mexico, DF: CIESS, 1987), 65–74, as cited in Gustavo Nigenda, "La práctica de la medicina tradicional en América Latina y el Caribe," *Salud Pública de México* 43, no. 1 (2001): 42.
20. In the 1840s, the partido of Mérida ranked third in the state behind Valladolid and Peto. By 1900, it had far surpassed all other urban centres in the state. Allen Wells and Gilbert M. Joseph, "Modernizing Visions, *Chilango* Blueprints, and Provincial Growing Pains: Mérida at the Turn of the Century," *Mexican Studies/Estudios Mexicanos*, vol. 8, no. 2 (1992): 181–185.
21. Arturo Erosa Barbachano, *La Escuela de Medicina de Mérida, Yucatán* (Mérida, Mexico: Ediciones de la Universidad Autónoma de Yucatán, 1997).
22. Eduardo L. Menéndez, *Poder, estratificación y salud: Analisis de las condiciones sociales y económicas de la enfermedad en Yucatán* (Mexico City: Ediciones de la Casa Chata, 1981), 237.
23. For an overview of institutionalized scientific medicine in this era, see Ibid., 235–245. See also Armando Solorzano, "The Rockefeller Foundation in Revolutionary Mexico: Yellow Fever in Yucatan and Veracruz," in *Missionaries of Science: The Rockefeller Foundation and Latin America*, ed. Marcos Cueto (Bloomington: Indiana University Press, 1994), 52–71.
24. A brief description is found in Robert Redfield, *The Folk Culture of Yucatan* (Chicago: University of Chicago Press, 1941), 317–323. See also José Juan Cervera Fernández, "Preceptos divinos y contradicciones racionales: el primer movimiento espiritista en Yucatán, 1869–1879," in *Los Aguafiestas: Desafíos a la hegemonía de la élite yucateca, 1867–1910*, coords. Piedad Peniche Rivero and Felipe Escalante Tió (Mérida, Mexico: Archivo General del Estado de Yucatán [AGEY], 2002), 193–238; and Kaja Finkler, "Sacred Healing and Biomedicine Compared," *Medical Anthropology Quarterly* 8, no. 2 (1994): 178–197.
25. The Carnegie Institution sponsored numerous scholars who produced a wealth of scholarship. These include Ralph Roy, *The Ethno-Botany of the Maya* (New Orleans: Tulane University, 1931); Redfield and Alfonso Villa Rojas, *Chan Kom: A Maya Village*, publication no. 448 (Washington, DC: Carnegie Institution of Washington, 1934); Redfield, *The Folk Culture of Yucatan*; and Villa Rojas, *The Maya of East Central Quintana Roo* (Washington, DC: Carnegie Institution of Washington, 1945). See also Asael T. Hansen and Juan R. Bastarrachea M., *Mérida; Su transformación: de capital colonial a naciente metropolis* (México, DF: Instituto Nacional de Antropología e Historia, 1984).
26. See, for example, Irwin Press, *Tradition and Adaptation: Life in a Modern Yucatan Maya Village* (Westport, CT: Greenwood Press, 1975); Menéndez, *Poder, estratificación y salud*, 343–358; Marianna Appel Kunow, *Maya Medicine: Traditional Healing in Yucatan* (Albuquerque: University of New Mexico Press, 2003). Kunow, *Maya Medicine*, 42–58, speaks of contemporary healers and their practices in the town of Pisté.
27. Kunow, *Maya Medicine*, 42.
28. Redfield, *The Folk Culture of Yucatan*, 390.
29. *Milpa* refers to the plot of land where Maya grew their corn, and implies the social and religious activities surrounding corn production. *Milpa* plots were used for two or three years, and then shifted as the soil lost its fertility. *Milpa* production was the mainstay of community economic life.

30. Redfield, *The Folk Culture of Yucatan*, 308–311; Menéndez, *Poder, estratificación y salud*, 238.
31. Kunow, *Maya Medicine*, 42–43.
32. Redfield, *The Folk Culture of Yucatan*, 313.
33. James Angus McLeod, "Public Health, Social Assistance and the Consolidation of the Mexican State: 1888–1940," Ph.D. diss., Tulane University, 1990, 158–188.
34. Illustrative of the literature on professionalization and the "othering" of non-scientific healers are: Diana Obregón, "Building National Medicine: Leprosy and Power in Colombia, 1870–1910," *Social History of Medicine* 15, no. 1 (2002): 89–108; Ricardo González Leandri, "La profesión médica en Buenos Aires, 1852–1870," in *Política, médica y enfermedades. Lecturas de historia de la salud en la Argentina*, ed. Mirta Zaida Lobato (Buenos Aires, Argentina: Editorial Biblos, 1996), 21–53; and S. E. D. Shortt, "Physicians, Science, and Status: Issues in the Professionalization of Anglo-American Medicine in the Nineteenth Century," *Medical History* 27 (1983): 51–68.
35. *La Emulación*, January 1873.
36. Ibid., June 1874.
37. Ibid., September 1874, January 1878.
38. Ibid., May 1874.
39. Ibid., November 1874.
40. Ibid., May 1874.
41. *La Revista Médica de Yucatán*, November 1905.
42. Ibid.
43. Ibid.
44. Ibid., June 1912.
45. *Boletín de Higiene*, 5 May 1895.
46. Jorge I. Castillo Canché and José E. Serrano Catzín, "Vigilar y normar el burdel: Legalización de la prostitución femenina en Yucatán durante el porfiriato," *Revista de la Universidad Autónoma de Yucatán* 198 (1994): 46–55.
47. *Boletín de Higiene*, 5 May 1895.
48. *Código sanitario del Estado de Yucatán* (Mérida, Mexico: Imprenta de la "Escuela Correccional de Artes y Oficios," 1911).
49. *La Higiene*, May 1918.
50. Gil Rojas to Governor, 16 Aug. 1918, , Fondo Poder Ejecutivo (FPE), Sección (Sec.) Beneficencia, Serie (Ser.) Salubridad, Sanidad, caja 642, AGEY; *La Higiene*, May 1918.
51. Gil Rojas to Enrique Wanovichtz, 10 Nov. 1917, FPE, Sec. Junta Superior de Sanidad, Ser. Copiador de Oficios, vol. 66, exp. 114, AGEY.
52. Rafael Colomé T., *La Escuela de Medicina Homeopática de Yucatán. Fundación, actuación, y clausura* (Mérida, Mexico: Talleres "Impresora Popular," 1938), 5–6; *Revista de Medicina Homeopática*, August 1921.
53. The request was made on 27 February and published in *La Higiene*, May 1919.
54. *La Higiene*, May 1919.
55. Menéndez, *Poder, estratificación y salud*, 241–242.
56. Colomé, *La Escuela de Medicina Homeopática*.
57. Gil Rojas to Governor, 11 Apr. 1922, FPE, Sec. Beneficencia y Sanidad, Ser. Correspondencia (Sanidad), caja 642, AGEY.
58. *La Revista Médica de Yucatán*, March 1933.
59. Ibid., April 1933.
60. May 29, 6 June 1929, FPE, Sec. Beneficiencia, Ser. Junta Superior de Sanidad, AGEY.

61. September 12, 13, 1929, FPE, Sec. Beneficiencia, Ser. Junta Superior de Sanidad, AGEY.
62. *La Revista Médica de Yucatán*, June 1931. The presentation was also published as *¿Cuales deben ser las medidas más adecuadas para prosequir la campaña contra el charlatanismo en sus diversas formas?* (Mérida, Mexico: Sociedad Médica Yucateca, 1931).
63. *La Revista Médica de Yucatán*, June 1931.
64. Ibid.
65. Ibid., June 1933.
66. Ibid., August 1933.
67. *La Revista Médica de Yucatán*, February 1933.
68. Ibid.
69. Ibid., May 1933.
70. *La Revista Médica de Yucatán*, February 1933.
71. Ibid.
72. Ibid.
73. Ibid., April 1933.
74. *Boletín Mensual del Sindicato de Médicos y Profesionistas Conexos de Yucatán*, July 1942.
75. Ibid.
76. Ibid.
77. Gustavo Nigenda-López, "The Medical Profession, the State and Health Policy in Mexico, 1917–1988" (Ph.D. thesis, London School of Economics and Political Science, 1995), 140.
78. May 23, 1927, FPE, Sec. Beneficencia, Ser. Junta Superior de Sanidad, Caja 899, AGEY. The newly formed *Departmento de Salubridad* issued this decree in 1923; clearly Yucatán did not hurry to comply with this federal statute. Nigenda-López, "The Medical Profession, the State and Health Policy in Mexico," 150–153.
79. May 23, 1927, FPE, Sec. Beneficencia, Ser. Junta Superior de Sanidad, Caja 899, AGEY.
80. The Association had been founded in 1922 with direct linkages to a body in Mexico City. It coordinated actions between federal and state levels. Jan. 27, 1922, FPE, Sec. Gobernación, Ser. Correspondencia, Peticiones, Informes, Renuncias, Memoriales y Reglamentos, caja 754, AGEY.
81. Oct. 31, 1934,Fondo Sanidad Pública (FSP), Sec. Ejercicio de la Medicina, caja 12, exp. 5, Archivo Histórico de la Secretaría de Salud (AHSSA).
82. Respicio Tirado to Governor, 22 Nov. 1934, FSP, Sec. Ejercicio de la Medicina, caja 12, exp. 5, AHSSA.
83. Menéndez, *Poder, estratificación y salud*, 244–246.
84. J. M. Esquivel and Luis Vega Loeza to the Jefe del Departamento del Salubridad Pública, 30 December 1934, FSP, Sec. Ejercicio de la Medicina, caja 12, exp. 5, AHSSA.
85. Correspondence from 11 Jan., 23 Feb., and 14 Mar. 1935, FSP, Sec. Ejercicio de la Medicina, caja 12, exp. 5, AHSSA.
86. José F. Díaz and Benjamín Gongora Triay, "La Higiene," in *Enciclopedia Yucatanese*, 2nd ed. (Mérida, Mexico: Edición Oficial del Gobierno de Yucatán, 1977), VI: 377–421.
87. Nigenda-López, *The Medical Profession, the State and Health Policy in Mexico*, 109.
88. Díaz and Gongora Tracy, "La Higiene," VI: 377; Menéndez, *Poder, estratificación y salud*, 244–250.

89. Alan R. Sandstrom, "Mesoamerican Healers and Medical Anthropology: Summary and Concluding Remarks," Sandstrom and Huber, *Mesoamerican Healers*, 309, 310.

90. Gustavo Nigenda, et al., "La Práctica de la medicina tradicional en América Latina y el Caribe: El dilema entre regulación y tolerancia," 41–51; Miguel A. Güémez Pineda, "De Comadronas a promotoras de salud y planificación familiar: Proceso de incorporación de las parteras empíricas yucatecas al sistema institucional de salud," in *Cambio cultural y resocialización en Yucatán*, coord. Estebán Krotz (Mérida: Ediciones de la Universidad Autónoma de Yucatán, 1997), 117–145.

5 A Benign Place of Healing?

The Contagious Diseases Hospital and Medical Discipline in Post-Slavery Barbados

Denise Challenger

The Bridgetown Contagious Diseases Hospital[1] (CDH) opened its doors in December 1869. The CDH confined and treated suspected female prostitutes who were infected with venereal diseases (VDs).[2] Built as a requirement of the Contagious Diseases Act (CDA) of 1868, the hospital detained women that medical authorities and police officers believed were most dangerous to the men of the British Army and Navy. The women were released from the hospital when the medical doctor determined that they no longer showed signs of VD. However, as an 1881 disturbance in the hospital shows, the women did not always wait on the doctor's approval to determine when they would leave. During a routine visit to oversee the operation of the hospital, the colony's Poor Law Inspector (PLI), Dr Hutson, observed that:

> [t]he inmates seem in open riot this evening . . . they are fighting and making a disgraceful [illegible]. Mrs. Reed thinks that this is likely to continue more or less all night, unless some of them are removed to the Police Cells. I hear the glass windows being smashed among other things. Three or four of them are walking round the buildings smashing glasses as they pass, and when the Policemen arrive four of them walk out to the front and meet them, evidently regarding the whole thing as a grand spree. I have never seen so disgraceful a scene anywhere in a Public Institution.[3]

Violence was a source of empowerment that the patients deployed to challenge the criminalization, confinement, and regulation of their bodies. Despite Dr Hutson's assessment of the situation as a 'grand spree', his account suggests that the riot and the women's interaction with the police was a calculated exit strategy. The women understood that any riotous behaviour resulted in their removal from the hospital to the prison. The actions of the women raise the question of whether the hospital had functioned as a benign place of healing and moral reformation by the time it closed its doors in 1887.

Bridget Brereton, in an insightful review of British Caribbean historical literature, asked, "What did emancipation mean for Afro-Caribbean women?"[4] She found that the scholarship on these women tended to focus on their lived experiences during the slave period. Scholars of post-slavery British Caribbean societies have begun to fill the lacuna that Brereton aptly noted.[5] Noticeably absent in the literature, however, are works that deal with medicine, gender, and sexual regulation as a determining factor in the post-emancipation experience of 'freedom' for women.[6] An in-depth study of the CDH addresses the concerns of Brereton in that it adds to our knowledge of the lived experiences of women in post slavery Barbados. Moreover, it also allows for a closer examination of how gender and power functioned in post slavery societies.

Within British Caribbean scholarship, the Contagious Diseases legislation has received limited treatment in a few works; however, an extensive consideration of the impact of the CDH and CDA on the lives of Afro-Barbadian women was not their main focus.[7] Scholarship on the CDA has expanded greatly since Judith Walkowitz's seminal text, *Prostitution and Victorian Society* (1980).[8] This chapter builds on the findings of Philippa Levine, whose illuminating *Prostitution, Race and Politics: Policing Venereal Disease in the British Empire* (2003) compared the application of the Acts throughout much of the empire, with the exception of the Caribbean. In doing so, it seeks to broaden our understanding of how the Act operated in one of Britain's older and formerly slave-based plantation colonies.

Throughout the colonies, CDHs, as Sarah Hodges has noted, "were emblematic sites where versions of colonial power and medical authority were produced and enacted." They "re-articulated a series of relationships that the larger Contagious Diseases Acts legislation sought to encompass— between coloniser and colonised, between state and subject, between men and women and between disease and diagnosis."[9] An in-depth study of the CDH is a fruitful way to illuminate the gendered and classed aspects of freedom in post-slavery societies. The struggles of Barbadian women touched by the Contagious Diseases legislation, which was enacted only thirty years after the declaration of legal freedom, should be seen within the wider context of the struggle for "full" freedom that marked nineteenth-century British Caribbean societies.[10] As Mimi Sheller noted, freedom was "a long term process of interaction between former slaves, former masters, and state personnel along with various brokers or mediators ranging from missionaries, to abolitionists, judges to overseers."[11] Thus, in a very real way, the Contagious Diseases legislation entangled medical doctors, matrons, and nurses as mediators of freedom. The medical practitioners of the CDH were central to shaping the autonomy that Afro-Barbadian women could experience in the newly freed society.

This chapter explores the dynamics of the relationships between the doctors, matrons, nurses, and the patients at the CDH. Doctors were central to the transformation of the women from 'patients' to 'prisoners', and to the refashioning of the hospital from a place of healing to a place of punishment. The central argument of this chapter is that although the patients were subject to the disciplinary techniques and coercive forms of power utilized by the male medical authorities, the nurses and matrons also subjected the patients to separate forms of power and discipline. The female practitioners brought their own ideas about discipline to the hospital, informed by their understandings of how punishment was administered in a former slave society. Moreover, the regularity by which the nurses and matrons deployed their authoritative power was equally shaped by the goals of the male doctors, as well as by their own material needs given the economic conditions. Therefore, the reformative aims of the hospital were haphazardly achieved due to the daily interactions among the nurses, matrons, and patients which both facilitated and hindered the ability of the doctor to establish his moral authority and operate the hospital as a disciplinary institution.

I

The Contagious Diseases legislation was designed to protect men serving in the British Army and Navy from contracting VDs both at home and abroad. Sexual regulation of mainly white male British bodies in racialized colonial environments reached new heights throughout the empire in the mid-nineteenth century due to the links made between VD and the poor performance of the British troops during the Crimean War (1853–1856). However, imperial scholars have recently demonstrated that prior to the Crimean War sexual regulation in colonial environments was a concern to military authorities in various colonial outposts and that these military doctors and officers were influential in shaping the Acts passed in Britain.[12] Thus, strategies of sexual regulation, of which the CDA was one, did not simply emanate from the British core and move to the colonial periphery.

The Barbados CDA was a gendered piece of sexual legislation. Men were exempt from the act. The CDA required police officers to issue a certificate to any woman they suspected of being a prostitute. Upon receipt of the certificate, a woman had a legal obligation to report to the CDH within seven days for a pelvic examination by a visiting surgeon. If the visiting surgeon found her to be infected with a VD, he issued her a medical certificate that required her to remain in the hospital until cured. Under the terms of each certificate, a woman could not exceed a three-month stay at the hospital, and the surgeon could only issue three consecutive certificates. Failure to comply with the Act could result in imprisonment for the woman for a period of one to three months.[13]

The majority of policemen were Afro-Barbadians who worked under the supervision of white officers.[14] The CDA empowered black men to regulate the sexual activities and economic options of poor women. If the activities of Barbadian police officers in Trinidad are any indication, one could speculate that Barbadian women were potentially vulnerable to the sexual advances of police officers. David Trotman found evidence that a Sergeant Holder, a Barbadian policeman working in Trinidad, routinely forced women to submit to his sexual advances and in return they did not have to visit the CDH. Holder was fired from the force and returned to Barbados.[15] The CDA ensured that for poor black women who engaged in sexual activity outside the sanctified spaces of Christian marriage or a long-term committed relationship, freedom meant sexual constraint, increased sexual vulnerability, and limited autonomy.[16] The Barbados CDA was based on the 1866 CDA passed in Britain. The British passed CDAs in 1864, 1866, and 1869.[17] The Contagious Diseases legislation was promulgated in parts of the empire that were seen to have high rates of VD. For the British Caribbean, the Act was first passed in Jamaica in 1867, in Barbados in 1868, and in Trinidad in 1869. By 1870, Contagious Diseases laws were in place in more than a dozen colonies and treaty ports where the British had commercial and naval interests.[18] One of the major differences between the operations of the CDA in Britain compared to its colonies was that the Act was never extended to the civilian population in Britain.[19] In Barbados, the CDA stipulated that the governor had the power to enforce the Act anywhere in the island he felt it necessary. The parishes outlined in the Act were those that the garrison community straddled, St Michael and Christ Church. There were no recorded changes to the Act to suggest its jurisdiction was extended; however, such changes may not have been necessary since the most populated urban centre, Bridgetown, was located in the parish of St Michael. Therefore, poor women drawn to the city for a variety of economic and social reasons, who may never have visited the garrison community, were within reach of the tentacles of the Act.

The CDA operated within an unfavourable social and economic climate for the labouring poor. During the last third of the nineteenth century, most Barbadian workers, in both rural and urban spaces, lived in near destitution. They faced lower wages and higher food costs, and increased unemployment particularly after the introduction of European beet sugar on the British market in 1857. Throughout the 1860s and 1870s, as Claude Levy noted, there were increased riots, and offences related to stealing food and looting on the estates. And although in 1870 there was a 30% increase in thefts related to food, the members of the local government in charge of poor relief were reluctant to dispense poor relief widely for fear it would encourage idleness amongst the workers.[20]

The socio economic situation was particularly difficult for poor women in the urban setting. The population of St. Michael increased by over 50% due to an increase in rural to urban migration, between 1871 and 1921.[21] And the job opportunities for women did not expand accordingly. Most women who left the low wages of the sugar plantations in search of alternate employment obtained jobs as domestics, seamstresses, washerwomen and hucksters in Bridgetown. However, these occupations increasingly became oversaturated. The 1875 Report of the Commission on Poor Relief vividly outlined the limited options available to women. It stated, "huckstering, needlework, laundry work and to a small extent confectionery, are their only resource; and it is needless to say that this will not supply work and wage enough for all women who are not engaged in field labour or domestic service."[22] During the period from 1861-1891, the number of women engaged in domestic service went from 9000 to 15000. As Jocelyn Massiah noted, the women faced a situation of underemployment as there were so many engaged in such a small market and many of the workers were living below their productive potential and earned less than a living wage.[23] The punitive and regulatory aspects of the Contagious Diseases legislation, therefore, contributed to the limited economic mobility that Afro-Barbadian women engaged in prostitution could experience in the post-slavery period. Moreover, the subjective nature through which women were sent to the hospital, by way of police identification, ensured that even those not engaged in the trade had to monitor their sexual behaviour.

II

In the slave period, particularly in the writings of anti-slavery imperialist and travel writers, Afro-Barbadian female bodies were deemed exploited sexual objects that the system of slavery had acted upon and morally corrupted.[24] However, in the post-slavery period, the CDA discourse contributed to a subtle shift in the depiction of poor Afro-Barbadian female bodies. They became subjects who acted upon the social system and, through their actions, infected the black and white members of the British West India Regiment and the British naval troops stationed on the island. The CDA discourse, therefore, posited poor black women as "dangerous" because they were autonomous subjects of a 'free' society versus the exploited objects of a slave society.

Military doctors in Barbados targeted female prostitutes as active transmitters of VD. For instance, when asked to consider the feasibility of the Act, Dr S.H. Fasson, the Deputy Surgeon General and Principal Medical Officer in the West Indies Military, stated that the primary concern of the military was that:

> ... diseased women whether taken for examination by the Police or voluntarily presenting themselves for examination in order to being received into the Hospital shall be admitted at once and shall not be left at liberty [as] "infected centres" free to distribute disease one moment longer than may be avoided ... that diseased women having been admitted into the Hospital, they shall not be discharged from the Hospital until being perfectly cured,[and]they are no longer "infected centers".[25]

Fasson's depiction of female prostitutes as imminent threats who needed regulation and confinement most likely grew from a combination of his personal experience in Barbados and India.[26] India had regulated its prostitutes who serviced military cantonments even prior to the CDA, and military officials stationed in India similarly held ideas about Indian prostitutes as active transmitters of diseases. Moreover, as Elizabeth B. van Heyningen noted, in the Cape Colony, doctors who had recently spent time in India were the most insistent in their demands for regulation.[27]

The ideas about Barbadian prostitutes generated in the CDA discourse were part of a wider medical discourse on women and VD. Doctors associated with the CDA in Britain were influenced by the medical literature of the day, which, as Mary Spongberg found, feminized VDs. The literature consistently represented men as victims of VD and women as its source.[28] For instance, at an enquiry about the effectiveness of the CDA in England, doctors in defence of its continued operation stressed the uniqueness of the prostitute's body and implied that only prostitutes could create 'true' venereal symptoms in men. Although the female body came to be treated as the organic cause of the disease, it was the prostitute's body in particular that medical authorities cited as most hazardous to society.[29]

The connections between female prostitutes and VD did not change in a colonial setting. There, only perceptions about the strain of VD changed. In Barbados, the women were transmitters of a virulent form of VD. In a letter that Governor Walker wrote to the imperial office, he explained that the strain of VD that was detected in the bodies of Navy and Army men underscored the necessity of the CDA. His letter stated:

> The returns of the Army Medical department at home will show that a vast majority of the cases in Hospital are of venereal disease, and many of them of a very *bad type* [italics mine]. It is not only therefore the garrison that is weakened, the men's constitutions are injured and often destroyed: and indeed to such a frightful state of things have we come that for the last twelve months the Officers commanding her Majesty's ships on this station have been obliged when giving general leave to the crew to repair to another island. [30]

Female prostitutes in Barbados, therefore, needed to be controlled and contained because the type of VD that they spread had the potential to destroy a man's physical strength and thereby emasculate him.[31]

Within the garrison community, the medical–political discourse racialized VD and framed it as a problem more closely associated with blacks. For instance, a committee in the Barbadian legislature consulted with the chief medical authorities of the Army and Navy stationed on the island to determine if the Act was necessary in Barbados.[32] Although the report contained statistics indicating that "venereal disease was the main reason for hospitalization amongst the troops both white and black", the findings were presented in a manner that stressed that VD was most prevalent within the black garrison community.[33] For example, in addition to the statistical evidence that demonstrated VD was prevalent amongst black and white men, the report included the Chief Medical Officer's remark that "the disease, I regret to say, appears to be on the increase, and especially among the Black Troops."[34] More importantly, the report also presented the spread of VD as a crisis in the civilian black community, yet ignored discussions of its occurrence in the white civilian community.

In the medical–political discourse, the spread of VD in the civilian community was an issue of race, sanitation, morality, and freedom. The committee's report noted:

> . . . the notorious fact that Syphilis in its various forms, prevails among our own people, leads your Committee to regard their sanitary condition as deserving of attention. 30 years ago Syphilis was a rare disease among the labouring classes, and its secondary form almost, if not altogether unknown. Lately it has gone on rapidly increasing year after year, until at the present day it affects a large percentage of our population whose habits tend greatly to its propagation.[35]

The medical–political authorities made links between the high rates of VD and the way in which black civilians behaved as free people.[36] In the absence of the slave system, the CDA operated as a regulatory mechanism that kept unfettered black sexuality in check. Therefore, it was not only the black prostitute but also the sexual practices of the black woman[37] not engaged in prostitution, along with the sexual behaviour of black men, which worked in tandem and caused rates of VD to be rife in the civilian community. However, the gendered aspects of the CDA legislation ensured that it was the bodies of females that would be examined, detained, and punished.

Despite the medical and political discourse, which justified the implementation of the CDA and the erection of the CDH, the actions of a new governor, John Pope Hennessy, placed the hospital under greater scrutiny. His arrival in 1876 greatly influenced how doctors and administrators managed the CDH and the lives of the women inside. Shortly after his arrival, Hennessy conducted an investigation into the state of the hospital and concluded that, within British naval circles, the hospital had "become a scandal throughout the West Indies."[38] He blamed its poor reputation on the incompetence of the Barbadian legislature, members of which comprised the Board of Directors in charge of the hospital.[39] In 1879, amendments were made to the 1868 Act. These amendments were designed to divide the administrative power of the hospital. As a result of the changes, the administration of the hospital fell under the purview of both the British colonial office and the Barbadian legislature. Previously, although the hospital was partially funded by the British colonial office, it was under the administrative control of the Board of Directors that was solely comprised of members of the Barbadian government. Hennessy's enquiry revealed that within its first ten years, the hospital operated as a neglected place of confinement rather than one of sound physical treatment and moral reformation.

The amendments ultimately had an impact on the experiences of the women inside since they directly influenced the role of the doctor. An investigation into the hospital, published in the *Globe* newspaper, revealed that the doctor on staff was too old and made infrequent visits to the hospital; that the one syringe on the premises was broken; that some women were dismissed before being cured; and that others who should have been dismissed remained in the hospital for too long.[40] After the 1879 amendments, the hospital's Board of Directors and the PLI, who also functioned as the Inspector of Hospitals, supervised the activities of the doctor and reported any irregularities to the governor.[41] The renewed attention given to the hospital was a double-edged sword for the women. One result of the changes was that the doctor was more systematic in his visits and, therefore, the women were subjected to greater surveillance and increased examinations.

III

On opening day of the hospital, according to Governor Rawson, seven women—five white and two coloured—volunteered to be examined. Only one was infected and confined, though Rawson did not specify which one.[42] The Inspector of the Hospitals, Dr Hutson, described the women rather bleakly when he stated, " . . . one cannot help being struck with the degradation of the women who are brought up under the Act. None but the lowest and most common as a rule being taken up."[43] Moreover, a member of the House of Assembly stated that "the inmates in that Hospital belonged, as was well known, to a most reckless and disorderly class of the population, and they were most impatient of any restraint, and by no means [a] menable to discipline."[44]

The women detained at the hospital were most likely poor young women who lacked material resources, had the least access to philanthropic and social services, and operated in public spaces (such as the streets or near wharves).[45] The 1881 PLI's report stated, "As an example of the early age at which prostitution begins in this Colony, I may say that out of 167 admissions in which the age is recorded, no less than 122 were under 20, many of them are noted as 14 and some even younger."[46] Within the first year of its operation, 358 women were examined at the hospital, 134 were detained, and 114 were dismissed as cured.[47] Between 1869 and 1878, there were 2194 women registered and examined at the hospital. In the same period, the daily average of women detained was 17.4,[48] and from 1879–1884, the daily average of women in the hospital at one time was 26.3.[49]

Although some women 'volunteered' to be examined when the hospital first opened, over time, that number shrank. According to the Visiting

Surgeon of the CDH, Dr William Clarke, by 1871—with the exception of eight women:

> all the women may be said to have been brought under the provisions of the Act by Police interference, and though at the commencement it was thought advisable to endeavour to obtain attendance by a simple warning by Police, latterly it has been found necessary to have recourse to Magisterial coercion in almost all cases.[50]

Thus, within the first two years of its operation, the CDH changed from a place women 'willingly' visited to a place they avoided.

The examination itself was a painful reminder to the women of the power that the doctors had over their bodies once they entered the hospital. Dr Browne's entry is the only record of the examination procedure. He noted:

> All that I have taken in today with the exception of three have gonor-rhoea. I search most carefully by the "urethra test" and if I find one speck of pus I keep them in as these women know well the test and wipe them-selves out before coming in and pass water so that any discharge in the urethra is washed out before they come in for examination and only what collects after they come in is found by careful squeezing of the urethra.[51]

The doctor—by virtue of his race, gender, and class—had the power, if he so desired, to control the women through the pain he exerted as he prodded their sexual parts for signs of VDs.

In addition to controlling the bodies of the women, the doctor attempted to control the emotional state of the patients with punitive measures. After their examinations, new patients to the hospital displayed a wide array of reactions upon learning that they were infected and would be detained. Some women cried, laughed, cursed, swore, or sang.[52] Even though the initial reactions of the incoming patients annoyed Dr Browne—he called the noise "something awful"—he only requested that those women be put a little farther away from the main examining room while they waited to be prepared for their indefinite stay.[53] However, Dr Browne displayed fewer leniencies with women who were already patients at the hospital and who reacted emotionally to the news that they would not be released. Dr Browne, who for a few weeks replaced the regular visiting surgeon, Dr Archer, was more interested in controlling the emotional outbursts of the women than was Dr Archer. Dr Browne ensured that the women, who "made a great noise in the Hospital"[54] or cursed him "to their hearts content" after their examinations,[55] were brought before the visiting magistrates.[56] Thus, to some extent, the level of subjugation the women experienced was depen-dent upon the doctor. However, the changes that occurred at the hospital suggest that all the doctors, and the Barbadian legislative members who supported their decisions, agreed that the hospital needed to increase its use of punitive and coercive measures to control the women. In the discourse, the women were viewed less like patients and more like criminals.

In order to function as an effective imperial and colonial tool for sexual regulation, the CDH was slowly transformed from a place of 'benign' healing to one of coercive discipline. The changes to the hospital were most evident in the attitude and actions of the Visiting Surgeon, subsequent legislative changes to the CDA, the addition of solitary confinement punishment cells to the institution, and the changing qualifications of the hospital matron.

Disciplinary matters arose within the first year of the hospital's operation. The doctor had the option to deal with infractions personally or to have the women appear before two visiting court magistrates and face more serious punishment. If the magistrates found the women guilty, the patients were sent to the general prison for women, District 'A'. During the first month of the hospital's operation, the Chief Medical Officer, Dr Clarke, felt certain in his ability to discipline the women and avoided sending them to the magistrates for punishment. He wrote confidently about his ability to handle the women:

> The conduct of the women in the Hospital had, on the whole, been tolerable satisfactory; and though as may have been expected amongst this class, some misdemeanors should be committed, these have been chiefly due to the impulsive temper of the black, and as yet I have been able to deal without magisterial interference.[57]

Despite his intentions of handling the matter personally, Dr Clarke's understandings of race shaped how he chose to respond to the patients' actions. He understood 'black' to mean irrational and short-tempered. The idea of these Afro-Barbadian women as individuals separate from their race and class had not yet emerged in the psyche of Dr Clarke. Thus his racialized response to these women does not appear to have caused him to be dismissive of their actions and may have frustrations rather than conciliatory and helpful.

By 1878, however, the use of the court magistrates to punish the women became routine. In that year, 44 percent of all women confined to the CDH were sent to District 'A' prison for various infractions.[58] By 1882, doctors sent women to the magistrate for infractions such as "bad conduct", "indecent language", "making noise", "fighting", "theft", and "attempting to contact persons outside of the Hospital."[59] The increased use of the magistrate to settle personal issues in the hospital signified the beginning of the transformation of the women and girls from patients to prisoners.

Regardless of the frequency with which the women saw the magistrates and were sent to prison, at times the magistrates protected the patients from the extreme disciplinary measures of the doctor. For instance, in March of 1882, Dr F.B. Archer, the Visiting Surgeon and chief authoritarian at the CDH, was frustrated at the magistrates' decision to over-rule and chastise him for actions he took against a "troublesome" and "notorious character," a patient named Louise Bryant. Bryant had previously spent two months in District 'A' Prison for previous instances of "bad conduct." According to Dr Archer, the matron reported to him that Bryant and two other women behaved "badly" and used very "indecent language," which was reason enough for him to have them tried before the magistrates. Before they were sent to the magistrates, however, Dr Archer locked the patients in the small ward. Ultimately, the magistrates dismissed the case against Bryant and the two women; however, what upset Dr Archer most was that the magistrates made it known to all of the patients that the actions he took to discipline Louise Bryant and the other women were extreme. Thus he saw the decision of the magistrates and their public condemnation of his behaviour as an assault on his moral authority and power. Dr Archer wrote:

> I fear I cannot improve the discipline if this is all the support I get. I will be glad to know if in future I can dare to take any such steps again to preserve good order in the institution. I do not wish to be harsh with any of the patients and in this particular case I insist I acted kindly to the girl and guarded her interests, while trying to keep the institution in a state of good discipline.[60]

Dr Archer, and to some extent, Dr Clarke, tended to hold similar attitudes with regards to their role in the hospital as doctors in other colonies. For instance, Elizabeth B. van Heyningen found that the hospital at the Cape Colony tended to attract doctors who saw "their function in moral as well as in medical terms and it was they above all who attempted to impose their own social values on the prostitutes."[61] However, despite this intervention on the part of the magistrates, most times they did not challenge the disciplinary decisions of Dr Archer.

In 1882, three solitary confinement cells were added to the hospital. The newly built cells did not improve discipline. Moreover, when those cells were full—which they often were—women were still sent to the District 'A' Prison or District 'C' Prison . The numerous comments of the PLI, Dr Hutson, captured the ineffectiveness of the newly built cells to instill order. In his fifth half yearly report of 14 June 1883, he wrote, "The punishment cells have been brought into use, and 7 women have during the half year been punished in them. These women are, some of them, the most incorrigible offenders and are not deterred even by these solitary cells."[62] In November of the same year, he wrote:

> It would appear that the prison discipline, in the cells here, is not sufficiently strict, the Inspector of Prisons often complaining that the prisoners do not accomplish their day's work of oakum picking.[63] The cells

have at times been full, and it has even been necessary to send patients to District 'A'.[64]

The addition of the cells, so many years after the hospital opened, suggests a strong commitment to coercive methods of discipline and an abandonment of any methods which may have encouraged the patients to change through personal bonds of attachment with either the doctors or female staff. Physical changes designed to improve the sanitary conditions in the hospital introduced prison-like elements to its structure and appearance. In 1884, the PLI commented that, "The windows of the upper wards have been fitted with iron bars and jalousie shutters, so arranged that they cannot very well be injured by the women. The wards will now be dark but thoroughly well ventilated and cool."[65] The iron bars served as a physical reminder to the patients that they were 'infected centers' who needed to be kept away from the rest of society like criminals.

In their continued efforts to produce obedient bodies, the medical authorities not only made changes to the structure of the hospital, but also to the magisterial protections granted to them under CDA legislation. In 1884, in an effort to improve discipline, the authorities took away the patients' ability to have their cases heard in an 'objective' judicial space. A bill was passed that reduced the number of magistrates required to hear a case from two to one. Previously, the women had the legal right to have their cases heard by two male magistrates.[66] Members of the House of Assembly argued that due to the amount of time it took to arrange for two judges to meet at the hospital at the same time to hear a case—sometimes this took days or weeks—the disciplinary action lost its effectiveness.[67] The major complaint was that, in many cases, by the time punishment was meted out, the offenders had already been discharged and were getting away "scot free."[68] However, discipline did not improve, despite this attempt at expediency. In the tenth half-yearly report, the PLI noted that, even after the 1884 amendment, he saw no improvement in discipline. "Offences are now promptly dealt with and punishment unsparingly administered, but with no deterrent effect apparently. At one time this half year we had actually more than half our numbers in prison."[69] Thus, despite the consolidated male power of the medical and political elite which worked to erode the women's access to legal protection, the patients refused to conform to the regulations of the institution and continued to protest their confinement.

A key indicator of the attitudinal shift in disciplinary methods for the women was the change in job qualifications for the matron's position. By 1881, Dr Hutson no longer believed that the patients could be morally reformed and disciplined solely through example. In a follow-up to his account of the 1881 riot, he wrote to the Board of Directors, "I feel bound to state that no matron in my opinion would have controlled by her influence the inmates I saw rioting that afternoon"[70] He added, "I believe that deeper, if not rougher methods of treatment, than a Matron's influence will have to be brought to bear on our Lock inmates before they become orderly."[71] The matron at the time of the riot, Elizabeth Reid retired shortly after the riot and Sarah Elizabeth Nurse replaced her. She held the post for fourteen months until the patients attacked and injured her in 1884.[72] The beating of Sarah Elizabeth Nurse convinced the medical–political authorities to abandon attempts at reformation based on conciliatory relationships between the female staff and the patients. The replacement matron was a woman from the prison system, thus completing the final symbolic transformation of the women from patients to prisoners.

The patients attempted to form connections with the auxiliary staff to combat the increased disciplinary measures. For instance, Dr Archer fired the carpenter, Mr Parris, once he found out that he brought in food for one of the patients. His justification was that, "All the carpenters were warned when they came to work here that they were in no account to have any conversation with the patients."[73] However, a year later, Archer found out that Parris had returned to work at the hospital. He not only removed Parris but also warned him that if he returned, he would be prosecuted. Archer was surprised to learn that Parris had worked at the hospital several times since their initial confrontation. He blamed a female staff member, Mrs [J] Tappin, for allowing Parris to enter the hospital gate. Dr Archer proceeded to ask the Colonial Secretary to contact Mr Parris's supervisor and ask him not to send Mr Parris to the hospital again.[74]

The patients not only became familiar with the staff that operated the hospital, they also familiarized themselves with the laws of the CDA. Some women attempted to gain control of their bodies through the law and used the legal provisions of the CDA to seek their release. Section XXV of the 1868 Act stated, in part, that a woman had the right to appear before a Justice to secure her release if she felt that she was free from disease and the visiting surgeon refused to release her.[75] It is not clear how many women took advantage of this provision; however, in 1883, there was at least one successful case, much to the chagrin of the Poor Law Inspector. He reported:

> At my visit in April the Medical Officer drew my attention to a patient who had that day 'claimed her discharge' in accordance with the provisions of the Act. The woman was uncured, but not incurable, and it seemed a misfortune that she should be allowed to leave the Asylum with the disease still on her. Some provision should be made against this in the proposed New Act.[76]

The ingenuity of this woman was notable given the lack of public attention paid to the CDH inmates. In comparison, in her study of the CDH in England, Judith Walkowitz found that some activities of the women in the hospital should be seen as part of a wider public protest led by women and men who wanted to repeal the Act and, therefore, were willing to inform the patients of their legal rights.[77] Unfortunately, the women in Barbados did not have a similar political support network of elite women.

Women may have developed a strategy that enabled them to present their bodies to the doctor as healthy. Hutson suspected that the women took advantage of his position as the temporary replacement for the regular visiting surgeon, Dr Archer, by attempting to "dupe" him during their physical examination. His 12 October entry noted, "Dismissed 19 patients. This seems a very large number but most of them were gonorrhoea patients who had been in for two weeks. I don't know if they played tricks on me but there was no trace of discharge from in the urethra."[78]

The fact that there was no discharge from the urethra leaves open the possibility that some women may have been in the hospital longer than necessary due to a misdiagnosis by Dr Archer. That possibility notwithstanding, if the patients did employ a 'trick' to get out of the hospital, it demonstrates the varied measures that women used to seek their freedom. The patients used support from the non-medical staff, members of the outside community, legal loopholes, and violence to combat the actions of the medical authorities. It was, however, their violent behaviour that received the most notice and led Dr Hutson to conclude, after one final riot in 1885, that "[n]either cells within the walls, nor yet imprisonments at District "C" [had] any deterrent effect on the lawlessness of these women." He believed that they made "light of the cells" and that they "positively prefer[red]" life in prison to "their Hospital life."[79] The medical establishment failed to consider seriously that perhaps most of these women were not 'lawless'; most likely, they wanted to free their bodies from routine male medical intrusion, and prison was a place they could do so.

The power struggle at the CDH was not a simple story of doctors imposing their authority in an attempt to produce disciplined bodies, and the patients resisting these attempts at their surveillance, incarceration, and control. As the beating of Sarah Elizabeth Nurse indicates, the nurses and matrons formed an important part of the power structure. However, the nurses had agendas separate from the disciplinary and regulatory measures that the medical–legislative establishment advocated. The competing agendas of the female practitioners and male doctors revealed themselves most clearly in their attitudes toward the patients.

Nurses often shaped the power dynamics of the hospital. The nurses introduced forms of punishment and regulations distinct from the institutionalized norms that the doctors and the legislature implemented. For instance, Dr Archer reprimanded Nurse Patterson for flogging young girls. He added, "I only discovered today that she has on two or three occasions taken this liberty."[80] Even though it is not clear how often other nurses used flogging as a method of control, the flogging incident demonstrates the presence of multiple forms of subjection and power within the hospital. The nurses were not empty vessels void of ideas about how to control and discipline bodies. Their ideas about corporal punishment, which they brought with them to the hospital, most likely stemmed from their experience of living in a former slave society.[81]

The nurses may have introduced their ideas about punishment to the hospital, but their authority and autonomy was limited as they functioned within a gendered power structure. Sometimes they attempted to protect the patients even if it meant undermining the authority of the doctors. For instance, Dr Archer fired Nurse Clarke because he believed that she lied to the magistrate in order to prevent two patients from being punished and sent to prison.[82] Thus, physicians could respond harshly to alliances between patients and nurses.

Doctors sometimes blamed the nurses for the violent outbreaks at the hospital. Dr Browne's 17 November 1883 entry revealed that he concurred with the magistrates' belief that a fight that occurred between patients would not have happened had a nurse been on duty at the ward. He wrote:

> I certainly think that there must be neglect on the fact of the Nurses here as I do not think all these fights could occur if the nurse was present in the wards while on duty. I have reprimanded her severely and I would not recommend her dismissal as she is I think on the whole a very good nurse.[83]

Doctors not only determined whether or not a nurse or matron would keep her job, but they also determined which job she would hold. For instance, in August of 1882, when a head nurse resigned, Dr Archer successfully blocked the promotion and wage increase that Nurse Ford was entitled to because he felt that she was incompetent. He stated:

> I would suggest that in making the next appointment, the new nurse be put in at the salary of the other two viz $4.00 per month and 1 s per day (one penny) for [dress]. The head nurse at present gets in addition to the above $2.00 per month. I see no reason for any distinction between the three nurses and were it to go by seniority in appointing, [Ford] would be the person and I consider her quite unfit to be <u>head</u>. [84]

Thus, it appears that the nurses needed to give at least some consideration to fulfilling their job duties when managing the patients. Dr Archer was willing to manoeuvre their job positions in an effort to ensure an orderly and well-maintained hospital.

Economic conditions played a part in how the nurses and matrons functioned within the hospital. In addition to dealing with the arbitrary system of job promotion, based in large part on the doctor's personal preferences, the nurses had to adjust to the modified wage structure that reduced the value of their incomes. Early in 1882, rather than receiving food rations as part of their compensation, nurses were given a food allowance of 14 cents a day.[85] This change doubtlessly reflected the current crisis in the sugar industry, which had an impact on the rest of the economy. Food costs were rising and the labouring class was increasingly impoverished and malnourished.[86] The female staff used their access to, and distribution of, food both as a tool for their economic survival and as a control mechanism.

Food became a currency of power at the hospital that the nurses and matrons utilized to control the patients and to enhance their own material well being. A dispute in 1883 between the head nurse and the matron revealed that an underground market of personal gain and exploitation operated at the CDH. Head Nurse Patterson told Dr Archer that the matron, Mrs Boyle, was neglecting to distribute the quantity of food rations to patients as ordered.[87] The cooks were aware of the activities of Mrs Boyle and substantiated the accusations of Nurse Patterson.[88] Dr Archer believed that the "discontent and ill feeling existing between the nurses and the matron" was "quite enough to prevent the successful working of any institution."[89] He responded by launching an enquiry to investigate the complaints that the nurses and matron made against one another. He concluded that "Nurse Squires ha[d] been guilty of grave misdemeanours in obtaining from some of the patients certain articles of food and provisions in exchange for money or other food." As a result of the enquiry, Dr Archer fired Boyle, Patterson, and Squires.[90] The underground market was emblematic of some of the ways that the female practitioners attempted to negotiate power in a gendered hierarchical system that gave the doctor complete control over their working lives. Moreover, the market also demonstrates that economic conditions influenced the way in which nurses and matrons used their authority and managed the patients.

Despite the actions of the nurses, the patients used the power of personal connections with people on the outside, or took matters into their own hands to contest their subjugation while detained at the hospital. For instance, in August 1882, Dr Archer reported that, "some of the articles of food were thrown over the wall to patients."[91] On Christmas Day in 1882, "one patient was caught stealing food and keys from Nurse Patterson's office."[92] In December 1883, Dr Archer reported that one patient hurt her hand as she tried "to climb over the railing to get in the 'cell yard'" to obtain "things of sor[t]" that "were thrown over the wall and dropped in the enclosure."[93]

The actions of the nurses and matrons highlight the multiple forms of power that shaped the dynamics of the hospital. At times, the female practitioners formed alliances with some patients that challenged the authority and disciplinary objectives of the doctors. At other times, the nurses and matrons subjected the patients to other forms of power that reflected the material realities of Barbadian socioeconomic conditions and their own ideas of punishment that were separate from the established goal of reformation and healing set by the hospital administrators.

The evidence about the background of the nurses and matrons who worked at the hospital is scant. The qualification distinctions suggest that class demarcations existed between the matrons and nurses. For instance, the 1883 advertisement for the position of the matron read:

> Wanted for this institution A MATRON, Salary £ 50 per annum. Application in writing addressed to Dr. Archer, at the Lock Hospital, enclosing two testimonials only, to be made not later than Monday the 12th instant. The selected Candidate must be prepared to assume her duties on Thursday morning, the 15th instant.
> By order,
> W.H. WHITEHALL,
> Clerk of Ex. Committee.[94]

Conversely, the advertisement for the position of the nurse read:

> Wanted—Two competent Nurses for the above Institution, on the 1st February next: Applications to be made at the Lock Hospital any day between the hours of 10 and 4 o'clock, when all information respecting duties, &c, can be obtained from the Matron.
> By order,
> W.H. Whitehall,
> Clerk of Executive Committee.[95]

Thus, the job duties required a certain level of education. Moreover, as the testimonial requirement suggests, the matron was expected to be a 'respected' member of the community. For the nurses, however, community-sanctioned 'respectability' and literacy were less decisive factors for their employment. Moreover, the legislative involvement in the financial well being of the matrons after they left the CDH suggests that they were respected members of the community. When the matron Elizabeth Reid retired, the legislature passed an Act that ensured that she received an annual pension of 12 pounds, 10 shillings until her death.[96] Also, the legislature passed a bill to provide Sarah Elizabeth Nurse with a one-time compensatory payment of 10 pounds after a physical altercation with some patients left her with a debilitating injury.[97]

The extent of white Barbadian female involvement at the CDH is uncertain. Planning for a nurse training school, which might have brought British nurses to staff the CDH, did not begin until 1889. The CDH closed in 1887. I am working with the assumption that the nurses were either black or coloured women given the absence of a nurse training school. The matron at the General Hospital, which opened in 1844, was a British woman.[98] The racialized social hierarchy that governed Barbados suggests that it is highly unlikely that white women would have worked under the supervision of black or coloured women. Thus, there is reason to assume that if white women worked at the CDH, they would also have done so in a supervisory capacity as matrons. However, I do not rule out the possibility that black or coloured women may have been chosen to work as matrons if white women could not be found to perform this role.

IV

The struggles of the nineteenth century for many Afro-Barbadians were, in large part, about access to greater cultural, economic, and social autonomy than was afforded to them in the slave period. The medical–legal discourse and practices of the CDA that constructed the female body as unruly and as an infected centre limited the opportunities that some women had to use their sexual bodies as sources of economic gain and material improvement. Therefore, "freedom" for some sexually autonomous Afro-Barbadian women included the criminalization, punishment, and isolation of their bodies.

This chapter illustrated the ways that Afro-Barbadian women, unable to avoid detection under the CDA, still continued to negotiate power within the CDH. The patients navigated their autonomy within the interstices of competing power systems: one governed by the male medical doctors and the colonial state, and the other governed by the female matrons and nurses. The patients used the legal system, outside community members, and violence to challenge the regulatory and disciplinary measures of the female staff, the male doctors, and the political elite. The competing and gendered forms of power that guided the hospital resulted in multiple forms of subjugation for the patients. The male medical authorities operated from gendered, racialized, and class-based assumptions about poor black women as 'dangerous' and 'infected centers' harmful to Barbadian men and those who represented the British empire. Thus, they responded to female protest through increased forms of surveillance, examination, and repression in an effort to produce obedient and healthy bodies.

The interactions between the nurses, matrons, and patients, however, limited the reformative capacity of the measures implemented by the medical-political elite. At various times, the nurses and matrons supported its disciplinary objectives. They even introduced, against the desires of the doctors, corporal punishment to ensure obedience. However, the nurses and matrons also functioned within a gendered power structure. The formation of an underground market was, in part, a response to the doctor's ability to reduce the earning capacity of the women. Thus, the female practitioners challenged the doctor's power and used the CDH as a place for their material gain at the expense of the patients' well being and autonomy. Despite the evidence of exploitation and punishment there is some evidence to suggest that, at times, the personal bonds of attachment that the matrons and nurses developed with the patients also worked to undermine state disciplinary objectives. Thus, any discussions of power in colonial institutions must take into consideration not only the discursive powers of the state, but also the material conditions and cultural assumptions of those who interacted with the patients on a daily basis.

NOTES

1. The CDH was also referred to as the Lock Hospital, and the terms are used interchangeably in this chapter.
2. The CDA stipulated that women were to receive some form of religious and moral instruction while detained at the hospital. There was no cure for venereal diseases in the nineteenth century, only painful treatments. Therefore the hospital isolated the women from outside society until they no longer showed signs of VD. For more discussions about the difficulty of diagnosis and treatment of VD in the nineteenth century, see Judith R. Walkowitz, *Prostitution and Victorian Society: Women, Class, and the State* (London: Cambridge University Press, 1980), 48–56.
3. "Memorandum by Dr. C. Hutson Poor Law Inspector," *Official Gazette* (OG), 2 January 1882.
4. Bridget Brereton, "General Problems and Issues in Studying the History of Women," in *Gender in Caribbean Development*, eds. Patricia Mohammed and Catherine Shepherd (Kingston, Jamaica: University of the West Indies Press, 1999).
5. For edited collections on gender and post-slavery societies, see B. W. Higman, Brian Moore, Carl Campbell, and Patrick Bryan, *Slavery, Freedom and Gender: The Dynamics of Caribbean Society* (Kingston: University of the West Indies Press, 2001); Pamela Scully and Diana Paton, eds., *Gender and Slave Emancipation in the Atlantic World* (Durham, NC: Duke University Press, 2005). For monographs that deal with gender issues in post-slavery societies in the British Caribbean, see Lara Putnam, *The Company They Kept: Migrants and the Politics of Gender in Caribbean Costa Rica, 1870–1960* (Chapel Hill: University of North Carolina Press, 2002); Juanita De Barros, *Order and Place in a Colonial City: Patterns of Struggle and Resistance in Georgetown, British Guiana, 1889–1924* (Montréal: McGill-Queen's University Press, 2003), Brian L. Moore and Michele A. Johnson, *Neither Led Nor Driven: Contesting British Cultural Imperialism in Jamaica, 1865–1920* (Kingston, Jamaica: University of the West Indies Press, 2004); Diana Paton, *No Bond but the Law: Punishment, Race, and Gender in Jamaican State Formation, 1780–1870* (Durham, NC: Duke University Press, 2004).
6. More work has been done in the Spanish Caribbean in this area. Most notably, Eileen J. Suárez Findlay, *Imposing Decency: The Politics of Sexuality and Race in Puerto Rico, 1870–1920* (Durham, NC: Duke University Press, 1999) and Laura Briggs, *Reproducing Empire: Race, Sex, Science, and U.S. Imperialism in Puerto Rico* (Berkeley: University of California Press, 2002).
7. See David Vincent Trotman, *Crime in Trinidad: Conflict and Control in a Plantation Society, 1838–1900* (Knoxville: University of Tennessee Press, 1987); Brian Moore and Michele Johnson, "'Fallen Sisters'? Attitudes to

Female Prostitution in Jamaica at the Turn of the Twentieth Century," *Journal of Caribbean History* 34 (2000): 46–70 and Anthony Phillips, "Politics in Barbados" (unpublished PhD thesis, University of the West Indies, 1990).

8. See also Kenneth Ballhatchet, *Race Sex and Class Under the Raj: Imperial Attitudes and Policies and Their Critics 1793–1905* (New York: St. Martin's Press, 1980); Elizabeth B. van Heyningen, "The Social Evil in the Cape Colony 1868–1902: Prostitution and the Contagious Diseases Acts," *Journal of Southern African Studies* 10 (1984) 170–197; Phillip Howell, "Prostitution and Racialized Sexuality: The Regulation of Prostitution in Britain and the British Empire before the Contagious Diseases Acts," *Environment and Planning D: Society and Space* 18 (2000): 321–339; Richard Phillips, "Imperialism and the Regulation of Sexuality: Colonial Legislation on Contagious Diseases and Ages of Consent," *Journal of Historical Geography* 28 (2002): 339–362; Sarah Hodges, "'Looting' the Lock Hospital in Colonial Madras during the Famine Years of the 1870s," *Social History of Medicine* 18, no. 3 (2005): 379–398.

9. Hodges, "'Looting' the Lock Hospital in Colonial Madras during the Famine Years of the 1870s," 384.

10. Some historical works that deal with the process of freedom in the British Caribbean include Gad Heuman and David V. Trotman, eds., *Contesting Freedom: Control and Resistance in the Post Emancipation Caribbean* (Oxford Macmillan Caribbean, 2005); Frank McGlynn and Seymour Drescher, eds., *The Meaning of Freedom: Economics, Politics, and Culture After Slavery* (Pittsburgh, PA: University of Pittsburgh Press, 1992); Bridget Brereton and Kevin A. Yelvington, eds., *The Colonial Caribbean in Transition: Essays on Postemancipation Social and Cultural History* (Jamaica: University of the West Indies Press, 1999); Frederick Cooper, Rebecca J. Scott, and Thomas C. Holt, *Beyond Slavery: Explorations of Race, Labor, and Citizenship in Postemancipation Societies* (Chapel Hill: University of North Carolina Press, 2000) and Thomas C. Holt, *The Problem of Freedom: Race, Labor, and Politics in Jamaica and Britain, 1832–1938* (Baltimore, MD: Johns Hopkins University Press, 1991).

11. Mimi Sheller, *Democracy After Slavery: Black Publics and Peasant Radicalism in Haiti and Jamaica* (Gainesville: University Press of Florida, 2000), 30.

12. See Phillip Howell, "Prostitution and Racialized Sexuality: The Regulation of Prostitution in Britain and the British Empire before the Contagious Diseases Acts," *Environment and Planning D: Society and Space* 18 (2000): 324–327; and Philippa Levine, *Prostitution, Race and Politics: Policing Venereal Disease in the British Empire* (London: Routledge, 2003), 38–40.

13. Bardados, *Laws of Barbados* (London: William Clowes and Sons, 1875), 277.

14. David Vincent Trotman, *Crime in Trinidad: Conflict and Control in a Plantation Society, 1838–1900* (Knoxville: University of Tennessee Press, 1987), 251.

15. Women who could prove that they were married or partnered with a man were exempt from examination.

16. The main difference between the 1866 Act and the 1864 Act was that the 1866 Act introduced a system of periodic fortnightly examinations of all known prostitutes, made compulsory under a well-organized system of medical police. Previously, only women identified as diseased prostitutes were solicited by the police for examination. Thus in 1866, women underwent a greater system of regulation and police surveillance. See Walkowitz, *Prostitution and Victorian Society*, 78.

17. Levine, *Prostitution Race and Politics*, 40.
18. Ibid., 56.
19. Claude Levy, *Emancipation, Sugar, and Federalism: Barbados and the West Indies, 1833–1876* (Gainesville: University Press of Florida, 1980), 130–134.
20. Woodville Marshall, "Villages and Plantation Sub-Division," in *Emancipation III. Aspects of the post-slavery experience of Barbados: Lectures Commemorating the 150th Anniversary of Emancipation, delivered in February and March 1987,* edited by Woodville Marshall (Bridgetown: Department of History, U.W.I., Cave Hill and National Cultural Foundation, 1988), 13
21. Report on Commission on Poor Relief Barbados 1875–1877, 12.
22. Unpublished Ph.D. Thesis, Joycelin Massiah, *The Population of Barbados: Demographic Development and Population Policy in a Small Island State* (Cave Hill: Faculty of Social Sciences University of the West Indies, 1981)14.
23. Levy, *Emancipation, Sugar, and Federalism:* 85.
30. Letter from Governor Walker to Lord Duke, 16 May 1867, Colonial Office (CO) 28/206, no. 602.
24. See Henrice Altink, *Representations of Slave Women in Discourses on Slavery and Abolition, 1780–1838* (London: Routledge, 2007), 78–87.
25. "Letter from Deputy Surgeon General and Principal Medical Officer to the Assistant Military Secretary: July 28, 1879," OG, 18 August 1879.
26. He noted in his letter that his time spent in India as a Deputy Surgeon General and as an Executive Officer, where he became acquainted with the Lock Hospitals in India, made him the most qualified to respond to administrative questions concerning the Lock Hospital in Barbados. See "Letter from Deputy Surgeon General and Principal Medical Officer to the Assistant Military Secretary: July 28, 1879," OG, 18 August 1879.
27. van Heyningen, "The Social Evil in the Cape Colony 1868–1902", 173.
28. Mary Spongberg, *Feminizing Venereal Disease: The Body of the Prostitute in Nineteenth-Century Medical Discourse* (New York: New York University Press, 1997), 3.
29. Ibid., 3.
31. Similarly, Philippa Levine found that medical doctors believed that the strain of venereal disease contracted in racialized environments was more dangerous than strains contracted elsewhere. Levine, *Prostitution, Race and Politics*, 66.
32. Letter from Governor Walker to Lord Duke, 16 May 1867, CO 28/206, no. 602.
33. Ibid.
34. Report from the Joint Committee of the Council and Assembly, 25 Jan. 1868, CO 28/206, 47.
35. Ibid. In 1868, upon consultation with the oral and documentary evidence of the chief medical authorities of the Army and Navy, the Joint Committee of Council and Assembly produced a report of their findings and submitted it to the governor. The Joint Committee of Council and Assembly was designed to investigate the issue of venereal diseases on the island. Letter from Governor Walker to Lord Duke, 16 May 1867, CO 28/206, no. 602.
36. Increasingly in the mid- to late nineteenth century, the medical discourse in Britain and the United States circulated ideas of VD as a disease that was rampant in the black community partly due to black sexual practices. See James H. Jones, *Bad Blood: The Tuskegee Syphilis Experiment* (New York: Free Press, 1981), 16–29; Jeremy C. Martens, "'Almost a Public Calamity': Prostitutes, 'Nurseboys', and Attempts to Control Venereal Diseases in Colonial Natal, 1886–1890," *South African Historical Journal* 45 (2001): 46.

37. Sander L. Gilman's fascinating article explores more closely how the world of medicine and art intertwined in a manner which represented the black female body in European visual culture as representative of syphilis, and thus the source of corruption and disease. Sander L. Gilman, "Black Bodies, White Bodies: Toward an Iconography of Female Sexuality in Late Nineteenth-Century Art, Medicine and Literature," *Critical Inquiry* 12 (1985): 231.
38. Letter from Governor Hennessy to Secretary of State Earl Carnarvon, 4 Nov. 1876, CO 321/11.
39. Enclosure No. 1, *Message from the Governor—To the Honorabale House of Assembly' Joint No. 18* , 4 Nov. 1876, CO 321/11, no. 233, 327.
40. *Globe*, 14 August 1879.
41. Ibid.
42. Letter from Governor Rawson to Secretary of State, 2 Dec. 1869, CO 28/209, no. 1000, 476. To date, a register which includes the name, age, and race of the women confined has not been found. Moreover, the clandestine nature of prostitution makes it difficult to determine the exact number of women involved in the trade. The only source of data includes information extracted from the governor's correspondence and the general Poor Law Inspector's and Visiting Surgeon's reports.
43. Extract of Report from Inspector of Hospitals, quarter ended June 30, 1879, OG, no. 1362, 9 October 1879.
44. Contagious Diseases Amendment Bill, *House of Assembly Debates*, 1884–1885, 16 December 1884.
45. I have been unable to find a register of prostitutes which documents the names, ages, or races of women who were either examined or detained.
46. Third Half-Yearly Report, July–December 1881, OG, no. 1700, 26 July 1882.
47. Report of the working of the Contagious Diseases Act, from December 1st, 1869 to December 31st, 1870, OG, no. 396, 23 January 1871.
48. Report of the Barbados Contagious Diseases Hospital from 2 Dec. 1869–31 Dec. 1878, OG, no. 1362, 9 October 1879.
49. Complied from table in Ninth Half-Yearly Report of Poor Law Inspector, OG, 2047, 21 May 1885.
50. Report of the working of the Contagious Diseases Act, from December 1st, 1869 to December 31st, 1870, OG, 1871, no. 396, 23 January 1871.
51. Visiting Surgeon's Logbook (hereafter VSLB), 28 November 1883.
52. VSLB, 21 November 1883.
53. Ibid.
54. VSLB, 16 November 1883.
55. VSLB, 28 November 1883.
56. VSLB, 16 November 1883 and VSLB, 28 November 1883.
57. Report from Dr. Clarke to Secretary of State, 19 Jan. 1870, CO 28/211, 94.
58. *Report on Gaols and Prisoners*, Barbados Blue Books, 1878.
59. A review of entries noted in VSLB, which only covered the period from 1882 to 1884.
60. VSLB, 20 March 1882.
61. van Heyningen, "The Social Evil in the Cape Colony 1868–1902", 196.
62. Fifth Half-Yearly Report, 14 June 1883, OG, no. 1808.
63. Oakum picking was the unpicking of old ropes for its fibres, work that was very hard on the hands. It was a task generally performed by slaves, poorhouse inmates, or prisoners. Raytheon Employees Wildlife Habitat Committee, "Portsmouth Asylum-Oakum and Idle Hands—Perfect Match?", http://rewhc.org/townfarmoakum.shtml,30 November 2006.

64. Sixth Half-Yearly Report January–June 1883, OG, no. 1856, 8 November 1883.
65. Ninth Half-Yearly Report July–December 1884, OG, no. 2047, 21 May 1885.
66. *House of Assembly Debates*, 1884–1885, 16 December 1884.
67. Ibid.
68. Ibid.
69. 10th Half Yearly Report January–June 1885, OG, no. 2095.
70. "Discipline at the Contagious Diseases Hospital", OG, no. 1640, 26 January 1882.
71. Ibid.
72. "Minutes House of Assembly", OG, no. 2077, 13 August 1885.
73. VSLB, 3 February 1882.
74. VSLB, 19 March 1883.
75. *A Bill for the Better Prevention of Contagious Diseases*, 29 April 1868, CO 28/206, 47.
76. Sixth Half-Yearly Report January–June 1883, OG, no. 1856, 8 Nov. 1883.
77. Judith R. Walkowitz and Daniel J. Walkowitz, "'We Are Not Beasts of the Field': Prostitution and the Poor in Plymouth and Southhampton under the Contagious Diseases Acts," *Feminist Studies* 1 (1973): 89.
78. VSLB, 12 October 1883.
79. Twelfth Half-Yearly Report Jan–June 1886, OG, no. 2226, 14 October 1886.
80. VSLB, 25 May 1883.
81. There are some similarities to the way power operated at the CDH that tend to support Diana Paton's assessment of how modern power operated in Caribbean workhouses and prisons. She showed that Jamaican prisoners were subjugated through both corporeal measures as well as through disciplinary techniques of examination and surveillance. Diana Paton, *No Bond but the Law: Punishment, Race, and Gender in Jamaican State Formation, 1780–1870* (Durham, NC: Duke University Press, 2004), 12.
82. VSLB, 21 May 1883.
83. VSLB, 17 November 1883.
84. VSLB, 30 August 1882.
85. VSLB, 8 February 1882.
86. Hilary Beckles, *Great House Rules: Landless Freedom and Black Protest in Barbados, 1834–1937* (Kingston: Ian Randle Publisher, 2003), 112.
87. VSLB, 17 August 1883.
88. Ibid.
89. VSLB, 31 August 1883.
90. VSLB, 5 September 1883.
91. VSLB, 31 August 1883.
92. VSLB, 25 December 1882.
93. VSLB, 10 December 1883.
94. "Notice. Lock Hospital," OG, 1 February 1883.
95. "Notice Lock Hospital," OG, 29 January 1883.
96. "A Bill entitled, An Act to authorize the payment from the public treasury of an annual pension to Elizabeth Reid, widow, the late matron of the Contagious Diseases Hospital," OG, 22 February 1883.
97. "Minutes House of Assembly." OG, no. 2077, 13 August 1885.
98. Eudeen Monica Ward Murray, "The Development of Nursing Education: Barbados with a Recommendation for an InterCaribben Curriculum" (EdD thesis, Columbia University, 1990), 39.

6 Tolerating Sex
Prostitution, Gender, and Governance in the Dominican Republic, 1880s–1924

April J. Mayes

On 19 November 1919, three years into the US occupation of the Dominican Republic, the city council (*ayuntamiento*) of San Pedro de Macorís convened a special session which included the Provincial Governor, Juan Félix Peguero, and US military officials, Provost Marshal Stack, in charge of security for the eastern district of the country, and Major Knoche of the Dominican National Police. The tension in the chambers must have been palpable. Stack and Knoche were angry and embarrassed: they wanted to hold the city council accountable for a nasty confrontation that had erupted on 18 November between US Marines and members of the Dominican National Police. Not surprisingly, a mixture of alcohol, youthful exuberance, and male competition over female prostitutes provoked an outlandish display of violence between Dominican law enforcers and US soldiers. As a result, the governor, Stack, and Knoche tried to convince the city council that closing down the city-licensed tolerance zone was the "only remedy" for preventing future clashes between Dominicans and US troops. Indeed, Knoche explained that he "had already made [a similar] . . . recommendation to the military governor." Despite the tide of opinion against them, San Pedro's city councilmen resisted this latest effort by the military government of the time to muscle its way into local affairs. They voted to keep the tolerance zone open; in a surprising move, the *ayuntamiento* outlawed the sale of liquor to all US Marines stationed in San Pedro and prohibited the consumption of alcohol within and around the red-light district. Theirs, however, was a last-ditch effort: in December 1919, the military governor signed Sanitation Law (*Ley de Sanidad*) which made prostitution and tolerance zones illegal.[1]

The city council minutes from November 1919 capture a multi-layered struggle between San Pedro's city council, provincial authorities, and US military officials over the parameters of local authority and the diverging visions of how commercial sex should be policed. As the meeting demonstrates, San Pedro's political elites had already developed strategies—among them the creation of the tolerance zone—for dealing with prostitution and problems associated with the sex trade such as loud noise, obnoxious behaviour, alcohol consumption, and venereal disease (VD).

From the 1890s until the occupation, the city council's efforts to cloak prostitution behind the invisible wall of the tolerance zone underscore Dorothy Porter's insight that "public health [is] an expression of the way different societies [address] questions of social order and nationhood."[2] Clearly, San Pedro's city councilmen understood the regulation of space as an important part of social order and as tangible evidence of sound and effective governance, not the failure to govern. Policing women, clients, and businesses within the tolerance zone enabled the city council to define and regulate the boundaries between refined society and the city's underclass, to protect male privilege and power, and to enhance authority over foreign-born residents.

Nevertheless, the quest for "social order and nationhood" in the Dominican Republic was complicated by United States imperialism in the Caribbean. As a result, the United States' military occupation disrupts a straightforward narrative in which the elaboration of public health policies smoothly parallels the rise of autonomous modern states. In US-occupied Dominican Republic as in Puerto Rico and the Philippines, public health reforms were crucial in the elaboration of the military's authority and for representing US rule as benevolent and necessary. Prior to the occupation, the absence of a national network of roads, railways, and telegraph lines nurtured regional autonomy and well-honed suspicions of centralized government. During US military rule, however, public health legislation, sanitary work done by trained professionals, and the construction of laboratories, hospitals, and clinics made the national state more visible and powerful. This new national authority sought to fulfill specific goals—eradicating syphilis and VDs—but was ultimately a foreign presence that ruled over a reluctant population and whose health officials viewed tolerance zones as abysmal failures for controlling and containing vice. Thus, between 1919 and 1923, the military government waged a campaign against prostitution. As Eileen Suárez Findlay and Laura Briggs have argued for Puerto Rico during the same period, the criminalization of prostitution by US officials provoked the anger of native political elites who used the occasion to protest the occupation. During that November meeting, then, San Pedro's city councilmen not only defended their public health strategies, they also called into question United States imperialism.[3]

Building on the insights of Suárez Findlay and Briggs, this chapter also argues that tolerance zones became a battleground where the United States' occupying force and Dominican political elites tried to assert their "ordered benevolence" and visions of social order over a population both groups considered in need of refinement "in the name of progress."[4] Dominican elites believed they could accomplish this by vigorously policing tolerance zones; US officials believed the opposite. Having much more to lose, US military authorities wanted to rid the country of tolerance zones to signal the effectiveness of moral reform and benevolent governance over recalcitrant populations. The differences between these two sets of authorities, however, should not be overdrawn. Implicit in the conversation during that November confrontation were key assumptions that military authorities and Dominican officials shared: they regarded tolerance zones as dens of vice and anti-social behaviour; they also presumed that all women who lived in or near tolerance zones sold sex and thus threatened respectable society; finally, they tacitly agreed that men's bad behaviour was somehow not their own fault, but could be blamed on other forces, such as alcohol.

As Suárez Findlay and Briggs have aptly shown, the implications of the elites' complicity with US rule and their efforts to resist elements of it were politically significant and influenced public health strategies. In addition to underscoring the ways in which public health officers and US military rule helped consolidate and buttress social hierarchies based on race, class, and gender, this chapter emphasizes the different meanings US and Dominican authorities attached to tolerance zones as spaces for male leisure. I argue that, despite agreeing over the fundamentals, US and Dominican officials disagreed over what the tolerance zone as a governable space represented. For Dominicans in San Pedro de Macorís, the tolerance zone signified elite hegemony over a multi-ethnic, multi-national, and multi-racial population. By creating tolerance zones and policing them, San Pedro's elites at once segregated neighbourhoods populated by Afro-Antillean and Puerto Rican migrants and integrated them into their vision of social order. In other words, regulating the tolerance zone allowed local political elites to maintain a social order based on male privilege and Dominican rule over foreign-born, at times darker-skinned, immigrants. In contrast, US officials believed that tolerance zones tolerated too much disorder. As spaces where interracial sex occurred and where Dominican men could physically (and sometimes successfully) challenge white US Marines, tolerance zones were places where white male authority was literally stripped and laid bare.

The chapter begins with a brief overview of San Pedro's public health regime, which developed in the 1870s and 1880s, just as San Pedro grew from a small *aldea* (town) on the shores of the Higuamo River into one of the Dominican Republic's busiest ports, thanks mostly to sugar production and immigration. In this first section, I argue that the city council's power was especially tested as San Pedro underwent tremendous demographic and economic changes during the last quarter of the nineteenth century. Sanitation work was a vehicle through which dominant elites crafted their identity as a moral vanguard and guardians of the *moral social* (moral community). Public health policy was also a mechanism the city council used to extend its authority over a diverse and growing population. The next section analyzes San Pedro's first prostitution crisis, which erupted in the 1890s. It argues that the crisis was the product of native-born elites who, anxious and uncomfortable with the influx of female and Afro-Antillean labour, initiated an effort to police public spaces and poor women. Elites' obsession with prostitution was somewhat aided by the city's effective and institutionalized public health regime. The concern over prostitution ebbed and flowed until the United States occupation in 1916. The US military government significantly altered Dominican public health, most notably through the centralization of public health work in the national government based in Santo Domingo. The third section briefly describes the military government's public health and sanitation policy, and analyzes the second prostitution crisis that erupted with the discussion and passage of the Sanitation Law in 1919.

The social history of public health in San Pedro is intimately connected with the story of the region's entrance into the global economy. In 1876, Juan Amechazurra built San Pedro's first mechanized sugar mill; by 1893, seven profitable mills surrounded the city. As a result, San Pedro became a key stop along hemispheric migration networks that brought North American investors, Cuban and Puerto Rican engineers, and Afro-Antillean cane cutters from Haiti and the British West Indies to the province. As mechanized sugar production took hold during the last quarter of the nineteenth century, San Pedro's political and economic elites faced the daunting task of meeting basic sanitation needs in a port city where the boom and bust rhythms of an agro-industrial economy, a growing population, and foreign immigration exerted unique pressures on the public's health. The transition to export-oriented agricultural production that occurred in San Pedro, and elsewhere throughout Latin America between 1870 and 1900, resulted in the creation of public health regimes designed to keep growing urban populations healthy, in part, to ready them for industrial work and to ensure the profitability of export-driven economies.[5] This was especially true in San Pedro where, after 1870, policing the public's health became an integral part of political elites' efforts to transform rural migrants living in the city into urbane residents who exemplified the values of progress, order, and modernity. Between 1870 and 1890, the city council became a more visible and powerful entity as police and sanitation officials waged campaigns against rabid dogs, loose farm animals, and the ever-encroaching marshlands described in the local paper, *El Cable*, as "a river of rotten mud whose fetidness infects the population and occasions terrible illnesses."[6]

As sugar production grew in significance for the national economy, San Pedro's political elites wanted to transform the town into a showcase city, worthy of a provincial capital. Public health policy and policing, as elsewhere in Latin America, "became an instrument for expanding the authority of the state" and masked the destruction of homes or the usurpation of private property as "ordered benevolence."[7] San Pedro's intellectual and political elites embraced an ideology of progress that was deeply paternalistic. They were heavily influenced by the Puerto Rican philosopher Eugenio María de Hostos, who regarded elites as a moral vanguard equipped to protect the *moral social* from the damaging effects of capitalism, urban growth, and cultural inertia.

For many intellectuals, Hostosian philosophy perfectly combined moderniza-tion through economic liberalism with a humane and optimistic role for elites as the protectors and teachers of the poor.[8] Sanitation policy became the ideal vehicle for dominant elites to exercise their vanguard role, make their vision of social order tangible, and secure the promise of modernity and develop-ment. Initially, San Pedro's city council took small steps, such as regulating food production and marketing. In the late 1880s, the council established a uniform standard for weights, rationed the amount of flour used in bread making, inspected meat scales and market stalls, and organized the slaughter of meat. These controls undermined speculation, curbed the negative affects of inflation on the local economy, and guaranteed *petromacorisanos* access to basic food items.[9] The regulatory apparatus of the city council demonstrates the elites' vision of themselves as a mediating force between a social body that needed their protection from the vagaries of a profit-driven and export-oriented economic system.

These small steps increased dramatically in the 1890s when San Pedro significantly diversified by class, ethnicity, and race, and when demography challenged the concept of the moral community as Dominican elites tried to assert their influence over a population that teemed with rural migrants, foreign immigrants, and black workers. San Pedro's population grew from a few hundred in the 1870s to nearly 8,000 in the 1890s, thanks to inter-nal and international migration.[10] By 1902, the population increased to approximately 11,000.[11] The city's streets were transformed by the pres-ence of Afro-Antillean men and women who dominated the local economy as cart drivers, marketers, laundresses, domestics, and prostitutes. In this social landscape, native-born elites competed with foreign-born immigrants for economic opportunities and access to space, whether housing, market stalls, or the sidewalk. Like their counterparts in Mexico during the same period, San Pedro's professionals, intellectuals, landlords, merchants, and propertied families responded to this challenge by crafting a "moral geog-raphy" to distinguish themselves and their respectable movements through the city's streets from the rough and tumble of the working poor.[12]

These social boundaries—based on national, racial, and class priv-ileges—were given spatial reality during the panic over prostitution that erupted in 1891.[13] The absence of evidence makes it difficult to determine just why a concern over prostitution erupted that year, but citizen's anxiety about commercial sex coincided with the *zafra* (sugar harvest), a period when the number of Afro-Antillean workers in the region would have increased dramatically the thousands who arrived to cut and process cane. Extant material from 1897 suggests that the debate over prostitution was the first in a series of anxieties over crime that were expressed in city council minutes and in the local newspaper. That year, for example, *El Cable* published several articles about violence in San Pedro, admitting that the *zafra* and the presence of foreign workers provoked mayhem in the city.[14] San Pedro's political and intellectual elite believed that a crime wave threatened to engulf the city, and since they could not control the influx of black workers to the region, they focused their energy on policing their neighbourhoods to assert their hegemony. In the fall of 1891, for example, petitioners living on Colón Street in downtown San Pedro requested that the city council remove a house of prostitution from their street. Manuel Richiez also bemoaned "the scandals that these women [cause] day and night with their bad conduct that [undermines] morality," and demanded that the city council regulate prostitutes' movements and their trade. In response, the city council resolved to fine and arrest those who organized and sponsored "bailes de rameras" (prostitute dances) where prostitutes congregated to solicit clients in residential neighbourhoods.[15] Clearly, San Pedro's elites imagined a city free of the scandals associated with commercial sex, even as they accepted prostitution as a form of male leisure.[16]

No wonder, then, that in 1893, the city council passed an ordinance that prohibited prostitutes from riding in coaches during the day. One writer in *El Cable* published a scathing critique of the law, arguing that the cover of darkness would only make prostitutes more dangerous to social morality. In dramatic language, he explained that the light of day "infused respect" among prostitutes and their clients, whereas beneath the shadow of night, their "imprudent whistles, burlesque peals of laughter, and drunken voices" would echo, unrestrained, throughout the city. The writer's aim was not to criminalize sex work; he simply wanted to humiliate "degenerate" women by forcing them to walk the streets, making their public lives even more public.[17]

The regulation, however, did not specify just who was a prostitute; forcing women into the tolerance zone did. As Kevin Mumford argues for early twentieth-century New York and Chicago, social boundaries were "constructed into the infrastructure" of San Pedro. The boundaries that emerged segregated respectable residents from others.[18] One such boundary was forcing some women to walk while others enjoyed a ride; another was physically removing businesses from certain neighbourhoods to other areas of the city. The creation of a tolerance zone seemingly appealed to everyone's desires—to define safe and genteel parts of the city by removing prostitution elsewhere while, at the same time, protecting male leisure. One interesting, if not surprising, tale from the period demonstrates that the city council played its moral vanguard role perfectly: Councilman Aybar moved to relocate the Hotel Venecia from its location near the port because, according to him, the brothel's employees flaunted their "immoral acts" and undermined public decency. In anticipation of Aybar's complaint, the city council president, the Police Commissioner, public health officials, and Venecia's madam collaborated to select another location for Venecia's workers, one that was far removed from residential areas.[19]

San Pedro's tolerance zones also symbolically represented, naturalized, and gave physical expression to political elites' vision of a social order based on honour, moral decorum, and male privilege. According to local lore, San Pedro's most notorious red-light district was located on the southern edge of town, near West Indian neighbourhoods. Residents called the area *La Draga*.[20] The verb, *dragar*, means "to dredge" and remove the accumulated debris and sludge from the harbour so that ships can enter the port easily. *Draga*, as a noun, is sludge, trash, and sewage removed from the seabed. Referring to the red-light district as *La Draga* was a powerfully negative indictment of prostitutes, anchored in the fear and suspicion with which Dominican elites held sexual commerce and, as a result of their physical nearness to this tolerance zone, foreign, black immigrants. Not only were prostitutes imagined as submissive to male sexual passion (since that which is dredged is passive), they were also regarded much like the city's swamplands—as rotted sites for the "discharge [of] humors, secretions, and excretions."[21] Such areas of danger, much like the marshlands feared by an earlier generation, had to be policed, fumigated, and contained. Since La Draga was located within Afro-Antillean neighbourhoods—an area already identified with foreignness and with the city's ties to the global market-policing its boundaries enabled the city council to incorporate commercial sex into the city's social order and exercise hegemony over immigrants and working women.

As in Puerto Rico during the same period, discourses about sex, morality, and respectability "were central to the construction of social and political orders" at a time of significant and dynamic change.[22] The increasingly moral tone of public health policy and concern over prostitution may have helped white and light-skinned native Dominicans forge a powerful alliance with white, moneyed immigrants from Spain, Cuba, and Puerto Rico and incorporate a foreign elite into the body politic. The *ayuntamiento*'s hiring of Dr Emilio Tió y Betances as Chief Medical Officer in 1900 was an important indication of this new power. A Spanish immigrant to San Pedro, Dr Tió arrived in the Dominican Republic with an approach to public health that blended miasmatic and bacterial theories of contagion, perhaps a result of his European training. Initially, Dr Tió focused his energies on the public market, which he often characterized as a "seed-bed of infection." Dr Tió also inserted himself into the lives of *petromacorisanos*: during his tenure, forced immunizations became regular features of the school year for San Pedro's children. The only way to avoid Dr Tió and his staff was to keep children at home, as one school principal complained: "some parents [did not want] their children to be vaccinated." Dr Tió also imposed mandatory *limpiezas*, general cleanings, of front porches and living spaces throughout the city. Sanitation officers did not usually wait for owners' permission to clean; when faced with resistance, they simply cleaned the area with water and disinfectant.[23] Forcing prostitutes to submit to regular "*limpiezas*" was not too far behind. During the last years of Dr Tió's career as Chief Medical Officer, Councilman James Brower, perhaps a West Indian, proposed obligatory, weekly examinations for "women of the bad life" to prevent the spread of syphilis throughout the population. The city council resolved to rent a house for the sole purpose of identifying, examining, and removing prostitutes from "the center of the population."[24] Then, in March of 1909, the *ayuntamiento* passed the city's first Prostitution Regulation—*Reglamento del Régimen de la Prostitución*.[25] The Regulation, among other things, required prostitutes to register with the city and have regular physical examinations at the public *gallera*—the cockfighting arena. The city then transferred syphilitic women to Santo Domingo for treatment.[26]

City council records do not fully explain why a formal prostitution regulation went into effect, but one might read its passage as the triumph of Dr Tió's leadership and the hegemony of bacteriology in San Pedro's approach to public health. The tolerance zone's popular moniker, *La Draga*, hints at this shift. Branded as *draga*, prostitutes were discursively imagined in both miasmatic and bacteriological terms, as the rot in which VD fermented and as vectors of disease. Tolerance for prostitution, then, may have declined in San Pedro as political elites and public health authorities reached a consensus in the debate over bacteriological and miasmatic theories of contagion.[27] Although the increased regulation of prostitutes, namely through the forced physical exams, points toward bacteriology's ascendancy, the continued use of miasmatic terms to describe La Draga rendered the transmission of VD mysterious and its vectors dangerous. As Laura Engelestein argues, in the case of Russia, ambiguity over the transmission and course of VD, particularly syphilis, made sexually transmitted infections, the regulation of prostitution, and the creation of tolerance zones "perfect vehicle[s] for the doctor's assertion of professional authority."[28]

During the prostitution panic, doctors needed as much authority as they could get because the Regulation failed in many respects. By 1911, the new health inspector, Dr Marchena, warned the city council that prostitutes were "finishing off with San Pedro's humanity" and claimed that there were "hundreds of infected women" who needed treatment.[29] Citywide inspections began 1 February, but within two weeks, a council member complained that few women were coming forward. He was right: two extant reports from March and April of 1911 show that only fifty women appeared for their required checkups. There were many reasons why women failed to submit to obligatory inspections. First, according to reports submitted by city officials, many women were Puerto Ricans or British West Indians who feared deportation. Also, some women avoided inspections because they did not want to appear on the city's tax rolls as prostitutes, especially if selling sex was just one of many income-generating activities they performed. Even Dr Marchena recognized this dilemma: "there are certain women who, during the day, present themselves as respectable women, but become prostitutes at night when they cannot be monitored by our staff or by the police. For this reason, it is difficult to classify them as prostitutes without sufficient proof."[30] Not surprisingly, the location of the examinations, the cockfighting arena, posed an additional problem. Women going to the arena faced public exposure and embarrassment, especially if, after being diagnosed with syphilis, they were hauled away in a health department vehicle toward Santo Domingo. Equally unattractive was the standard treatment for VD: doctors recommended an extensive cleaning of the genital areas with soap, water, and a mercury-based douche injected into the urethra.[31]

Much like market inspections, city-wide *limpiezas*, and vaccination drives, herding prostitutes into the *gallera* and processing them through obligatory physical exams was a spectacle that expressed the city council's power. These public health strategies, moreover, were designed to combat disease without addressing how poverty, poor housing, or political disenfranchisement affected residents' health. The tiny sample obtained from three medical reports sustain Dr Marchena's claim that prostitutes suffered from myriad venereal and vaginal diseases, resulting mostly from poor hygiene and diet. During the three weeks for which there is data, doctors diagnosed twelve women with gonorrhea and sent two to Santo Domingo for syphilis treatments. Eleven women received clean bills of health, while forty-one women were diagnosed with chronic metritis (inflammation of the uterus), vaginitis, scabies, and other illnesses of the vulva.[32] Dr Marchena was forced to admit that the Prostitution Regulation failed. Instead, he claimed, women needed access to gynaecological care and suggested the opening of a specialized hospital for women to address this problem. Nothing, however, resulted from his prescient and sympathetic recommendation. Even though the city's own evidence suggested that San Pedro's prostitutes were not spreading syphilis at dangerous rates, the cultural presumption that loose women posed a health threat and the spectacle of bringing women to their physical exams buttressed the pervasive idea that sexually active women were sources of syphilis. This assumption persisted within the international medical community as well. For instance, an article published in the Pan American Sanitary Bureau's magazine presumed that men contracted syphilis from commercial or clandestine prostitutes, but did not transmit the disease to them.[33]

To be sure, by focusing on women and not men as the transmitters of syphilis, health officials in San Pedro institutionalized gender and racial inequality into public health discourse and policy.[34] The edges of the city's moral topography were found on poor women's bodies and their sexual activities. Removing prostitutes, their catcalls, and clients from certain areas of town was necessary for crafting a social and moral order in the city. At the same time, by policing women's movements, San Pedro's political elites protected sites of male leisure in a society that privileged

male sexual pleasure and men's ability to freely transgress the boundaries between respectable and dishonourable *petromacorisano* society.
Perhaps, too, the panic over syphilis resulted from men's unease about
women's participation in a market economy and the commodification
of pleasure. In the late nineteenth century, European and North American intellectuals and doctors blamed syphilis' rapid dissemination on
overcrowded conditions which encouraged looser social mores governing
sexual activity.[35] In the Americas, as elsewhere, the problem with syphilis was linked to women, and the syphilitic prostitute became emblematic
of social ills that pertained to urban growth, economic expansion, and
social change.

Moreover, one man's "nightly scandals" might have been how women
(and some men) conducted their business on the city's streets, whether or
not it involved sex. Sparse evidence suggests that by the first decade of the
twentieth century, Afro-Antilleans were overrepresented in San Pedro's
police ledgers, often fined or jailed for scandalous behaviour, which could
include fighting or verbal abuse. For example, records from the criminal
court indicate that in the period before the occupation, between 1915 and
1916, twenty-nine Dominicans (seventeen men and twelve women) stood
accused of scandalous behaviour and "mistreatment," while sixty-eight
West Indians (fifty-one men and seventeen women) were charged with the
same crime.[36] To be sure, some *petromacorisanos* wanted the city council
to police commercial sex, but the higher numbers of West Indians in court
suggest that "measures of morality" not only kept illicit sex far from the
homes of respectable citizens, but also kept the growing Afro-Antillean
working classes a safe distance from Dominican society.[37] Therefore, in
addition to interpreting the Prostitution Regulation as a product of political elites' fears regarding poor, migrant women and their paternalistic
commitment to refining San Pedro's residents, the Regulation also constituted the city council's efforts to re-craft the *moral social* in light of
Afro-Antilleans' importance in the local economy.

Finally, the Prostitution Regulation symbolized the advancement of bacteriology in public health policy in San Pedro. After 1900, this new ideology of contagion, which privileged regulation and intervention, provided
elites with even greater tools to police racial and sexual boundaries in the
city, and was a mechanism for incorporating foreign male elites into the
city's power structure. This is suggested by the presence of James Brower
on the city council, a man who, despite his possible connections to the
West Indian community in San Pedro, supported legislation that probably
obligated many of his co-subjects into forced physical exams. As Megan
Vaughan has argued in the case of colonial East Central Africa, the battle over prostitution in the name of combating syphilis united native- and
foreign-born men over the problem of poor women's sexuality, a problem
defined as men's lessened control over women.[38] Onto and into the bodies
of prostitutes, "through the rhetorics of gender and race," the local state

not only broadened the scope of its power, but a new political elite came into power.[39]

Whereas the debate over prostitution and tolerance zones facilitated certain male alliances in the 1890s and early 1900s, the same struggle to contain commercial sex failed to unite Dominican political elites and US military authorities during the occupation, which began in 1916. Instead, the bodies of prostitutes and the sites of their labour became battlegrounds over which two kinds of male authorities tried to claim dominance. Initially, US military authorities accepted the status quo, permitted municipalities to run their own affairs, and tolerated legal prostitution. When Capitan Harry S. Knapp established military rule in 1916, he reassured Dominicans that the occupation was not "undertaken with [the] immediate or ulterior object of destroying the sovereignty of the Republic of Santo Domingo, but . . . [was] designed to give aid to that country in returning to a condition of internal order." [40] This state of affairs changed, however, in 1917 when United States military authorities suspended congressional sessions and elections, eliminated both the executive and legislative branches of the Dominican government, and replaced a civilian administration with military officers. Although Dominicans retained control over their city councils, the Dominican state was essentially administered by the United States Navy.[41]

The elaboration of public health policy by the US Navy tightened the military's hold on the national government. Military officials regarded protecting and enhancing Dominicans' well-being a centrepiece of the US's civilizing mission in the Dominican Republic and throughout the Caribbean basin: as one medical authority insisted, the eradication and prevention of epidemic disease was an "imperative obligation". As it was a territory under US occupation, US authorities enacted a national health policy and established sanitation standards in the Dominican Republic, a feat not even possible in the United States, where state governments resisted the creation of a federal public health authority. Most important, public health policies in the Dominican Republic resulted from years of US empire-building and scientific research in tropical medicine that took place in Cuba, Puerto Rico, the Philippines, and Panama. Military personnel moved from one colonial context to the next, as was the case of P. E. Garrison, who honed his skills in the Philippines before arriving to the Dominican Republic, where he became the country's first Chief Sanitation Inspector in 1917. In his report to the governor, Admiral Harry Knapp, Garrison argued that public health and sanitation reform would allow Dominicans to "enjoy and profit" from their status as a free people living in a capitalist democracy; he also implored, "Santo Domingo must not harbor infectious diseases to the menace of . . . its many neighbors." Garrison insisted that Santo Domingo had an "obligation surely comparable to those of financial integrity and internal order" to prevent and treat contagion before it could threaten another country.[42]

Garrison crafted an extensive and invasive approach to public health that became the occupation government's official sanitation policy. Initially, military officers left tolerance zones intact and the regulation of prostitution remained in the hands of municipal officials. Until 1920, the status quo permitted US military officials to maintain the fiction of not subverting Dominican sovereignty even as the occupation government fundamentally changed the Dominican national state. Admiral Thomas Snowden, who replaced Admiral Knapp as governor, echoed the sentiments of his predecessor when he insisted that the "Dominican Republic [was] not a colony, therefore, its laws [had] to be respected." This apparently included tolerance zones. In October of 1919, Snowden argued that the military government did not have the authority to overturn the decision of Santo Domingo's city council to create tolerance zones. In fact, Snowden claimed, segregating prostitution had "improved the moral health of the entire community since decent people . . . no longer confront[ed] prostitutes on a regular basis."[43] As a result, US military officials provided assistance to anti-prostitution efforts led by Dominicans. For example, in August of 1918, surgeon Reynolds Hayden encouraged Major Ross S. Kingsley to strictly regulate prostitution following precedence established by Dominicans: as in San Pedro de Macorís, prostitutes in the capital city, Santo Domingo, were required to remain in segregated areas; they were only allowed to leave if they were diagnosed with VD, at which point public health officials transferred them to the Dominican Military Hospital. Prostitutes were also required to carry an identification book and endorsements of good health. Prostitution regulations, however, did not address the prevalence of VD among US soldiers. Hayden wanted more vigilance because, as he reported, over 50 percent of Marine hospitalizations were the results of VD.[44] Garrison questioned the efficacy of Santo Domingo's anti-prostitution strategy, arguing that the city was unable to deal with the proliferation of prostitution because, as he vaguely surmised, "some [were] personally invested in the question." Garrison claimed that 10 percent of enlisted forces in the capital contracted VD because, he reasoned, nearly half of those prostitutes examined had sexually transmitted diseases. Again, rather than outlaw prostitution entirely, Garrison proposed increased vigilance, more money, and the help of Marine commanders in enforcing sanitary regulations.[45]

Tolerance for the tolerance zone declined, however, once the United States entered World War I and as Progressives launched a full-scale campaign against prostitution in the hopes of preventing the spread of syphilis and other VD among soldiers.[46] Backed by a new sanitary officer, Reynolds Hayden, the *Ley de Sanidad* (Sanitary Law) became law in December of 1919, and was fully implemented in January of 1920. Critics described the *Ley de Sanidad* as too ambitious: Thomas Jackson, who once served as director of the national laboratories in the Dominican Republic, argued that the sanitary code was "too elaborate for a country as primitive as the Dominican Republic."[47] Significantly, as Rebecca Lord shows, unlike during the previous administration, the Sanitary Law was written without input from Dominican doctors and:

> reproduced the same tropes [of US–Dominican relations]—that Dominicans were childlike, unable to manage their own governance, and had to be directed in order to fulfill their international obligations. These in turn were built on essentialist notions of racial inferiority, tropical weakness, and cultural difference.[48]

Most important, the Sanitary Law shifted the focus of public health work to syphilis eradication, a move which promised to inject money and personnel into a project some Dominican elites considered worthy of dedicated effort. Nevertheless, the evidence showed that endemic diseases, like malaria, afflicted Dominicans with deadlier precision than syphilis, especially in sugar-growing regions such as Santo Domingo and San Pedro de Macorís. For example, in 1919, there were 9,555 cases of malaria with 760 fatalities; the disease claimed 888 lives in 1920. During the same time period, only forty people died from syphilis.[49] Malaria, and tuberculosis, were diseases of poverty, poor living conditions, and poor access to health care. The military government, for its part, defined these illnesses as naturally occurring ailments that affected tropical nations and African-descended people. Since these diseases were regarded as part of the natural landscape and inherent to certain races, US authorities believed them beyond the parameters of the Dominican Department of Sanitation, as they did in Cuba, the Philippines, Puerto Rico, and Panama, where endemic diseases also received scant attention.[50] The military government's syphilis eradication program was more ideological than practical, designed to protect the lives of white, US Marines, and their wives or lovers waiting for them back home.

While the military government pursued commercial sex as a criminal activity that had to be eradicated by prohibition, Dominicans tended to regard prostitution as a challenge that still could be managed by removing commercial sex to particular areas of the city and by policing tolerance zones with greater vigilance. In 1918, for instance, Major James McLean of the National Guard reported that San Pedro's "Santa Fe Port [bordello]" operated "with absolute disregard for municipal regulations." He recommended shutting down the business. Council member Antonio Marmolezo concurred that the house often "held dances on work days" and "large mêlées frequently broke out," but he blamed this on "poor police vigilance."[51] When Isaac Curiel sent his letter of protest against "those nightly scandals that took place on the corner of September 10th and President Henríquez Streets," in the heart of downtown San Pedro, he demanded more policing, not prohibition.[52] As in the 1890s, those who submitted complaints about prostitution during the US occupation did not want to criminalize prostitution; rather, they preferred to see it removed from respectable society. This time, however, their demands reached the ears of an occupying force that, fresh from the experiences of dealing with VD in the trenches of World War I and in other tropical colonies, responded by outlawing prostitution.

Just as the elaboration of tolerance zones enabled municipal elites in San Pedro and Santo Domingo to assert their political hegemony over growing cities, destroying them symbolized the loss of Dominican sovereignty and put the occupation force in full power. Admiral Snowden justified the criminalization of prostitution and the destruction of the tolerance zone because Washington politicians had expressed a "strong desire" to promulgate such a law. As a result, the prohibition banning commercial sex led to a full-scale campaign against "clandestine" prostitution from 1920 until 1923. Perhaps this heightened concern over commercial sex was the result of research which showed that a significant number of naval personnel were infected with VDs.[53] Although most military officials assumed that prostitutes in the Dominican Republic infected US soldiers, it is just as likely that many of these soldiers acquired their illnesses at home or during stints in other countries also under US occupation. Physical examinations revealed that 12.5 percent of naval personnel had a VD; in the Dominican Republic, the incidence of sexually transmitted illnesses among US Marines was even higher. For example, military doctors discovered that 45 percent of Marines encamped near Puerto Plata, a town that lacked a prostitution regulation, were infected with a VD.[54]

The military government acted swiftly and comprehensively to resolve the threat posed to troops by jailing prostitutes and imposing egregious fines. Between 1920 and 1923, the period for which there is available evidence, San Pedro's prostitutes paid the highest amount in fines, second only to those accused of robbery. On average, prostitutes paid $25, but they handed over $1,285 to the city treasury, an amount just a few hundred dollars less than the total sum paid in health code violations.[55] For instance, between 26 May and 25 August 1920, the police arrested fifty women, and the courts levied hefty fines against them, ranging from $15 to $50. Some were even sentenced to the local jail: Margot Cortera was brought to trial in June of 1920 for selling sex and was fined $25 with additional jail time; a group of five prostitutes, all with Spanish names and perhaps working out of the same house, were arrested a few weeks after Cortera and were fined $40 each with an additional forty days behind bars.[56]

Whereas evidence from the 1890s only suggested that many women selling sex were immigrants, police records from the occupation confirm that prostitutes were a mobile, multi-national, and multi-racial segment of San Pedro's urban workforce. For instance, Celina Ortiz and Amalia Cruz were Puerto Rican immigrants arrested for prostitution in December of 1921 and sentenced with deportation. Luckily, Celina's father, Manuel Ortiz, intervened and promised authorities to "keep his daughter away from immoral conduct" if she were allowed to remain in the country. The military government granted his request, but deported Amalia Cruz.[57] Court records from San Pedro also suggest that British subjects worked in the sex trade. Leticia Richardson from Nevis, Fernanda Williams, from St. Thomas, and Carmelita Balcanil from St. Kitts, were among those charged with clandestine prostitution in the 1920s.[58] Clearly, San Pedro's dynamic economy and the overwhelming presence of men—whether US soldiers or cane cutters—conspired to transform the city into a golden opportunity for tenacious, female migrants.

Since the Sanitation Law was one of several pieces of legislation that most symbolized the loss of Dominican sovereignty to an occupying force, the Dominican reaction to the anti-prostitution campaign was dramatic. City council members were reluctant to comply since that meant giving up power. This was apparently the case with Provost Marshal Kincade's attempt to appoint Lucas Espinal as San Pedro's Police Commissioner; San Pedro's city council and the provincial governor rejected his candidacy for the position. Some Dominicans seem to have been uncomfortable with policing commercial sex without provision for poor women's future. Once the occupation ended, a writer in the country's major newspaper, the *Listín Diario*, opined that the military government's prostitution policy was both morally wrong and ineffective. According to the anonymous author, the role of the state was to help those who could not help themselves, including so-called "fallen women." The writer argued that prostitution should be addressed with education and health care. The *moral social*, the article proclaimed, could only be restored when all members of society felt that the state acted in their best interests.[59]

As the *Listín* writer noted, the military government's policy regarding prostitution was in no way concerned with the moral community, but rather with exercising power. Dominican elites viewed tolerance zones as an important strategy in the elaboration of their political hegemony and their role as a paternalist, moral vanguard; in contrast, US military officials considered red-light districts as dangerous inter-zones, defined by Kevin Mumford as "areas of cultural, sexual, and social interchange." As in urban areas in the United States, these "interzones created a new complex of racial and gendered politics," in which foreign-born immigrants, Dominican men, and US soldiers competed over foreign-born women, many of them of African descent.[60] These were not spaces that exemplified social order; tolerance zones could, in the minds of US authorities, upend social hierarchies based on race and gender and upset the US's imperial project. Bars, brothels, dances, and sex districts were dangerous spaces where the superiority of white, North American men and their imperial masculinity, on which the United States established its empire across the Caribbean, was tested. US superiority over Dominican subjects could not be sustained in a brothel or on the streets, where Dominican men felt empowered enough to challenge US Marines over "their" women.[61]

Evidence for this takes us back to Celina Ortiz, the Puerto Rican-born woman threatened with deportation after her arrest for clandestine prostitution. Her complicated love life suggests that some women accused of prostitution may not have ever sold sex commercially and that Dominican men and US Marines competed for women's affection. Ortiz resided downtown, but lived in such crowded conditions that investigators noted her address as: "10 September Street in the tall [red] house between numbers 5 and 7. Just in the court in front of number 6 house." According to Ortiz, she had lived in the Dominican Republic from the age of six and had "a child, mother, and sister to look after for they [were] unable to maintain a living." In 1921, Ortiz was arrested for prostitution, but a memo submitted by the Provost Marshall noted that a "crooked intelligence agent from the PND (*Policía Nacional Dominicana*—Dominican National Police)" accused her of selling sex after he witnessed Ortiz interacting with a US Marine. In an unsigned letter translated into or rendered in poor English, a police agent pointed out that Ortiz was living with a Marine even though she was married to Lico, a fellow PND officer: "Interview I had with one of them friend she have, learn me that, Celina . . . live with an American USMC. I don't know if [he] is a general, corporal, sergeant [sic] or officer." One early morning, the PND agent saw Ortiz in "a great conversation with a person who was in the automobile form buick" and afterward told Lico about the confrontation. The report closed noting how, "Liquito is [her] sincere [husband] who she love[s] . . . more than Christ." Nevertheless, Ortiz's relationship with Lico was fraught with problems. As the informant continued, "the man don't give her nothing, not a cent, only some strokes"; instead, he added, "Celina give him money when he *necesita* [needs it]."[62]

Celina Ortiz may have sold sex; more likely she exploited a relationship with a US Marine for economic advantage to support her family and her partner, Lico. The truth may never be fully understood, but as a poor, female immigrant, Celina Ortiz and many others were located at the centre of a contentious debate between Dominican political elites and US military authorities over the nature of governance and the role of public health and sanitation in making concrete particular visions of social, moral, and imperial orders. In important ways, US and Dominican officials' thinking converged. Both Dominican and US military officials regarded women like Ortiz, and the crowded tenements and courtyards where they lived and worked, as bodies and spaces in need of policing; they believed that prostitutes were vectors of disease; that syphilis and VD warranted greater attention than illnesses associated with poverty; and that reasonable strategies to eradicate syphilis included policing, inspection, and some form of removal.

Nevertheless, public health policy served different understandings of social and political order and the ways in which space reflected hierarchy and order. For Dominican officials, prostitutes threatened the moral community, but such a threat could be managed by an elite vanguard that could protect respectable society from commercial sex through the construction of tolerance zones. Prostitutes' integration into the moral order, by policing their movements through and in space, resulted in public health policies that placed poor women and immigrants under great scrutiny, and instituted sanitation procedures that were invasive and humiliating. For Dominican elites, then, the tolerance zone represented moral direction and social order. Precisely the opposite was the case for US officials who regarded tolerance zones and clandestine prostitutes as signs of disorder, danger, and contagion. Prostitutes threatened the healthiness of troops and, as we have seen in the Ortiz case and in the November confrontation that opened this chapter, tolerance zones and slum districts were also spaces where US Marines could be financially exploited, or where violent confrontations between Marines and Dominican police officers over women took place. Although one kind of "paternalist master narrative" lost to the other, public health policy became a vehicle for Dominican elites to confront and question US imperialism in the circum-Caribbean region.[63]

NOTES

1. The author wishes to thank Julia Kramer for her research assistance, and also acknowledges Rebecca Lord, whose dissertation about public health in the Dominican Republic under US military rule has made a significant contribution to the social and cultural history of public health and US imperialism. Ayuntamiento de San Pedro de Macorís, *Libros de Actas de Sesiones*, libro 13, 8 Sept. 1919 to 2 Feb. 1922 (Session dates: 24 Oct. 1919; 19 Nov. 1919; 27 Nov. 1919; 29 Dec. 1919). Hereafter, *Libros de Actas de Sesiones*.
2. Dorothy Porter, *Health, Civilization and the State: A History of Public Health from Ancient to Modern Times* (London: Routledge, 1999), 16.
3. Eileen J. Suárez Findlay, *Imposing Decency: The Politics of Sexuality and Race in Puerto Rico, 1870–1902* (Durham, NC: Duke University Press, 1999), 8, and especially, 77–109; and Laura Briggs, *Reproducing Empire. Race, Sex, Science, and US Imperialism in Puerto Rico* (Berkeley: University of California Press, 2002), 46–74.
4. Christopher Abel, "Health, Hygiene, and Sanitation in Latin America c.1870 to c.1950," Working paper: Institute of Latin American Studies, 3, 7.
5. See the collection of Everardo Duarte Nunes, ed., *Juan César Garcia: Pensamento social em saúde na América Latina* (São Paulo, Brazil: Cortez Editora, 1989). For a discussion of the modernization process in the Dominican Republic during this period, see Jaime Dominguez, *La Dictadura de Heureaux* (Santo Domingo, Dominican Republic: UASD, 1986).
6. "Ciénega," *El Cable*, 24 April 1893, p. 1. For various public health initiatives, see *Libros de Actas de Sesiones*, libro 1, from 1886–1888 (11 Mar. 1887); libro 5, from Jan. 1897 to Nov. 1898 (17 Feb. 1897); libro 11, 24 Nov. 1913 to 27 July 1917 (29 July 1916).
7. Abel, "Health, Hygiene, and Sanitation in Latin America," 6–7.

8. Raymundo González, "Hostos y la conciencia moderna en República Domini-cana," in *Política, identidad y pensamiento social en la República Dominicana (Siglos XIX y XX)*, eds. Raymundo González, Michiel Baud, Pedro L. San Miguel, and Roberto Cassá (Madrid: Doce Calles, 2003), 95–104; citation here refers to p. 99; Teresita Martínez-Vergne, *Nation and Citizen in the Dominican Republic, 1880–1919* (Chapel Hill: University of North Carolina Press, 2005), 11; April Mayes, "Sugar's Metropolis: The Politics and Culture of Progress in San Pedro de Macorís, Dominican Republic, 1870–1930" (PhD diss., University of Michigan, 2003), pp. 1–15.

9. *Libros de Actas de Sesiones*, libro 1, 1886–1888 (23 Jan. 1887) and libro 2, 25 Sept. 1888 until 14 May 1891 (4 Jan. 1889). Health officials fined meat and bread vendors who sold their goods without using the proper scales.

10. H. Hoetink, *El pueblo dominicano* (Santo Domingo, Dominican Republic: Editora de Colores, 1986), 87–90. See also Hoetink, "Materiales para el estudio de la República Dominicana en la segunda mitad del siglo XX," *Caribbean Studies* 5, no. 3 (October 1965): 3–21; citation here refers to p. 18. Hoetink does not cite the source of his census information.

11. Guillermo Atiles Santos, *Guía Local y de comercio de la ciudad de San Pedro de Macorís* (Santo Domingo, Dominican Republic: n.p., 1902), 20.

12. I borrow the term "moral geography" from William French, *A Peaceful and Working People: Manners, Morals, and Class Formation in Northern Mexico* (Albuquerque: University of New Mexico Press, 1996), 5.

13. As early as 1855, Dominican legislators passed the "Repression of Idleness and Vagrancy" law which stipulated that women without "honest occupations" or who "lived their lives in a scandalous manner" were to be confined to government-run homes where they would be "kept busy and respectable". See Elpido E. Ricart, "Historia de la sanidad en Santo Domingo," in *Congreso Médico Dominicano del Centenario. Memoria* (Ciudad Trujillo, Dominican Republic: Congreso Médico Dominicano, 1944), 162.

14. See, for instance, "Ruido," *El Cable*, 8 April 1897.

15. President of the Ayuntamiento to Treasurer, 9 Oct. 1891; and Manuel S. Richiez, et al., to President of Ayuntamiento [San Pedro de Macorís], 23 Nov. 1891, Ayuntamiento de San Pedro de Macorís, legajo 5, 601 (7), año 1891, Archvio General de la Nación (AGN).

16. Robert B. Hoernel, "Sugar and Social Change in Oriente, Cuba, 1898–1946," *Journal of Latin American Studies* 8, no. 2 (1976): 236–237.

17. "Mezclilla," *El Cable*, 13 May 1893, p. 1.

18. Kevin Mumford, *Interzones. Black/White Sex Districts in Chicago and New York in the Early Twentieth Century* (New York: Columbia University Press, 1997), xvii. For discussions on the connection between social improvement, race, and health, see Sidney Chalhoub, "The Politics of Disease Control: Yellow Fever and Race in Nineteenth Century Rio de Janeiro," *Journal of Latin American Studies* 35 (1993): 441–463; and Nancy Stepan, *The Hour of Eugenics. Race, Gender, and Nation in Latin America* (Ithaca, NY: Cornell University Press, 1991).

19. *Libros de Actas de Sesiones*, Libro 8, 1 May 1903 to 31 July 1908 (14 August 1906).

20. Interview with Bishop Telésforo Isaac, Santo Domingo, Dominican Republic, 9 October 1999.

21. Alain Corbin, "Commercial Sexuality in Nineteenth-Century France: A System of Images and Regulations," in *The Making of the Modern Body*, eds. Catherine Gallagher and Thomas Laqueur (Berkeley: University of California Press, 1987), 209–220, quote is taken from 211. See also Margareth Rago, *Os prazeres da noite. Prostituição e códigos da sexualidade*

feminine em São Paolo, 1890–1930 (Rio de Janeiro, Brazil: Paz e Terra, 1991).

22. Findlay, *Imposing Decency*, 8, 77–109. Also Donna J. Guy, *Sex and Danger in Buenos Aires. Prostitution, Family, and Nation in Argentina* (Lincoln: University of Nebraska Press, 1991).

23. The information here is taken from various city council session minutes. The sources are listed in the order they appear in the narrative: *Libros de Actas de Sesiones*, libro 8, 1 May 1903 to 31 July 1908 (19 Jan. 1906); libro 7, 23 May 1901 to 27 Apr. 1903 (21 Oct. 1904); libro 6, 10 Nov. 1898 to 19 May 1901 (8 Apr. 1901); and libro 7, 23 May 1901 to 27 April 1903 (24 Jan. 1902).

24. *Libros de Actas de Sesiones*, libro 8, 1 May 1903 to 31 July 1908 (15 July 1908 and 20 July 1908).

25. The council secretary references the regulation in his notes from 1 March 1909. *Libros de Actas de Sesiones*, libro 9, 30 Jan. 1909 to 17 Apr. 1909 (1 Mar. 1909). Also, *Libros de Actas de Sesiones*, libro 13, 8 Sept. 1919 to 2 Feb. 1922 (24 Oct. 1919).

26. *Libros de Actas de Sesiones*, libro 8, 1 May 1903 to 31 July 1908 (8 May 1908); and libro 10, (5 Dec. 1910).

27. For a discussion on the debate between miasmatists and bacteriologists, see George Rosen, *A History of Public Health* (New York: MD Publications, Inc., 1958), 324.

28. Laura Engelstein, "Morality and the Wooden Spoon: Russian Doctors View Syphilis, Social Class, and Sexual Behavior," in *The Making of the Modern Body*, eds. Gallagher and Laqueur, 169–208, here 176.

29. Dr J. Marchena to Ayuntamiento de San Pedro de Macorís, 27 Jan. 1911, Ayuntamiento de San Pedro de Macorís, legajo 5, 524, exp., 37, año 1911, AGN.

30. Hygiene Inspector to Ayuntamiento de San Pedro de Macorís, 2 January 1911, "Informe de la Salud Pública, 1910," Ayuntamiento de San Pedro de Macorís, legajo 5, 524, exp., 37, año 1911, AGN; and *Libro de Actas de Sesiones*, libro 10 (13 Feb. 1911).

31. Dr. Joseph Earle Moore, et. al, "El Cuidado de la sífilis en la practica general," *Oficina Sanitaria Panamericana* 22 (December 1929): 1–17, citation here refers to 2–3.

32. Dr. Emilio Tió y Betances to Ayuntamiento de San Pedro de Macorís, Health Reports for March and April of 1911, Ayuntamiento de San Pedro de Macorís, legajo 5, 524, exp., 37, año 1911, AGN.

33. Moore, "El Cuidado de la sífilis," 4.

34. Kristen Luker makes a similar argument regarding anti-prostitute campaigns in the United States: Kristen Luker, "Sex, Social Hygiene, and the State: The Double-Edged Sword of Social Reform," *Theory and Society* 37 (1998): 601–634.

35. Engelestein, "Morality and the Wooden Spoon," 171.

36. *Alcaldía de San Pedro de Macorís*, libro 31 (1 Feb. 1915 to 26 Mar. 1916), AGN.

37. *Libros de Actas de Sesiones*, libro 11, 27 Nov. 1913 to 27 July 1917 (5 July 1915).

38. Megan Vaughan, "Syphilis in Colonial East Central Africa: The Social Construction of an Epidemic," in *Epidemics and Ideas: Essays on the Historical Perception of Pestilence*, eds. Terence Ranger and Paul Slack (Cambridge: Cambridge University Press, 1992), 269–302, here 299.

39. Briggs, *Reproducing Empire*, 73.

40. Quoted in Bruce Calder, *The Impact of Intervention: The Dominican Republic during the US Occupation of 1916–1924* (Austin: University of Texas Press, 1984), 17.

41. Ibid., 17–25.
42. Quoted in Rebecca Ann Lord, "'An Imperative Obligation': Public Health and the United States Military Occupation of the Dominican Republic, 1916–1924" (PhD diss., University of Maryland, College Park, 2002), 4, 89, 96–97.
43. Thomas Snowden to Commander Mayo, 21 October 1919 Gobierno Militar, legajo sin número, Correspondencia Cruzada con la Secretaría del Estado de Justicia e Instrucción Pública, AGN. Placing female prostitutes in quarantine or in prison, however, was nothing new. European countries had, since the eighteenth century, placed restrictions on sex work, and in the nineteenth century, sent many women to prison hospitals and jails under the aegis of reform. See Luker, "Sex, Social Hygiene, and the State," 601–634.
44. "Record of Proceedings of a Board Investigation Convened at Marine Barracks in Santo Domingo City," 6 August 1918, Gobierno Militar, legajo sin número, Correspondencia Cruzadas con la Secretaría del Estado de Justica e Instrucción Pública, AGN, pp. 2–3. These numbers are highly questionable since the report does not provide any information about the study which produced these results.
45. P.E. Garrison, Chief Sanitary Officer, to Brigade Commander, 17 October 1917, Gobierno Militar, legajo 24, Correspondencia de la Secretaría del Estado de lo Interior y Policía, 1917, AGN.
46. Lord, "An Imperative Obligation," 185–187. As Lord points out, in 1917, the Secretary of War created the Committee on Training Camp Activities designed to provide alternative pastimes for men otherwise tempted by the lure of nearby prostitutes. Authorities relied on two strategies to keep troops syphilis-free: the use of prophylaxes and the creation of prostitute-free zones around military encampments.
47. Thomas W. Jackson, "Public Health in the Dominican Republic," *The United States Naval Medical Bulletin* 1, no. 6 (1907): 331–349, here 334.
48. Lord, "An Imperative Obligation," 115, 132–143; quote is taken from p. 143. Also, Calder, *The Impact of Intervention*, 40–50. The structure of the public health regime in the Dominican Republic was similar to that in the Philippines. The Ley de Sanidad divided the country into ten sanitary districts, each governed by a District Sanitation Officer, who reported to the Chief Sanitation Officer in Santo Domingo. A Department of Sanitation and Beneficence, headed by a Secretary of Sanitation who held a cabinet position in the government, was also created. See Mary C. Gillett, "U.S. Army Medical Officers and Public Health in the Wake of the Spanish-American War, 1898–1905," *Bulletin of the History of Medicine* 64, no. 4 (1990): 567–587.
49. In 1919, for example, of the 760 people who succumbed to malaria, 450 were Dominicans, but tuberculosis killed 424 Dominicans as well. In 1920, meanwhile, malaria claimed 888 lives and tuberculosis, 612. Even more telling were findings from the sugar zones where malaria was supposed to be a particular problem. Similarly, in Barahona, 487 deaths were attributed to malaria, but *bubas* (plague) claimed 339 lives: Secretaría del Estado de Sanidad y Beneficencia, "Relación de los Presos Asistidos en el Hospital Militar de Santo Domingo durante el año 1919," *Informe que el Secretario de Sanidad y Beneficencia presenta al Presidente Provisional de la República*, and "Relación de los casos de enfermedades trasmisibles en la República Dominicana durante el año 1919" (Santo Domingo, Dominican Republic: J.R. Viuda Garcia, 1923), n.p.
50. Lord, "'An Imperative Obligation,'" 103. Interestingly, some medical officials regarded syphilis as an endemic disease in Haiti, also under US occupation. N.T. McLean, who served as Chief of the Public Health Service in Haiti,

claimed that 90 percent of blood samples tested positive for syphilis, but also found "little evidence of active syphilitic infection", a fact he attributed to a "'survival of the fittest' elimination" that carried away the weakest and made the strongest immune to the effects of syphilis. McLean's science affirmed for many in the white medical establishment that people of African descent were "natural" carriers of venereal diseases: N.T McLean, "Public Health Problems of the Southern Countries," *The United States Naval Medical Bulletin* 2, no. 1 (1922): 25–39.

51. *Libros de Actas de Sesiones*, libro 12, 27 July 1917 to 8 Sept. 1919 (6 Dec. 1918).
52. Ibid., libro 14, 6 Feb. 1922 to 11 Feb. 1924 (3 Apr. 1922).
53. Admiral Thomas Snowden, Occupation Governor, "Prostitution Regulation," 21 Oct. 1919, Gobierno Militar, legajo sin número, Correspondencia Cruzadas con la Secretaría del Estado de Justicia y Instrucción Pública, AGN.
54. Lord, "'An Imperative Obligation,'" 196, 199.
55. Alcaldía de San Pedro de Macorís, Penales, libro 40, año 1920, AGN. The Alcaldía books include court statistics from the following periods: 2 January to 30 August 1920; 1 November to 19 December 1923; and 1 August to 20 December 1924. The dollar amounts are in Dominican *pesos* which, at the time, equaled the US dollar.
56. Alcaldía de San Pedro de Macorís, Penales, libro 40, (1–10 June 1920, case no. 25; 16–25 June 1920, cases 89–92), año 1920, AGN. Military government records suggest that US Marines or Dominicans trained by Marines coordinated these raids. The Provost Marshall submitted reports to the occupation government regarding arrests of prostitutes. See *Libros de Actas de Sesiones*, libro 13, 8 Sept. 1919 to 2 Feb. 1922 (29 Dec. 1919); and C. H. Lyman (District Commander) to Commanding General, 11 April 1922, Gobierno Militar, legajo 122, Interior y Policía, AGN.
57. R. Warfield to Colonel Ramsey, "Memo from Agricultura y Inmigración," 5 Jan. 1922, Gobierno Militar, legajo 20, Secretaría del Estado de Justicia y Instrucción Pública, AGN.
58. Alcaldía de San Pedro de Macorís, libro 40, case no. 135,pp. 86–87 (29 Apr. 1920); case no. 15, p. 90 (7 June 1920); case no. 18, p. 108 (6 July 1920); and case no. 205, p. 164 (11 Dec. 1923), año 1920, AGN.
59. Conde, "Urge una medida," *Listín Diario*, 4 September 1925.
60. Mumford, *Interzones*, 20, 21.
61. Kelvin Santiago-Valles, *"Subject People" and Colonial Discourses: Economic Transformation and Social Disorder in Puerto Rico, 1898–1947* (Albany: State University of New York Press, 1994), 4–5.
62. All of the following documents can be found in Gobierno Militar, legajo 20, Correspondencia de la Secretaría del Estado de la Justicia e Instrucción Pública, AGN: Unsigned and undated letter; Celina Ortiz to Provost Marshal Stack, 19 Dec. 1921; Memo from the Office of Provost Marshall Major Kincade to Captain García, PND, no date; and Memo from Agricultura y Inmigración, Ron Warfield to Col. Ramsey, 5 Jan. 1922.
63. Mary Renda, *Taking Haiti. Military Occupation and the Culture of US Imperialism, 1915–1940* (Chapel Hill: University of North Carolina Press, 2001), 28–29.

7 The Politics of Professionalization

Puerto Rican Physicians during the Transition from Spanish to US Colonialism

Nicole Trujillo-Pagán

Under Spanish colonial rule, many Puerto Rican physicians were active among the liberal elite and espoused a version of modernity that both challenged colonial dominance and buttressed their political authority on the island. Many had been educated in the medical schools of a politically tumultuous Spain, which led them to envision a broad social regeneration based on scientific principles.[1] They worked to expose Spanish colonial authority as traditional and a source of deficiency, degeneration, and decay at both individual and institutional levels. Physicians defined themselves as "modern" professionals, differentiated themselves from the Spanish conception of colonial modernity, and used their status to justify their political involvement and social leadership. They also used their professional status to radicalize other liberal elites' claims for political autonomy, economic liberalization, and social reform. As leaders of a struggle for greater political autonomy under Spanish colonial rule, physicians articulated an identity that treated the political and the professional as inseparable.

After 1898, under US colonial rule, Puerto Rican physicians' political strategy and professional identity shifted. Physicians' status and leadership were undermined by a U.S.-directed modernization that questioned their "professionalism", doubted their qualifications, and found everything "Spanish"—including the political–professional role that Puerto Rican physicians had crafted—prone to corruption and political self-interest. As many physicians were excluded from direct political participation, they strategically asserted their ascribed status as Puerto Ricans to promote their professional authority and political influence. However, physicians found that this approach limited their professional authority. They quickly revised this strategy, abandoned the independence of their recently developed professional association, and narrowed their emphasis to pursue professional, rather than broader political, autonomy.

The shifting nature of physicians' strategy and identity raises central questions about the profession's relationship to the state. The following study asks how and why establishing themselves as "professionals" became an extra-professional and *political* strategy for turn-of-the-nineteenth-century Puerto Rican physicians? This question cannot be answered without addressing the related question of how members of a status group could imagine themselves to be furthering an emergent "national" cause while protecting their own class interests? In order to answer these questions, this chapter treats the end of the Spanish-American War in 1898 as an event marking a fundamental transformation in the relationship between professionals and the state. It compares Puerto Rican physicians' political and professional involvements under late-Spanish and early-US colonial governments and addresses the political and professional tensions introduced by shifting colonial orders.

The chapter assesses Puerto Rican physicians' struggle for professional status and autonomy from the colonial state in four ways. First, in order to distinguish between state- and market-related aspects of this struggle, it compares the ideological meanings supporting physicians' struggle for professional status under Spanish and US colonial rule. Second, it elucidates the intra-professional challenges to physicians' markets and status that increased significantly in the years following the 1898 military invasion. Third, it considers how the terms of institutional conflict and competition between physicians and the state shifted from the Spanish to the US colonial state. Finally, it emphasizes physicians' actions to support their professional status by discussing how they articulated their ethnic difference, formed an independent medical association, and subsequently incorporated this association into the American Medical Association. The study concludes with a discussion of the implications these fundamental transformations had on the subsequent development of medicine and public health in Puerto Rico. I argue that Puerto Rican physicians' professionalization involved struggles for market control, social mobility, and a political–professional status that initially challenged the structure of the colonial state and its discriminatory institutions.

THE CONTEXT

Most of Latin America had achieved independence from Spain during the early nineteenth century. Puerto Rico remained one of three colonies that struggled toward greater autonomy under the Spanish empire. Ironically, independence movements did not enjoy stable support. For instance, the 1868 *Grito de Lares* has been understood as a call for independence and as a class-based struggle resulting from rapid economic change and social repression.[2] Rather than widespread support for independence, the creole (island-born residents who claimed pure Spanish lineage) elites' struggle for autonomy was a political and economic reaction that stemmed from both "economic contraction after auspicious growth [and] political repression to compensate for Spain's earlier fragile hold on the rest of its colonies."[3] Creole elites worked to establish a political structure that could facilitate the island's social and economic modernization. These elites included creole physicians who were heavily influenced by Spanish liberalism, such as Dr Ramón Emeterio Betances, who led the revolt for independence.

Historians have generally believed that Spanish liberalism influenced the series of political changes that occurred after 1868, when the Liberal and Conservative parties formed. Initially, liberals pushed for two political status options under Spanish authority: autonomy, with decentralized control, or assimilation as an equal peninsular province. Astrid Cubano-Iguina has argued that these options represented the liberal creole elite's promotion of a "rhetoric of harmonious negotiation" and that, from this early date, they "attempted to integrate the native-born inhabitants of the colony by constructing a single ethnic identity for the island." Nonetheless, this Puerto Rican identity was neither a direct challenge to Spanish colonialism, nor even to the "paternalist social relations then prevailing on estates of the interior. . . ."[4] Rather than a direct political and/or economic challenge, the creole elite used this identity to inform a framework that included a diverse population and could bolster the elites' struggle for greater political freedoms under Spain.

By the late 1890s, despite important internal divisions, autonomists had gained the support of the majority of the population. The Spanish crown issued three decrees in late 1897 that established the island's political autonomy under its authority and the first transitional cabinet that took office in February 1898. A month after elections were held, in April of 1898, the United States declared war against Spain. By October, the Treaty of Paris had ceded Puerto Rico to the United States. The ensuing period from 1898 through 1912 witnessed a rapid dispossession of the island's agricultural classes and a shift in the status of physicians. The military government lasted eighteen months, during which time Hurricane San Ciriaco hit the island in 1899. This event had two important consequences. The military government appointed US Army physician, Bailey K. Ashford, to establish a provisional tent hospital to facilitate medical relief efforts. It was in this provisional hospital that Ashford began his hookworm campaign, which would have international repercussions. Following the hurricane, and intensified by rapid economic changes, physicians who had operated in rural districts migrated to urban areas in search of work. These economic changes were amplified by the Foraker Act, passed in 1900, which not only established a US-appointed civil government for the colony, but also devalued the Spanish peso relative to the US dollar. Creole physicians faced increased competition from US physicans' research on the island, demographic shifts, and decreased spending power. Although an increasing number of physicians would become involved in Ashford's campaign against the hookworm, many creole physicians found their influence undermined by the unfolding colonial political culture. By 1912, of the five founders of the Independence Party were licensed physicians, but they had become atypical in their profession because of their explicit political involvement.

PHYSICIANS' POLITICAL–PROFESSIONAL
STATUS CONSTRAINTS

During the latter half of the nineteenth century, physicians' collective identity was closely related to their class position. Although they were professionals, physicians identified with other Puerto Rican elites who similarly strove to reform their long-standing status as colonial subjects. Within their struggle for political autonomy, physicians became notable actors because their education and social status afforded them greater access to political networks and activities. For instance, many physicians, such as José Gómez Brioso and Santiago Veve y Calzada, distinguished themselves through their work within the Autonomist Party. Other medical doctors, like Francisco del Valle Atiles, Manuel Zeno Gandía, and Cayetano Coll y Toste, strongly influenced reformist elites through their literary and historical writings.[5] Physicians like Dr Ramón Emeterio Betances developed a radical, separatist political ideology surrounding the 1868 *Grito de Lares* rebellion, which almost gained autonomy for Puerto Rico as a concession from the Spanish colonial state.[6]

Physicians attempted to mediate Spain's tumultuous transition to a modern state by locating political control within the colony. They considered colonialism antithetical to their own economic, political, and professional autonomy. For example, they argued that, "to stay far from that struggle was an indignity for those who considered that politics was a *science* for the men of good faith".[7] As they construed political involvements as both professional and patriotic duties, they also regarded their professional work as political because they negotiated it within a political structure they saw as prejudicial. They defined their healing mission broadly and considered themselves social servants whose responsibilities included promoting Puerto Ricans' "moral and material" interests. They caucused secretly with other elites to strategize against Spanish colonialism and exercised political influence within their meetings.

The medical elite used their education to position themselves as a vanguard within the autonomist movement, but this education also made their vision of broad social reform more radical than that of many other liberal reformists.[8] Impelled by late nineteenth-century scientific advances, many believed they could use their education to organize Puerto Rico along scientific principles and cure its "social ills". For these physicians, eradicating social ills meant defending the collective social body against a broader moral decay that included alcoholism, "disenfranchised eroticism", suicide, homicide, and robbery. They used the notion of "disease" to articulate what they saw as the consequences of colonialism. They believed that by reforming the political environment, they could eradicate illness and regenerate Puerto Ricans as modern and productive citizens fit for equality with their Spanish counterparts. In guiding Puerto Rican society's regeneration, physicians saw themselves as playing a central role within a broader social transformation.

As medical practitioners struggled for political reforms, they not only conflated their own interests with those of all Puerto Ricans, they also promoted their vision of modernization. For instance, in the 1890s, they pushed Spain for institutional reforms that included administrative shifts in the insane asylum (*Casa De Beneficiencia*) so that they could effect their classification and separation of patients, which included women, children, and the poor. Because this was a site where the Spanish colonial state promoted modernity in Puerto Rico, physicians tried to use their local autonomy and status to "finish the asylum, organizing it under scientific principles, to offer a hope of healing the unfortunate that inhabit it."[9] Thus, in urban areas like San Juan, where the insane asylum was located, liberal physicians' discourse reflected their desire to control modern institutions and stratify urban social boundaries, distance themselves from elements within it they saw as threatening, and place themselves at the top of a social hierarchy.[10]

Physicians viewed the Spanish colonial government as an obstacle to their version of modernity, which included their professional and political autonomy. They argued that Spain created a political structure that frustrated their attempts to heal what they saw as Puerto Ricans' social pathologies. Ultimately, their advocacy of autonomy, rather than independence, influenced Spain's decision to concede political autonomy to the island through the Autonomic Charter of 1897. As professionals, physicians would have enjoyed greater eligibility for political office, increased their influence over a reformist legislature, and expanded their local influence within municipalities. Unfortunately, they were not able to realize this political influence because the US military landed in Puerto Rico, established a military government, and began centralizing medicine under a new colonial government in 1898.

Perhaps ironically, the same physicians that had promoted political autonomy under Spain's colonial rule initially joined other elites in welcoming the US military's arrival in Puerto Rico in 1898. Physicians shared the widespread belief that US intervention would "eradicate" colonialism and foster favourable trading terms for Puerto Rican markets. They responded positively to a survey, commissioned by a US president, of conditions on the island, and complained about Spanish colonialism to Henry Carroll, the report's author. Although physicians joined a broad cross-section of Puerto Ricans who also responded to Carroll's interviews, they seemed confident that their ideas for reform would be crucial to planning Puerto Rico's future development, and that US intervention would bring about the modernizing reforms they had envisioned for medicine.

Puerto Rican physicians' initial enthusiasm quickly dissipated. Their status was undermined by the US colonial government and its representatives, which included US Army medics, who began competing for legitimacy. Puerto Rican physicians found themselves almost immediately sidelined in decisions regarding a new compulsory smallpox campaign in

1898, even though they had performed smallpox vaccinations throughout the nineteenth century.[11] They were demoted by US military officers, who worked directly with municipal mayors to appoint physicians and organize the work. Their work was appropriated by Major John Van R. Hoff, who did not laud the physicians carrying out the work, but rather stressed that his impossible administrative task had been made "possible only through military agency."[12] Although the campaign drew the physicians into unpopular work that included denying public access to "schools, theatres, and public transportation to all who had not undergone the procedure," US colonial administrators privileged their own efforts as both efficient and educational.[13]

Physicians' disappointment with the US military government coincided with other threats to their market position and professional status that followed in the wake of the San Ciriaco hurricane of 1899. Their markets of wealthy and middle-class patients were destabilized as they competed with a heterogeneous group of medical practitioners who had migrated to urban areas in search of work. In addition, their scientific presentation and competence were undermined by the US military's relief efforts, which included a provisional tent hospital where US Army medic, Dr Bailey K. Ashford, claimed to discover the true scientific cause of anaemia in the hookworm. Although Puerto Rican physicians, including the award-winning Dr Agustín Stahl, had worked on anaemia and explained its origin in iron and nutritional deficiencies, Ashford dismissed these explanations as unscientific.[14] Puerto Rican physicians' competence was still in question more than thirty years later when Ashford wrote in his biography that "only the bedrabbled old *curandera,* or medicine-woman of the town, with her stringy hair and one remaining tooth, was held competent when it came to curing this terrible disease."[15]

Although physicians were disappointed by these initial changes, their loss of professional status was more definitively evident when the 1900 Foraker Act created a civil government structure that ignored public health and medical care. Elite Puerto Rican physicians had attempted to protect their professional identity by promoting political autonomy, but the Foraker Act made it plainly evident that their status would change under US tutelage. Their hopes that US colonial government's spending on the smallpox campaign, the provisional hospital, and sanitation would be positive developments for their professional autonomy quickly dissipated when these changes ignored their professional authority. They also found that US colonial administrators considered their training inadequate and their medical explanations "unscientific". Puerto Rican physicians were increasingly alarmed that they would not have a significant role in in medical developments because US colonial administrators considered them incompetent and corrupt. Their identity as uniquely qualified leaders was undermined by a US colonial state that did not distinguish them from other medical practitioners.

Finally, Puerto Rican physicians' status was also undermined by a shifting medical structure. Within the new and developing institutions that Ashford influenced, Puerto Rican physicians' sense of order and change was challenged by a shifting relationship to treating the island's poor. For instance, Ashford highlighted Puerto Rican physicians' seeming disregard for public health in the way he described Stahl's involvement in the early stages of his research and relationship to the poor that visited the clinic. "One of them had been unsuccessfully trying to get Dr. Stahl to pay a professional visit to his bedridden wife . . . Stahl suddenly veered round in purple rage."[16] Ashford's research on hookworm not only shifted attention away from Puerto Rican physicians' emphasis on the political and economic influences on disease, but also created the idea that Ashford could do more to solve medical problems than Puerto Rican physicians could on their own.

PROFESSIONAL IDENTITY AND STATUS

Under Spanish colonialism, Puerto Rican physicians tied their professional identity almost exclusively to their class position. As a result, their work was often indistinguishable from that of other practitioners, including non-elite practitioners who were trained outside of Europe, such as pharmacists, surgeons, *practicantes* (medical and surgeon assistants), *parteras* (midwives), *curiosos* (those curious about solutions), and *curanderos* (folk healers). Their work also overlapped with that of other specialists who used various forms of medicine, including blood-letting, leeching, cupping, and caustic healing, although these methods had rapidly declined in popularity by the end of the century.

Physicians outside of Puerto Rico fostered a collective identity through institutions like education, but physicians in Puerto Rico lacked a medical school. A select group of physicians offered courses at the *Ateneo* but their efforts had only recently developed after 1888, and students still had to complete their medical education outside of Puerto Rico. Similarly, other institutions they could have used to define and maintain their professional identity, such as hospitals, were weak and required significant improvements. As a result, class played a more significant but indirect role in defining physicians' status than any direct attempts on the part of physicians to restrict entry to the profession in order to maximize their influence and market. As a result, a relatively small and elite group of physicians who had received academic training in Europe (and increasingly, the United States) enjoyed the highest social status.[17]

Because Puerto Rican physicians felt reasonably secure in their class position, and because they could not control the medical profession's boundaries or membership, they were likely to collaborate with other medical practitioners. For instance, Puerto Rican physicians acquired the smallpox vaccine from the neighbouring island of St. Thomas before the Spanish medical team arrived with it in 1804,[18] and they took on *curanderos* as their assistants during the cholera epidemic of 1855.[19] In 1888, Drs Gabriel Ferrer and José Baralt illegally performed anatomical dissections in the cemetery's autopsy room to train practitioners. The existence of a separate and frequently mentioned category of practitioners well into the twentieth century, the *curiosos,* also indicates their regularized apprenticeships with academically trained physicians.

The single most important source of competition for all practitioners came from pharmacists. Pharmacists prescribed and prepared medicine without a physicians' prescription, despite Spanish legislation that prohibited this practice. Pharmacists also ignored Spanish authorities' attempts to control the "secret" compounds used in preparing medications, including poisons, opiates, and abortifacients. They performed "illegal" procedures, including abortions, deliveries, and caesareans. Thus, many Puerto Ricans avoided physicians and their fees altogether by buying drugs directly from pharmacists.

Ultimately, physicians used geographic and social factors to bolster their professional status and limit collaboration and competition under Spanish colonialism. Most elite physicians worked in growing urban areas on the coast, where their private practices catered to a wealthy clientele that could afford their services. Some academically trained, non-elite physicians sought out wealthy clients in urban areas, but most worked with the urban middle class in towns. *Curanderos* served the poor and, because trained physicians had little incentive to visit the sick of the countryside for little or no pay, they were often the only medical practitioners available in isolated rural environments. *Parteras,* women who were perhaps the least segregated of the medical practitioners, aided other women in their deliveries. The gendered character of their work meant that deliveries were poorly remunerated and were less interesting to trained physicians. Thus, rather than competing with academically trained physicians for the same clients, alternative practitioners served clients and practiced in areas that trained physicians found undesirable.

Despite instances of collaboration, competition among practitioners drastically intensified in the years following 1898. The Spanish colonial state had not usurped physicians' authority. Although the effects of a new colonial government on institutional growth would only gradually become apparent, immediate factors arose that threatened elite physicians' markets and status. Medical education offered at the *Ateneo* ceased immediately upon the inception of the Spanish-American War, the US military government ignored physicians' work and undermined their qualifications, the San Ciriaco hurricane threatened physicians' markets, and Ashford's emergent campaign crippled elite physicians' "scientific" presentation.

INSTITUTIONAL SITES OF CONFLICT AND COMPETITION

Physicians' class position heavily influenced their identity, which impeded their attempts to mobilize other academically trained, non-elite physicians as "rank-and-file" members of the profession. The following sections will demonstrate how elite physicians' status was threatened under US colonial rule by using licensing and municipal (rank-and-file) physicians as case studies. These case studies demonstrate that institutions were sites of conflict and competition for elite physicians who tried to consolidate their professional status within shifting colonial contexts. More specifically, these cases show that physicians attempted to compensate for their inability to control the medical profession's boundaries and membership by emphasizing institutions where they could gain control under the US colonial state, even though colonial state politics repeatedly undermined these efforts.

Many scholars view licensing as a form of state regulation and treat physicians' influence in regulating access to the practice of medicine as a first step toward professionalization. In both the Spanish and the US colonial contexts, however, the colonial administrations firmly held the profession's regulatory functions, and licensing remained outside of Puerto Rican physicians' control. Spain had created a governmental body, the *Real Subdelegación de Medicina,* to control the highly heterogeneous collection of practitioners working in municipalities. The *Subdelegación* was unable to control the variety of medical practitioners operating in Puerto Rico for a number of reasons. First, those who did not work for the Spanish colonial government had greater flexibility in their practice and therefore could elude governmental regulations. Second, advances in medicine increased demands for medical attention, which undermined Spanish legislative attempts to control particular practitioners and their practices. Third, practitioners occupied distinct niches in the market, which limited competition, and elite physicians were less inclined to pressure the Spanish colonial government for improved licensing measures. As intra-professional tensions increased, the *Real's Subdelegación* fruitless efforts compromised elite physicians' ability to formulate a collective identity, control access to the profession, and standardize medical practice. Elite physicians confronted the Spanish colonial state as an obstacle in their efforts to standardize medical practice, develop training opportunities, and create a modern bureaucratic structure to support their development of institutions, such as training hospitals, that could control access to the profession.

Although the *Real Subdelegación* had created an opening for physicians to develop a collective identity and mobilize the profession, physicians' efforts in this regard were squelched by the dramatic shift to US colonial rule. The US military government re-established Puerto Rican physicians as colonial subjects when it reorganized and renamed the *Real Subdelegación de Medicina* as the Superior Board of Health (SBOH) in 1899.[20] Two Puerto Rican physicians, Drs Gabriel Ferrer and Ricardo Hernandez, were directly involved in the SBOH, but because they were appointed, they were subject to the US colonial administrator's dictates.[21] More importantly, elite physicians' professional status was recast as unscientific because the profession was unregulated.[22] Some physicians' qualifications were "tolerated" by US colonialism, but many physicians who had not obtained a license under the Spanish colonial state now faced a new US colonial government that would regulate the profession along similarly arbitrary standards and with a similarly small, elite, and insulated board of colonial officers.[23] Other elite physicians had little influence over the SBOH and were not included in selecting examination committees for a new licensing exam, which the SBOH introduced and modeled on the one then in use at New York State University.[24] As elite physicians lost control over licensing, they also lost control over the ability to standardize the knowledge base of medicine and control access to the profession.

Physicians knew there was still little basis for distinguishing physicians based on the quality of their medical education and that US colonial administrators were discriminating against their competence because, even in the United States, medical education would not be standardized until after the 1910 Flexner Report.[25] Their frustration intensified because neither the SBOH nor the US colonial government made any provisions for helping Puerto Rican physicians meet these new licensing requirements; there were no immediate plans to set up a medical school in Puerto Rico, and no funds were set aside to help physicians study in the mainland United States. Physicians felt US control over licensing undermined the value of their medical knowledge. They saw that the SBOH would impose new standards and norms onto licensing exams and control the medical profession through what they considered a "foreign culture, language, and standard of work". They insisted that the profession had entered into a "hybrid process . . . [of] inevitable and fatal crisis."[26] Elite physicians began to consider themselves a "class" that could no longer claim its unique position among elites in leading Puerto Rico's modernization.

MUNICIPAL PHYSICIANS AS "RANK-AND-FILE" PROFESSIONALS AND STATE CONTROL

Under both Spanish and US colonial rule, there was no clearer evidence of state competition than in the case of municipal physicians. Under Spanish colonial rule, elite physicians saw their municipal counterparts as a significant obstacle to their professional status and attempts to gain autonomy from the state. Although elite physicians' understanding of the nature of the problem changed with the shift from Spanish to US colonialism, their inability to control municipal physicians' appointments, work, and compensation consistently compromised their ability to negotiate on the profession's behalf and gain broader autonomy. Elite physicians were not completely "free" to control their work because Spanish colonial legislation required they provide medical attention to the poor in areas where there was no municipal physician. On the one hand, elite physicians' work was constrained by this law, which represented one way in which the Spanish colonial state attempted to use physicians and their medical qualifications to promote its own political interests.[27] On the other hand, elite physicians' concerns were mediated by the lack of a concerted effort to provide the poor with medical attention. As a result, many trained physicians saw municipal appointments as an opportunity to increase the likelihood that they would be paid for providing medical attention to the poor and to charge those who were not "poor" for their services. Despite the benefits, elite physicians saw municipal appointments as an obstacle to promoting their status because many of the appointed physicians had inadequate qualifications, which undermined physicians' legitimacy. Physicians envied the ability to appoint municipal physicians, because it would put them in a better position to negotiate their autonomy from the Spanish colonial state and within municipal governments. Their inability to control municipal physicians' appointments limited their ability to assert their status claims with many other rank-and-file members. Thus, a major goal for physicians' professional autonomy was administrative autonomy from municipal governments.

Although physicians were certain that the US government would take their concerns seriously, and although they found that Henry Carroll's 1898 survey recognized their concerns about municipal appointments and municipal work, they also found that the same report ignored their concerns about compensation. Instead, elite and municipal physicians were not distinguished in Carroll's report, which held all physicians equally responsible for public criticism. One physician's testimony that "scarcely one in a hundred of the poor who die has the attendance of a physician" fit neatly within this criticism, because Carroll pointed out that the poor distrusted "town doctors . . . [who] would not visit the sick and poor without pay." Elite physicians' professionalism was summarily dismissed along with that of municipal physicians because Carroll portrayed both groups as self-serving and irresponsible.

US colonial administrators again ignored elite physicians' concerns when the 1900 Foraker Act established a civil government but ignored medicine, leaving these matters to local legislatures.[28] Elite physicians' failure to gain formal political power in the civil government meant that their only opportunity to present their concerns before the US government was neatly contained within Carroll's report. Rather than authors of modernization, elite physicians were reduced to respondents within a report that would promote US colonial administrators' emphasis on sanitation and reproduce physicians' subservience to state-directed work. They also found that the US colonial government used sanitation to promote its own priorities: instead of addressing their vision of modernization, the US government was more interested in using sanitation to protect its soldiers' health and promote infrastructural and institutional development not directly related to medicine.[29]

Physicians also found their authority and vision of modernization quickly displaced by the US military government, which restructured the SBOH and gave it more centralized (insular) control over municipal governments than its Spanish predecessor had enjoyed. Their hope of using the problems of municipal physicians to promote their own status before the US colonial government was displaced by the SBOH, which drew municipal physicians increasingly toward US colonial state-directed work, as it required them to collect demographic statistics that it could use to further regulate urban areas (urban hygiene), private properties (codes regarding painting, construction materials, distance from floor to ground, latrine construction, and the like), and social hygiene (the "hygiene of prostitution").[30] Elite physicians' desire to modernize urban spaces was similarly undermined by the SBOH, which introduced a new colonial agenda of restructuring areas like San Juan by addressing water bottling at street crossings and improving hygienic conditions in public schools and the condemnable houses adjoining the US General Hospital.[31] Despite these changes, elite physicians' concerns about municipal physicians persisted, and the SBOH experienced significant resistance and trouble enforcing sanitary legislation. As a result, the SBOH was largely ineffective.[32]

Although they did not have professional autonomy within municipal governments, physicians were blamed for the failures of SBOH centralization. US colonial governor, William Henry Hunt, recognized that municipal government was "as bad as the central," but insisted that "the habit of dependence upon the central government is yet deeply seated in the character of the people."[33] US colonial administrators, who argued that US "tutelage" would build Puerto Ricans' self-reliant character, summarily ignored elite physicians' desire for professional autonomy from municipal politics. Rather than conceding elite physicians' autonomy from municipal physicians' appointments and work, the US colonial government passed a set of laws in 1902 that reduced municipal autonomy on sanitary matters because it found municipal physicians "without adequate experience in such matters."[34]

Physicians were also culturally displaced when Governor Hunt noted that the legislation "does not depart too radically from what was good in the former system, but blends with it much that is American of an approved character."[35] Elite physicians did not significantly influence the new legislation that centralized sanitation, increased the SBOH's legislative control, and appointed an Insular Director of Sanitation accountable only to the US colonial governor.[36] They were further distanced from municipal physicians, who were increasingly embedded within the US colonial order. The legislation also expanded municipal physicians' work to chemical laboratories that could analyze forensic evidence, thus turning municipal physician's police and laboratory work into an activity that complemented US colonial rule. Their attempts to craft a more coordinated relationship with municipal physicians were displaced by the SBOH, which, rather than excluding political affiliations from physicians' work, promoted their political support for the US colonial administration. Elite physicians would be further marginalized when the Director's power expanded from merely advising municipal physicians to appointing a new cadre of "sanitary inspectors" in January 1903.[37]

The new legislation demonstrated that the US colonial administration would address problems in medicine, but not in the way Puerto Rican physicians had hoped. Elite physicians recognized that the reduction of municipal physicians' local autonomy further reduced the possibility that colonial state work could promote physicians' broader autonomy, and the legislation aggravated elite physicians' subservience to SBOH-directed licensing. While Ashford's campaign had grown and expanded the state's control over medicine, Puerto Rican physicians gained little credit for these developments.[38] Instead, Ashford and other US colonial administrators continued to malign Puerto Rican physicians' political involvements, insisting that such involvements were self-serving attempts to gain power at the expense of people's health. These events confirmed that elite physicians' ideas about how medicine should progress were sidelined, and that the increasingly disparaging remarks about their political involvements would affect their future status. These events also led elite physicians to form Puerto Rico's first independent medical society, the *Asociación Médica de Puerto Rico* (AMPR), in 1902.[39]

THE EMERGENCE OF PUERTO RICO'S FIRST MEDICAL ASSOCIATION

Elite medical practitioners sought to achieve a political status that could influence the US colonial state. More specifically, as the following sections will show, physicians' underlying motives for turning themselves into professionals, and their attempts to negotiate and maintain their special position, originally challenged the colonial state's threat to their social location. In this challenge, the AMPR fashioned an ideology that preceded similar political developments in favour of Puerto Rican autonomy. Initially, the AMPR opposed the US colonial state as a "conqueror of race, language, laws, customs, and banner"; insisted it "constrained"; "invaded"; "strikes and implants . . . all official channels of new and regulated activities". The AMPR distinguished its "culture, language, and standard of work".[40] The early history of the AMPR included professional struggles to gain a special location within the economic order, which influenced the character of social stratification in Puerto Rico.

One important spokesperson for this ideology and for physicians was the AMPR's first president, Dr Manuel Quevedo Báez. He received his medical education in Spain and was involved in a series of important medical institutions, including the *Boletín Médico,* the Board of Medical Examiners, and the *Academia de Medicina.* He was also involved in cultural institutions, and served as the president of *Ateneo Puertorriqueño,* a member of the Antillian Academy of Languages, director of a children's magazine, and president and professor at the *Instituto Universitario José de Diego.* He founded the AMPR and presided over the AMPR's inaugural session before the *Cámara de Delegados* (House of Representatives) in San Juan.

The AMPR formed on 21 September 1902 at around the same time that Rosendo Matienzo Cintrón began a campaign to defend the "Puertorrican personality" within US colonial politics. Trained physicians concurred with Cintrón's idea that there was something both unique and in crisis about being a Puerto Rican. Like the Unionist Party that would soon result from Cintrón's campaign, and that would continue struggling for greater political autonomy, the AMPR sought a political legitimacy that physicians tied to their professional status and autonomy from the US colonial state. Their strategy was similarly based on elucidating the difference of the "Puertorrican personality", which physicians based on "culture, language, and standard of work". They hoped to clarify the "scientific and social problems" corresponding to pathology and hygiene and, in this way, influence Puerto Rican politics.

To pursue their goals, the AMPR obliged all associates to practice "absolute fidelity, discipline, and observance of statutes which include support of bodies that could one day help the AMPR," including the SBOH. Although it was debated within the AMPR, the association's support for the SBOH was part of a defensive strategy to protect elite physicians' material interests.[42] Its emphasis was evident when Quevedo Báez stated that the new medical association's primary objective and purpose was "none other than the defense of the material interests of the class first, performing as many gestures as necessary for those close to official spheres, and later, to study and discover other means that may exist for this defense". Similarly, the invitation sent to physicians construed physicians as a class when it proclaimed their participation in "the interests of the class in general." These statements reflected the elite's immediate attempt to gain legitimacy within the US colonial administration, to continue pursuing alternate methods for promoting their economic position beyond the US colonial state, and to revive their status through the profession.

The new policy of supporting the colonial state was influenced by successful developments within the Puerto Rican labour movement, which was in the process of formally affiliating itself with the American Federation of Labor to promote its demands. Unlike the labour movement, which increasingly supported Puerto Rican statehood, elite physicians did not initially promote the AMPR's affiliation with a mainland-US organization like the American Medical Association (AMA). Instead, elite physicians promoted

Puerto Rico's political autonomy in much the same way that Cintrón called on all Puerto Ricans to put aside their differences, such as class and political affiliation. Elite physicians presented themselves as advocates of rank-and-file practitioners, generalized their interests to the entire profession, and attempted to revive their social position by organizing the AMPR and mobilizing non-elite practitioners' support for professional autonomy.

The AMPR's ethics promoted an autonomous professional identity that demonstrated elite physicians' emphasis on material interests and class. In general, ethics allow a profession to establish a collective identity and promote its status, but unlike other codifications designed to develop domestic legitimacy, the AMPR's *moral médica* explicitly emphasized physicians' control over markets and their interest in social mobility within a changing colonial context. Although inter-professional conflicts were not evident at the time the AMPR was established, elite physicians recognized that they remained alienated from the rank-and-file members of the profession, and this alienation undermined their influence within the colonial government. AMPR-affiliated physicians tied physicians' general alienation from one another to medicine's subservience within municipal politics and seized upon the problem as a focus of mobilization.

This strategy reflected several considerations. First, the 1902 legislation drew local medicine into insular politics and remained physicians' only legitimate and uncontested link to political power. Second, the lack of trained physicians on the island gave them some degree of immunity from local political affiliations. Third, elite physicians still did not control municipal appointments, which continued to threaten their professional status. AMPR-affiliated elite physicians turned municipal physicians' position into an opportunity for gaining legislative power within the new colonial government. They championed the cause of all municipal physicians and insisted that their lack of status and power within municipal governments impeded their medical work and the enforcement of sanitary regulations. More specifically, AMPR physicians began to argue that physicians lost power because of local politics. Quevedo Báez argued that "a *majority* of the time, [municipal physicians] disobeyed orders that implied a great social benefit because of mayors' imposition".[42] In their new strategy, AMPR physicians reproduced a colonial discourse that construed explicit political involvements as impediments to medical progress. What distinguished the colonial discourse from the AMPR's strategy was that AMPR-affiliated physicians hoped to gain independence from local government and redirect their political participation from a privileged space of professional sovereignty.

Although AMPR-affiliated elite physicians sought to promote their own interests vis-à-vis municipal physicians, these interests were not mutually exclusive from those of rank-and-file practitioners. The only other option open to non-affiliated practitioners was to participate in US-directed changes within the administration of sanitation. Two critical decisions in

1904 demonstrated that the US colonial administrators would promote medical progress only to the extent that it benefited US interests, which did not preclude promoting physicians' support for the US colonial state's political influence. One was in the area of rural sanitation. Elite physicians' interventions on Puerto Rican bodies were redirected by a critical administrative decision in 1904, when Governor Hunt approved funds for the Puerto Rico Anemia Commission, thereby establishing a more permanent rural sanitation campaign that introduced a new way of regenerating rural *jíbaros*. Ashford—who highlighted the central economic importance of anaemia and workers' efficiency within US colonial interests, and emphasized a specific aetiology[43]—usurped the physicians' broader concerns about prevalent diseases and social issues (such as hunger and malnutrition) on the island.

Physicians obviously lacked Ashford's political and professional status and could not compensate for the training opportunities and institutional development that Ashford's "scientific" campaign offered. Physicians found their scientific and professional presentation displaced by the Puerto Rico Anemia Commission, which emphasized and expanded the use of the microscope in diagnosis. Elite physicians' former claims to expertise and authority based on clinical observation were undermined by the increasing influence of the microscope, which meant elite physicians' control over standardizing medicine was displaced by Ashford's campaign. More importantly, physicians worried about how they could mobilize the many rank-and-file physicians who worked with Ashford's campaign and the microscope and who, as a result, were increasingly distanced from elite physicians' politics.[44]

As more rank-and-file physicians were drawn into the US colonial administration, elite physicians found themselves losing many of these members to the anaemia campaign's work. Elite physicians' calls for greater political and professional autonomy were ignored by the US colonial state. Many physicians were aligning with those of the US colonial state, which was simultaneously centralizing their work within the US colonial bureaucracy. As a result, many physicians saw their attempts to gain professional status and autonomy from both municipal and colonial-state governments as largely unsuccessful. For example, at the end of 1902, Quevedo Báez had mourned the position of any physician who remained "an instrument of all political egoisms". He restated this problem as late as 1948, when he argued that municipal physicians' "abstruse and misunderstood problem" continued to make the medical profession suffer. Quevedo Báez extrapolated beyond municipal physicians, however, and mourned what he saw as the lamentable state of physicians who had to haggle for compensation. Physicians recognized the influence of the anaemia campaign on the medical profession and envied the gains labourers had made within the US colonial administration, industrial societies, and commercial trusts. According to Quevedo Báez, physicians working with the campaign had

given in to labour's "strong and agitated muscle" to maintain social harmony, but they had not been able to peer over the summits of their position
to "breathe the more beautiful air of a life of greater liberty". Physicians,
he argued, remained a class "enslaved" to society and the political power
of others.

Demoralized by its inability to control licensing and direct municipal
medicine, the AMPR continued to defend its material "class" interests by
emphasizing physicians' role in promoting Puerto Rico's productive efficiency. Quevedo Báez led the AMPR's new emphasis on Ashford's "scientific" campaign, seeing it as an opportunity to develop professional status
by participating in the construction of a new Puerto Rico, whose "labor
was more efficacious and better suited to enjoy liberty". He encouraged
physicians to work toward developing "the people's' [physical] energies to
feel liberty because "liberty without fruit and efficacy" was like a "lumi-
nous radiance painted on the imagination of brains *somnolientos* [sleepy
and drowsy] and sick, visionaries of a conquest they would never possess." Although Quevedo Báez sought to "use science to give [Puerto Rico]
better fruits from labor", he underemphasized scientific advancement in
physicians' struggle for status. Instead, he encouraged other physicians to
develop their status by using all available means to accomplish the mission
the profession had established. Rather than a concern over broad domestic
legitimacy, he articulated the AMPR's emphasis on authority by encouraging all physicians to develop their work at the regional level, winning
authority first and confidence later. Quevedo Báez also encouraged physicians to develop the "moral condition of their professional class" through
solidarity with one another, trusting in the AMPR to guarantee each individual's scientific character.[46]

INCORPORATION[47]

The AMPR's inability to gain control over municipal physicians and licensing regulations demoralized physicians, and the organization began to
see that the best solution was to accommodate US medicine.[48] Forgoing
the physicians' original strategy of forming a "medical body with its *own
personality*", the AMPR struggled with the decision to incorporate itself
within the AMA. In fact, debate among AMPR members reached such
heights that its activities stopped for a period in 1909. To resolve the stand-
off, the AMPR held an extraordinary session in Ponce on 14 August 1910,
where its president, sociologist–physician, Dr Eliseo Font y Guillot, seemed
to deliver a eulogy, as he called upon all Puerto Rican physicians to unite,
"strong and firm", within a single body because they:

> had demonstrated [through] bitter and inconsolable experiences that
> isolated and individually [physicians] could not maintain respect and
> considerations that physicians deserved, while united [they] will con-

stitute a great social force, perhaps the most intense of the country, [a] force that will be felt in all public bodies.[49]

The AMPR's radical about-face reflected elite physicians' attempt to reformulate their political and professional identity. On the one hand, many physicians were Spanish, or of direct Spanish descent, and considered themselves "outside" the US government in political, ethnic, and professional terms. On the other hand, they wanted the professional status that Ashford enjoyed, the technological modernity that the microscope represented, and the metropolitan representation and status that their political accommodation of US colonialism could afford.[50] In crafting their role in producing workers who were "more efficacious and better suited to enjoy liberty", Puerto Rican physicians also negotiated their position as a class of intermediaries between the colonizers and the millions that they governed.

The AMPR's desire for autonomy and its eventual incorporation into the AMA paralleled the increasing political divisions in the period from 1909 to 1912. Divisions within the Unionist Party led most physicians to abandon their hopes for independence, feeling it was no longer politically feasible, while others like Zeno Gandía worked to establish the Independence Party. The Puerto Rican AMPR, choosing political affiliation in favour of the profession, voted unanimously for incorporation on 17 December 1910. Physicians postponed their hopes for political autonomy indefinitely after incorporating these hopes into the AMA, while subsequent changes suggested these hopes had, in fact, died.

IMPLICATIONS AND DISCUSSION

In the years following the AMPR's incorporation into the AMA, elite physicians were further subsumed by their alliance with the US colonial state, but they continued to resist discriminatory US colonial state interventions. Physicians found their collective identity and professional status developing in relation to their US-physician counterparts and to the US colonial state. For instance, the number of physicians seeking licenses increased from four in 1900 to twenty-six by 1915. Licensing exams also demonstrate that more physicians were being trained in the United States and fewer received their training in Spanish or Venezuelan medical schools. Meanwhile, Ashford's successful campaign led him to propose establishing an Institute for Tropical Medicine in 1911, which would become the present-day School of Tropical Medicine.[51] Under this organization, Puerto Rican physicians promoted aggressive programs to regulate prostitutes and control poor women's reproduction.[52]

Early twentieth-century Puerto Rican physicians used professionalization as a political strategy to gain an autonomy that the US colonial state threatened. The terms of this professionalism largely resulted from physicians' unsuccessful competition with the US colonial state. This chapter explored physicians' attempts to define the terms of professionalism and to promote their political–professional status. Puerto Rican physicians had a minimal role in decisions affecting the growth of medicine and could neither compete nor gain autonomy from colonial state interests in medical work. Thus, in the "messy reality of the interactions between the . . . state and the professions," the US colonial state transformed elite physicians' political strategies and professional identities.[51] Elite physicians' pursuit of professionalism included reviving the status they enjoyed under the Spanish colonial state, advancing their position within a shifting economic order, and challenging the US colonial state's threat to their social position. Their struggles for professional status also influenced social stratification because elite physicians' political opportunities shifted from protesting Spanish colonial legislation and its negative consequences for the nutrition of the poor, to promoting US colonial interests in developing labour's efficiency and productivity. The ideological meanings supporting the elite physicians' "professional project" also shifted, as Puerto Rican physicians articulated their cultural difference under early US colonial rule. Elite physicians opposed US colonial-state control as a "conqueror and distinguish their own standard of work."[53] Professionalization implied developing an ideology around a national identity that resisted colonial-state control.

Although sociologists most frequently understand professionalization as a struggle for market control and social mobility, the case of Puerto Rican physicians demonstrates that the process can include developing a politicized identity that challenges the structure of the colonial state and the discriminatory institutions it establishes. This chapter found that professionalization among Puerto Rican physicians included imagining a new, modern "nation", presenting themselves as its patriots, and making claims on behalf of Puerto Rico's political autonomy. However, this chapter also showed that the Puerto Rican physicians' class location impeded their ability to develop a populist base that could support their claims. In short, status consciousness drove political pragmatism. This chapter has demonstrated that, on the one hand, elite Puerto Rican physicians were critical of the US colonial-state formation, and, in turn, the US colonial state was instrumental in developing the medical profession. On the other hand, US policies undermined the working of this relationship, limited professional autonomy, and subsumed physicians' work to colonial interests. This continues to undermine Puerto Rican professionals' ability to take an active role in the state.

NOTES

1. L. Guerra, *Popular Expression and National Identity in Puerto Rico: The Struggle for Self, Community and Nation.* (Gainesville: University Press of Florida, 1998); G. Nouzeilles, "La Espinge De Monstruo: Modernidad e Higiene Racial en La Charca de Zeno Gandía," *Latin American Literary*

Review 25, no. 50 (1997): 89–107; F.A. Scarano, "The Jíbaro Masquerade and the Subaltern Politics of Creole Identity Formation in Puerto Rico, 1745–1823," *The American Historical Review* 10 (1996): 1398–1431; B. Trigo, "Anemia and Vampires: Figures to Govern the Colony, Puerto Rico, 1880–1904," *Comparative Studies in Society and History* 41, no. 1 (1999): 104–123.

2. O.J. Wagenheim, *Puerto Rico's Revolt for Independence* (1993); L. Bergad, "Toward Puerto Rico's Grito de Lares," *Hispanic American Historical Review,* 60 (1980): 617–642.

3. Teresita Martínez-Vergne, *Shaping the Discourse on Space: Charity and Its Wards in Nineteenth-Century San Juan, Puerto Rico* (Austin: University of Texas Press, 1999), 5.

4. Astrid Cubano-Iguina, "Political Culture and Male Mass-Party Formation in Late-Nineteenth-Century Puerto Rico," *Hispanic American Historical Review* 78, no. 4 (1998): 635.

5. F. Atiles, *Cartilla de higiene* (Puerto Rico: Imp. José González Font, 1886); C. Coll y Toste, *Repertorio histórico de Puerto Rico,* 1(1) (Puerto Rico: Sucesion de J.J. Acosta, 1896); M. Zeno Gandia, *La Charca: Crónicas de un Mundo Enfermo* (Ponce, Puerto Rico: Est. Tip. de M. López, 1894).

6. L.Figueroa Mercado, *Brief History of Puerto Rico: from the Beginning to 1892* (New York: Anaya Book Co., 1972). Rather than outright independence, most liberal autonomists struggled to have Puerto Rico recognized as a Spanish province, on equal footing with the other Spanish provinces.

7. A.S. Pedreira, *Un Hombre Del Pueblo* (San Juan, Puerto Rico: Imprenta Venezuela, 1937), 1: 39.

8. Liberal *criollo* physicians were mobilized by their educational experiences in revolutionary and Restoration Spain, where there was an "overwhelming sense that a society is being rapidly constructed, consciously and from scratch, in all its institutions, and that simultaneous participation in many cultural orders is vital in this project" W. Ríos-Font, "El crimen de la calle de San Vicente: Crime Writing and Bourgeosis Liberalism in Restoration Spain," *MLN,* 120, no. 2 2005: 335-354.

9. M. Quevedo Báez, *historia De La medicina y cirugia en Puerto Rico* (San Juan: Puerto Rico Asociación Médica de Puerto Rico, 1946), 1: 474.

10. Martinez-Vergne, *Shaping the Discourse on Space.*

11. J.G. Rigau-Perez, "The Introduction of Smallpox Vaccine in 1803 and the Adoption of Immunization as a Government Function in Puerto Rico," *Hispanic American Historical Review* 69 (1989): 393–323; S. Arana-Soto, *Historia De La Medicina Puertorriqueña* (Barcelona: Artes Gráficas Medinaceli, S.A, 1974).

12. M.C. Gillett, *The Army Medical Department, 1865–1917* (Washington, DC: Center of Military History, 1995).

13. On "efficient and educational", see L. P. Davison, *U.S. Public Health Service* 14, no. 16 (1899): 549.

14. B. Ashford, *A Soldier in Science: The Autobiography of Bailey K. Ashford* (New York: Grosset & Dunlap, 1934), 55.

15. Ibid., 67.

16. Ibid.

17. Guerra finds that there were only 100 physicians for a population of 750,000 Puerto Ricans. F. Guerra, Epidemiologia americana y filipina, 1492-1898 (Madrid: Ministerio de Sanidad y Cansuma, 1999).

18. J.G. Rigau-Pérez, "The Introduction of Smallpox Vaccine."

19. S. Arana-Soto, *La Sanidad en Puerto Rico hasta el 1898* (San Juan, Puerto Rico: Academia Puertorriqueña de la Historia, 1978).

20. The extent of the reorganization was such that many US colonial officers ignored the SBOH's institutional history and referred to it in their correspondence as a new organization.
21. Military Governor of Porto Rico, "Report of the Superior Board of Health", First Annual Report of the Governor of Purto Rico (Washington: Government Printing Office 1901).
22. US officials found that "quackery of every conceivable sort" flourished as a "natural consequence" of structural weaknesses within the medical profession. Letter dated 22 March 1901 signed by Hernández, President of the SBOH and Fawcett Smith, Secretary, attached to the 1st Annual Report of Charles H. Allen Covering the Period From the 1st of May 1900 to the 1st of May 1901, RG 59, National Archives (NA).
23. Although the SBOH used the policy of "toleration . . . [for] those who had a diploma or other equal evidence of attainment granted by a teaching body, but who had failed to obtain a license for the Spanish Government in Porto [sic] Rico", it evaluated new licenses on a case-by-case basis and retained complete authority over evaluating acceptable educational attainment. For instance, the SBOH did not accept Dr J. K. Konek's licensing examination results from Costa Rica. See Appendices to the First Annual Report of the Military Governor, p. 501.
24. At the end of an eleven-day examination period, four physicians, seven pharmacists, and one *practicante* in minor surgery had passed the first licensing exam. No dentists, midwives, or nurses presented for the licensing exam. In his first annual report, Hernández wrote that several of the [pharmacist] candidates displayed an ignorance that was phenomenal in its depth and comprehensiveness". Letter dated 22 March 1901, signed by Hernández, President of the SBOH and Fawcett Smith, Secretary, attached to the 1st Annual Report of Charles H. Allen Covering the Period From the 1st of May 1900 to the 1st of May 1901, RG 59, NA. Quevedo Báez argued that nurses' failure to present for the exam was one of the earliest efforts to professionalize women's work. American Red Cross and Rockefeller Foundation archival documents also detail their introduction of "training" for the new cadres.
25. P. Starr, *The Social Transformation of American Medicine* (New York: Basic Books, 1982).
26. M. Quevedo Báez, *Historia de la medicina y cirugía de Puerto Rico,* vol. 2 (San Juan, Puerto Rico Asociación Médica de Puerto Rico, 1949).
27. Dispensaries developed only after Ashford's campaign and, although they limited their medical efforts to anaemia, they provided some medical attention to the poor in rural areas.
28. Post did not see the Foraker Act's omission of state regulation in medicine as an error and instead believed that responsibility should be left to the local legislature. "This cannot have been an oversight on the part of Congress; they were perfectly aware of the importance of these duties, and especially in the tropics, of that of health." In a letter dated 25 March 1904 from Regis H. Post, Auditor of PR, to Attorney General of Washington, DC, SEN58A-F19, box 80, RG 46, NA.
29. Puerto Rican physicians had worked on hygiene, but were not immediately concerned with improving sanitation. Vincent Cirillo, *Bullets and Bacilli: The Spanish-American War and Military Medicine* (New Brunswick, NJ: Rutgers University Press, 2004) notes that the experience of a typhoid epidemic during the Spanish-American War demonstrated the importance of sanitation to US military officers. Rates of soldiers with venereal disease in Puerto Rico were 467.8 per 1,000 in 1898, while on the mainland, the rate in 1897 was 84.59 per 1,000 (E. Garver and E. Fincher, *Puerto Rico:*

Unsolved Problem (Elgin, IL: The Elgin Press, 1945). Station logs demonstrated US administrators' concerns over soldiers' health, which centered on sexually transmitted diseases and waste from buildings surrounding military barracks; see entry 547, RG 94, 92.4.4 (Records of the Adjunct General's Office). Sanitation was also important to the development of institutions that could support the consolidation of US colonial rule, for instance, in the case of education Aida Negrón de Mantilla, *Americanization in Purto Rico and the Public School System* (Barcelona: Editorial Universitoria, 1975).

30. US War Department, *Report of the Governor of Porto Rico* (Washington, DC: US Government Printing Office, 1901), 32.

31. Documentos Municipales, San Juan, leg. 126, Archivo General de Puerto Rico (AGPR). See exp. 181 on street crossing; exp. 206 on public schools (1899); and exp. 174 for a letter to Alcalde from Captain and Assistant Surgeon in charge of hospital, dated 19 April 1899. US colonial administrators considered the poor condition of houses a menace to the welfare of patients. They also saw the schools' poor hygienic condition as a problem for San Juan because visitors observed them.

32. The SBOH introduced unpopular sanitary legislation and had become more effective in sanctioning individuals for minor infractions, including littering. See Documentos Municipales, San Juan, leg. 107, exp. 160, AGPR for fine to an individual, Juan Alvarez; or Exp. 150b, 155, or 157 for fines to businesses.

33. W.H. Hunt, *Second Annual Report of the Governor of Porto Rico Covering the Period From May 1, 1901 to July 1, 1902* (Washington, DC: US Government Printing Office, 1902), 57.

34. Rowe argued that the climate in Puerto Rico required "more careful administration of sanitary regulations than is necessary in northern latitudes", and that sanitation required a centralized administration. Proposal from Commissioner Rowe, The Insular Director of Sanitation and The Advisory Board of Health, SEN 57A-F21, box 108, RG 46, NA.

35. Hunt, *Second Annual Report*, 58.

36. For an example of municipal government's protest, see the newspaper clipping from *El Machete* dated 22 March 1904, titled "Sanidad y Beneficiencia Municipal," in Fondo: Oficina del Gobernador, Correspondencia General, Clemencias Ejecutivas, Publicaciones, Sanidad, Caja 226 (Julio 1903–1907), AGPR.

37. Many municipal physicians were still appointed as political favours after 1898, while technical qualifications for sanitary officers were relaxed. See the Mayor of San Juan's report where he argues that health officers are over-represented in the Puerta da Tierra, where "for every worker there was an inspector who is paid $107.75 daily!" He implies that the thirty-four inspectors were named for political reasons, and they included "simple children of people in high places . . . none of who ever saw the work for whose inspection they were paid" (translation mine). R.H. Todd, *Informe al pueblo de San Juan y al honorable gobernador de Puerto Rico, Año Económico de 1924–25* (San Juan, Puerto Rico: The Times Publishing Company, 1925).

38. Dr Pedro Gutierrez Igaravidez worked closely with Ashford, but was subordinate to Ashford's authority and rarely received credit for his work. Ashford also noted that Igaravidez had severed "all of those professional relations which would have made him to-day the wealthiest physician in San Juan" and that Igaravidez's association with "the first Porto [sic] Rico Anemia Commission invited the criticism and even the ridicule of those who constituted the society in which he lived." Ashford, *Soldier in Science*, 56. Although physicians gained training opportunities through Ashford's campaign, they could

neither control rural clinics nor direct the work because ultimate authority remained with Ashford and the US colonial government.

39. According to Salvador Arana-Soto *La Academia de Medicina Puertorrigueña* (Barcelona: Artes Grafica Medicinal, 1979), the Association for Mutual Medical Assistance (*Asociación de Auxilio Médico Mutuo*) was founded in 1883, but the organization's efforts seemed limited to medical attention for its members, and even these limited activities were restricted to those physicians living in San Juan.

40. M. Quevedo Báez, *Historia de la medicina Y cirugia de Puerto Rico*, vol. 2.

41. The only debates in the AMPR's inaugural session involved establishing rules on its members' political associations, the 34th statute stipulating, "affairs that are not professional, that some relation to politics and religion have, are beyond its jurisdiction" was eliminated. Similarly, the 10th statute that members "carrying out charges related to Board require not being very significant in local or regional politics" was reformulated. This statute was significantly debated because some members (Drs Saldaña and Dobal) argued that it limited the "rights" of the AMPR's associates (Báez 1949).

42. Quevedo Báez, *Historia de la medicina y cirugia de Puerto Rico*, 2: 53–54.

43. R. Dubos, *Mirage of Health: Utopias, Progress, and Biological Change* (New York: Harper Torchbooks, 1959); S.N. Tesh, *Hidden Arguments: Political Ideology and Disease Prevention Policy* (New Brunswick, NJ: Rutgers University Press, 1988).

44. S.J. Reiser, *Medicine and the Reign of Technology* (Cambridge: Cambridge University Press, 1978).

45. The AMPR referred to its affiliation with the AMA as "incorporation", but the AMA referred to the AMPR as a "constituent assembly".

46. Quevedo Báez, *Historia de la Medicina*, 16.

47. AMPR physicians approached the AMA on the issue of incorporation as early as 1905, after their political losses and before their involvement in Ashford's campaign. See American Medical Association archives and House of Delegates, "Proceedings of the American Medical Association Meeting in Portland, Oregon, July 10-14, 1905," Journal of the AMerican Medical Association, July 22, 1905, 255-258. (1905) July 22, 1905, 285.

48. Puerto Rican physicians sought to be recognized as equals within the profession and gain metropolitan representation and status through the AMA.

49. Quevedo Báez, *Historia de la Medicina*, 130.

50. The Institute became a school under the auspices of Columbia University in 1926. Ashford became the AMPR president in 1914.

51. Laura Briggs, *Reproducing Empire: Race, Sex, Science, and U.S. Imperialism in Puerto Rico* (Berkeley: University of California Press, 2002); H. Rodriguez-Trias, "The Women's Health Movement: Women Take Power," in *Reforming Medicine: Lessons of the Last Quarter Century*, eds. V. W. Sidel and R. Sidel (New York: Pantheon Books, 1984), 107–126.

52. K. Macdonald, *The Sociology of the Professions* (London: SAGE Publications, 1995), 100.

53. Quevedo Báez, *Historia de la medicina y cirugia de Puerto Rico*, vol. 2.

8 "Improving the Standards of Motherhood"

Infant Welfare in Post-Slavery British Guiana[1]

Juanita De Barros

In 1921, a group of Caribbean-based physicians—some European-born and others of Caribbean origin—met in Georgetown, British Guiana, to discuss the health problems afflicting their respective colonies. For about two weeks, they exchanged information about the causes and cures of various diseases and illnesses, the nature of local public health training programs, and the prospects for a pan-Caribbean medical infrastructure. Delegates ended the conference by crafting a wish list of some twenty-two measures they wanted to see implemented. At the top, they placed a statement about the importance of infant welfare, calling on governments to take "every possible means" to preserve the lives of children and mothers. Its inclusion and privileged position reflected contemporary concerns about the consequences of high rates of infant mortality in the Caribbean. Similar worries were frequently expressed elsewhere, including Britain and its empire, where infant welfare measures resembled those developed in the British Caribbean. Although Britain's system of home visitors and infant clinics provided an institutional model for the British Caribbean, in this region, discussions about infant mortality and the best ways to deal with it emerged from colonial attitudes toward race and gender. Non-white women, whether as mothers or as informally trained midwives, were blamed for high rates of infant mortality and condemned for their "uncivilized" behaviour which was seen as putting the lives of infants at risk.

This chapter first explores these ideas in the late nineteenth- and early twentieth-century British Caribbean, arguing that they resonated with perceptions of the "failure" of emancipation that were expressed in both the colonies and the metropole in the post-slavery period. It then examines the kind of institutional responses constructed in one particular colony, British Guiana. The source materials for this subject are very rich for this colony, but its significance is greater than this: British Guiana provided a model for approaches to infant welfare work elsewhere in the region. With its emphasis on training local "respectable" women as midwives and health visitors to educate "ignorant" non-white mothers, British Guiana's infant welfare system demonstrates the influence of colonial ideas about race and gender on the nature of infant welfare work in the post-slavery British Caribbean, as well as the varied roles that men and women of different ethnic backgrounds and social classes played. But in showing the continuing presence of "traditional" midwives in this government-run system, this chapter suggests the ways in which colonial social welfare systems were never fully completed structures; the women most involved in their day-to-day operation ensured its accommodation to the realities of local life.[2]

THE PROBLEM OF INFANT HEALTH IN THE POST-EMANCIPATION BRITISH CARIBBEAN

In the late nineteenth and early twentieth centuries, politicians and medical professionals in Europe and the Americas discussed infant mortality and health, frequently expressing concern about their social consequences, particularly in terms of the moral and physical well being of populations as a whole.[3] In Great Britain, such worries resulted in the development of milk depots, infant welfare clinics, maternal education initiatives, and health visiting—all were part of a wider pro-natalist project which aimed to ensure the survival of infants and the health of their mothers. Although a range of environmental and social factors were identified as responsible, such as poor housing and the general effects of poverty, "'bad mothering'" earned much of the blame.[4] Consequently, the "mothercraft campaign" reflected a tendency to hold "incompetent" (and often poor) mothers responsible for high rates of infant mortality.[5] As Deborah Dwork has argued, "infant welfare work was increasingly seen as a maternal problem or a question of motherhood: the instruction and well being of the mother was the first objective."[6] These sentiments were expressed in Britain's colonies. In South Africa, as Susanne Klausen has maintained, white physicians linked anxieties about population size and motherhood to eugenics and called for maternal-education schemes. But Klausen shows that in early twentieth-century South Africa, physicians were overwhelmingly concerned with that colony's white population ("the quality and quantity of the white race," as she puts it), specifically with educating white women to be better mothers in an effort to ensure the health of white infants.[7] In contrast, in predominantly non-white "tropical" colonies, such as Fiji and Malaya, concerns centred on reproduction of labourers and the poor mothering skills of non-white women. They became the subjects of maternal education programs which were shaped by a combination of British influences and local factors.[8]

Similarly, in the British Caribbean, early twentieth-century infant welfare measures were not directed toward white women; instead, the African- and South Asian-descended populations were their primary targets. Worries about the health of infants and their "ignorant" mothers resonated with racially based views expressed during the period of slavery. Black women in American slave societies were regularly condemned as "unfit" mothers, and the British Caribbean was no exception.[9] Elite commentators represented Afro-Creole mothers as neglectful and indifferent.[10] After slavery's end, these sentiments continued to be expressed in the British Caribbean, but they were employed as evidence of the perceived physical and moral "regression" of former slaves, and indeed of the purported "failure" of emancipation itself. The initial official optimism with which emancipation was greeted quickly gave way to pessimism, as former slaves throughout the region showed themselves to be determined to control their own working lives as free people. Although they continued to work on the estates, their unwillingness to provide the hours of work demanded by planters convinced British imperial officials and West Indian planters that they were uncivilized and not fit for freedom. Sources produced in the second half of the nineteenth century by government officials in Britain and the Caribbean and other "elite" commentators repeatedly condemned the moral "regression" of the emancipated population, often highlighting former slaves' purported neglect of their children as proof. For example, during the cholera epidemic which attacked the region in the 1850s, the Secretary of State for the colonies, Earl Grey, complained that former slaves had not sufficiently "advance[d] in civilization and morality," pointing as evidence to their "bad management" of their children when sick and the resulting high rates of infant mortality.[11] By the early 1870s, British Guiana's governor considered that former slaves had "cruelly disappointed the hopes of their well-wishers," citing their "indiffer[ence] to the welfare of their children" to support his claim.[12] Such sentiments continued to be expressed in the late nineteenth and early twentieth centuries and were articulated by other commentators. In 1894, British Guiana's Revd J. G. Pearson, in an article published in a local journal, argued that the now-free population in the British Caribbean had failed to live up to the demands of "civilization [and] citizenship" and was therefore becoming a "scourge to [their] own and other people." Although declaring that he was not advocating a return of slavery, he called for "such a modification of its wholesome methods as [would] secure for the ex-slaves' descendants such a measure of justice as [would] secure his babe from the present risk of passive infanticide."[13] Almost ten years later, testifying before a 1905 Guianese inquiry investigating the causes of infant mortality, British Guiana's Revd Ritchie blamed infant mortality on the population's "primitive[ness]," their ignorance of "the domestic virtues involved in freedom," and their inability to "bear the burden of such social obligations."[14]

By the early twentieth century, like their counterparts elsewhere, British Caribbean-based physicians pointed to a combination of social and medical factors as causing infant deaths: poor sanitary facilities, intestinal illnesses, diseases such as malaria, and maternal ignorance. They emphasized that "ignorant" mothers were ill-informed about such matters as hygiene and the "proper" feeding of their infants, giving them "paps" and "teas" rather than nursing them.[15] Poor feeding, they argued, led to intestinal illnesses which could be fatal.[16] These physicians' acceptance of contemporary British medical views is not surprising, given their education. British Caribbean physicians were a diverse group; many were born in Britain, but growing numbers were born in the region and were of African, British, Portuguese, European, South Asian, and Chinese descent.

Regardless of their race and nationality, most had trained in British medical schools, and some had practiced there for many years.[17]

But physicians also identified the social and cultural practices of the non-white population as being responsible for infant deaths. They "racialized" infant morality. Women's "ignorance" was seen as representing the racial failings of a population trapped by an unthinking obedience to the customs of the past. As the long-standing medical officer of health for Georgetown, British Guiana, William de Weaver Wishart observed, the "physical, social, and economic conditions of the community" were important contributory factors, but infant mortality was also "[r]ooted in a remote ancestry."[18] The Guianese-born physician, Andrew J. Craigen, lamented that although British Guiana's "excessive" rate of infant mortality could be "reduced," it might never fall as low as that in places like New Zealand and Australia, which he described as "more temperate and healthy localities" inhabited by "more intelligent and educated people."[19] The efforts of two Barbados-based physicians, J. W. Hawkins and A. J. Hanschell, to explain why that colony's infant mortality rate was higher than Britain's led them to a similar conclusion: they pointed to Barbados' greater population density and to the fact that its population was "poorer and blacker."[20] They blamed infant deaths on social and cultural factors that they tied to colonial ideas about race and civilization.[21] This link between infant mortality and culture was particularly apparent in discussions about the impact of illegitimacy. In the post-slavery British Caribbean, physicians and other members of the social and political elites maintained that low marriage rates among Afro-Creoles "proved" that they were uncivilized and were to blame for a variety of social ills, including infant mortality.[22] Angus Macdonald, the medical officer of health for Kingston, Jamaica, listed illegitimacy as among the four "general causes" of infant deaths, after "industrial conditions" but before "defective death certificates" and "improper feeding."[23] Indeed, the deleterious health effects of Caribbean mating patterns was not only a subject of discussion for physicians, but was also addressed in more popular sources, such as newspapers.[24]

"Traditional" midwives and their "barbaric" customs were also blamed for infant deaths. Historians have noted the extent to which informally trained midwives were denigrated in England and elsewhere—they were frequently condemned as incompetent and dangerous to mothers and infants alike.[25] But Deacon's conclusion for the Cape Colony—where a "neat combination of the European image of the 'untrained' midwife as a dirty, ignorant, drunk and gossipy old woman" intersected with racist colonial views of black women[26]—suggests the impact of ideas about race in places inhabited by non-whites. This was the case in the post-slavery British Caribbean, where similar views were held of informally trained midwives. Local women of African and South Asian descent who were mothers themselves were often the only source of assistance available. Physicians and other members of the local political and social elites in the late nineteenth and early twentieth centuries regularly condemned these "Granny" mid-wives—regardless of their ethnic background—as unskilled and incompetent, qualified only by their own reproductive history.[27] In British Guiana in the 1880s, commentators such as the magistrate Henry Kirke castigated them as "stupid, ignorant, and superstitious," a view echoed by many of his contemporaries.[28] They were also believed to provide erroneous and often fatal advice to new mothers, notably with regards to infant feeding.[29] British Guiana's Surgeon General and the president of the British Guiana branch of the British Medical Association, J. E. Godfrey, characterized untrained midwives as sources of "ignorance, prejudice, and superstition," women whose "habits and customs [had been] handed down from generation to generation."[30]

Dr Ethel M. Minett, the medical officer for the British Guiana Baby Saving League, expressed some of these attitudes in her presentation at the 1921 Caribbean Medical Conference.[31] Established in 1914 with the encouragement of the governor's wife, Lady Egerton, and supported by government funds and volunteer efforts, the League attempted to reduce infant deaths by educating women. At the conference, Minett described dangerous childbirth practices in British Guiana. She noted that often the cord and infants' eyes were bathed with milk or urine and that "East Indians" rubbed a mixture of butter and "lamp-black" around and into the eyes of newborns. "[T]ight strings were tied around the abdomen of the new mother and "amulets and assafoetids" around the babies themselves.[32] Minett characterized such practices as "superstitions" originating in the "ignorance of the people" and the "main cause" of infant deaths. They were also, she declared, "remnants . . . of some old form of propitiatory and secret devil worship."[33] In the discussion after her talk, Jamaica's medical officer of health, E. D. Gideon, agreed with Minett and argued that "ignorance and superstition . . . thwart[ed] efforts in the direction of child welfare"; the "native mind," he maintained, did not "readily adapt itself to altered conditions or altered ideas."[34] The League's inspector of midwives, Violet E. Nurse, echoed Minett's conclusions, describing the "grannies" as exercising a "sinister influence in advising the mothers in the use of bush medicines."[35] The language used by Minett and Nurse—"devil worship" and "bush medicine"—suggests they were alluding to *obeah*, an Afro-Creole medical/religious practice in the British Caribbean with its roots in the period of slavery.[36] Widely condemned by Europeans, obeah was identified by some early twentieth-century commentators as practiced by South Asians in British Guiana and Trinidad. This representation of the childbirth practices of Afro- and Indo-Creole midwives demonstrates the seriousness with which these customs were regarded; far from harmless superstitions, they were instead seen as the barbaric rituals of an uncivilized people. Yet the sources hint that they may have served an important purpose for women during childbirth. Offering them amulets doubtless promised protection, and tying strings around their abdomens—as "traditional" birth attendants in nineteenth-century India did—may have been seen as familiar by many South Asian women in British Guiana.[37]

The attention paid to infant mortality in the British Caribbean was rooted in perceptions of its serious social and economic consequences. Contemporary concepts of race and degeneration provided a language for physicians to express these concerns. Kingston, Jamaica's medical officer of health in the early twentieth century, James Ogilvie, saw infant mortality as "affect[ing] the life and best interest of the community" and the "very existence of the race."[38] Some physicians were clearly familiar with current British thinking on this subject. Wishart, for example, included a quotation from George Newman's *Infantile Mortality* in his 1914 report. Newman was a medical officer of health in early twentieth-century England and, according to Dwork, an "expert on infant mortality." To emphasize the significance of infant morality as a social problem, Wishart quoted Newman: '[a]s a nation grows out of its children and its children die in thousands in infancy, it means that the sources of a nation's population are being sapped, and further that the conditions which kill such a large proportion of infants injure many of those which survive.'[39]

But G. B. Mason (a magistrate and district medical officer in St Vincent and the Leeward Islands), in including the often-used quotation that a "nation's health [was] a nation's wealth" in his discussion of this problem, emphasized the practical significance of these sentiments in the context of the post-slavery British Caribbean. He argued that this phrase was nowhere "more true" than in this region, where "prosperity [was] as largely dependent on the health and efficiency of the field labourers as it [was] on the introduction of capital."[40] Although it is impossible to reduce concerns about health matters such as infant mortality to a single factor, in British Guiana, at least, perceptions of the size and health of the labouring population were clearly significant. Unlike colonies such as Barbados, with its large population, in British Guiana, complaints about inadequate supplies of labour for the sugar industry were common in the late nineteenth and early twentieth centuries. This was the rationale behind the decision to introduce several hundred thousand indentured South Asian workers into the colony between 1834 and 1917, more than to any other British West Indian colony. With the end of indentureship in the late 1910s, the labour question seemed even more pressing. As the author of the 1918 report of the Baby Saving League noted, the colony had a "crying need" for more people to "develop" the mineral industry in the interior and to "maintain the industries that [were] already established on the coast." In British Guiana, African-descended men dominated the mineral and other extractive industries in the colony's interior, and South Asians dominated the coastal sugar industry. As a result, the report continued, the "State" was obliged to "preserve every single birth and to rear it in its most virile form, so that a more numerous and stronger manhood [would] be the result."[41] Wishart echoed these sentiments, arguing that children were an "invaluable asset, especially in a colony whose urgent need [was] population."[42] Perhaps these factors account for the decision of British Guiana's Governor Hodgson to hold an inquiry into the causes of infant and general mortality in 1905.[43]

These discussions about infant mortality in the British Caribbean were part of a transatlantic conversation between officials in the British Colonial Office and in the Caribbean itself. British officials regularly drew conclusions and devised recommendations based on the regular reports from the colonies produced by colonial officials, generally the governors, themselves influenced by information relayed from colonial medical officers and surgeons general. London-based officials then prompted colonial officials to respond. In the case of infant mortality, colonial reports convinced imperial officials, who were themselves doubtless aware of this subject's significance in the British context, that infant mortality rates were "appalling" and "one of the most important of the current West Indian questions," blaming "ignorance" and "the neglect of the mothers" for the "sacrifice of infant life."[44] Imperial officials pushed those in the colonies to act, but with mixed success. The dire state of many colonies' economies made co-operation difficult, and the British government seemed to have little more than moral suasion to offer. But some actions in the colonies can be linked to imperial encouragement. From the early twentieth century, public health and medical reports in the British Caribbean began to include regular updates on infant mortality rates and calls for ameliorative measures.[45] After the early 1900s, Caribbean-based officials began to regularly tabulate and publish rates of infant mortality in the British Caribbean, although some individual colonies had collected these figures in the late nineteenth century.[46] Moreover, the 1921 Caribbean medical conference was the result of a Colonial Office suggestion.[47]

Colonial Office officials assessed the responses of the individual colonies, criticizing those seen as doing too little—such as Barbados—and praising others—such as British Guiana—perceived as more active in this area, and it acted as a conduit for information about developments in other colonies. It disseminated information about British Guiana's infant and maternal welfare services to British Caribbean and other "tropical" colonies, holding them up as a model.[48] British officials described British Guiana as "an object lesson for the rest of the West Indies" for holding an inquiry into the causes of infant mortality in 1905, and the "pioneer in taking [infant mortality] seriously" when the Baby Saving League was founded in 1914, sending a copy of its first annual report to British colonies in the Caribbean and elsewhere.[49] But information was spread through other channels as well. Approaches to public health were disseminated at Caribbean-wide gatherings in the early twentieth century, such as conferences on quarantine regulations and tuberculosis and the 1921 Medical Conference, but also via the *British Guiana Medical Annual*, the publication of the British Guiana branch of the British Medical Association. It was published in British Guiana but, according to Barbados' public health inspector, John Hutson, it occasionally made its way there.[50] Although British Caribbean physicians (especially the medical officers of health) were familiar with British approaches to infant welfare work and often developed policies explicitly modeled on those operating in the United Kingdom, the sources suggest that they were influenced by British Guiana in this respect.[51] A Colonial Office official and Trinidad's governor, Lord Chancellor, described Trinidad's Baby Welfare League as modeled on British Guiana's Baby Saving League.[52] And, during the 1921 Caribbean Medical Conference, medical officers of health from St Lucia, Trinidad, Barbados, and Grenada praised British Guiana's efforts, holding up its Baby Saving League as a model for other territories; indeed, St Lucia's government charged its chief medical officer, Dr H. E. Sutherland Richards, with reporting on British Guiana's programs.[53]

Drawing inspiration from these varied sources, philanthropists, physicians, and government officials throughout the British Caribbean established maternity clinics and healthy baby organizations in the 1910s and 1920s. The scarcity of published work on this subject makes it difficult to detail the nature of some of these initiatives, but some conclusions can be drawn.[54] Between 1914 and 1929, members of the local and foreign-born middle and professional classes founded healthy baby organizations in a number of colonies, including British Guiana (1914), Grenada (1914), Jamaica (1916), Trinidad (1918), St Kitts (1920), Belize (1920), Barbados (1921), and St Lucia (1929).[55] A combination of state and private involvement invariably characterized these West Indian initiatives. The philanthropic organizations often worked closely with governments either at the local or central level which provided funding and logistical and administrative support. In some colonies, such as British Guiana and Trinidad, charitable groups ran mother and infant clinics attached to local hospitals; in others (in Jamaica, but also in British Guiana and Trinidad), the state and charitable groups shared responsibility for providing trained medical staff (physicians, nurses, and midwives) dedicated to working with infants and new mothers.

INFANT WORK IN BRITISH GUIANA

The remainder of this chapter will concentrate on the infant welfare system developed in British Guiana in the first three decades of the twentieth century. As in Britain and elsewhere in the empire, in British Guiana, government officials and physicians stressed the education and surveillance of poor women. Local "respectable" women were trained as midwives and "health visitors" were employed to visit new mothers in their homes with the goal of improving the "standard of motherhood." The methods used reflected the views of non-white women discussed earlier in this chapter. But despite official rhetoric that condemned informally trained midwives, the actions of non-white women and the realities of colonial life interfered, resulting in a measure of accommodation.

From its start in the late 1880s, government-directed infant welfare work in British Guiana emphasized the importance of midwives.[56] In her work on Malaya, Lenore Manderson characterized them as "gatekeepers," women whose "support or resistance to Western health services would determine community acceptance and compliance," and certainly they seemed to play a similar role in British Guiana.[57] The observation by the Baby Saving League's inspector of midwives, Violet Nurse, that formally trained midwives were the "chief means of preventing the spread of the practice of midwifery by uncertified women," neatly sums up the dominant view.[58] Legislation passed in 1886 to establish a government medical service provided for the establishment of midwifery training at the Georgetown Public Hospital.[59] By at least 1895, such a program was open for business to "respectable" women. Within a few years, the colonial government began subsidizing the employment of trained and "certified" midwives in a number of districts, with the aim of replacing "ignorant" midwives with "educated women" who could be "scatter[ed] . . . throughout the villages." [60] Pregnant women's reluctance to employ these government-provided "strangers" instead of the familiar, local midwives seemed to doom this attempt.[61] It was replaced in 1906 by a scheme incorporating local women. Under this new system, "intelligent women" from throughout British Guiana were encouraged to attend midwifery-training programs and then return to "practice among their own people."[62] The colonial government defrayed the costs of some of the women's expenses while they were undergoing training and temporarily subsidized their salaries.[63] Those who successfully completed the program received certificates and "sign-plates" attesting that they were "'certified by Government examination.'"[64] The hospital-based training program, which eventually spread to other public hospitals in the colony, included lectures and practical work in the wards and initially ran for six months; it was lengthened to eight months, and, by the early 1920s, to two years.[65] Graduates found work in rural medical districts, in estate and public hospitals, and, as of 1908, as outdoor midwives based at the Georgetown Public Hospital.[66] The British Guiana Baby Saving League employed them as well. The League subsidized the employment of trained and certified midwives in its clinics in Georgetown and smaller towns and villages. Renamed the Infant Welfare and Maternity League of British Guiana in 1924 (but still referred to as "the League"), its Georgetown operations (including a crèche) were taken over by the city's mayor and town council the same year, leaving the League based in the country areas.[67]

Female health visitors comprised the other element of the colony's infant welfare system, and the two were closely intertwined. Modeled on the British system of health visitors, home visits as a means to instruct the poor in hygiene and public health began in British Guiana in 1912 by the British Guiana Society for the Prevention and Treatment of Tuberculosis.[68] The

Georgetown Town Council used this approach to educate local women about childbirth and hygienic child rearing; in 1913, it hired two female health visitors for infant welfare work, and two more were hired the following year.[69] The town council worked closely with the Baby Saving League on this initiative, which saw the League pay the salary of one of the city's health visitors, and the visitors themselves encouraging new mothers to visit League clinics.[70] Facilitated by the city's adoption of the Early Notification of Births Ordinance in 1913, Georgetown's medical officer of health notified the health visitors of births; they, in turn, were to make fortnightly visits to the homes of newborns, up to the end of their first year, in sections of Georgetown to which they were appointed. In practice, however, the visitors concentrated on poor women, most of whom were non-white. As Wishart noted, "[i]n some cases people of the better class did not desire the Health Visitors to visit them."[71]

All but one of the first group of Georgetown health visitors had some kind of formal training and accreditation, and most acquired this in the colony. Initially, no "qualified" health visitors were available; the first woman hired by the Georgetown town council in 1913, Miss E. Tennent, was described on her retirement as qualified only by her "valuable knowledge in the school of experience." She was soon joined by Miss J. G. Lawrence, who possessed a National Health Society certificate which she had earned in England.[72] Subsequent appointments, however, had earned health visitors' certificates in British Guiana, and most had trained and worked as nurses, midwives, or health visitors in the colony.[73] By the late 1910s, women health visitors could receive Royal Sanitary Institute certificates following the successful completion of an examination offered by a Board of Examiners which rotated through Trinidad, Barbados, and British Guiana.[74] The example of Uranie E. D. Goulding is illustrative in this respect. Goulding, who was hired as a health visitor by the city of Georgetown in 1923, possessed the necessary health visitor's certificate and had worked as a temporary replacement health visitor for both the Tuberculosis Society and Georgetown's public health department.[75] Even Ethel Minett had been employed by the Tuberculosis Society before she began working for the Baby Saving League.[76] Their cases demonstrate not only the availability of local medical training, but also the extent to which women could move from position to position in the public health sector, in both its public and charitable manifestations. By the mid-1920s, women who applied for these positions without the necessary qualifications were refused employment.[77]

Like their British counterparts, British Guiana's health visitors were charged with educating new mothers.[78] Wishart believed that instructions provided to health visitors in London, which stated that they were to advise mothers about "the proper nurture, care and management of young children, and the promotion of cleanliness," provided a useful model in a colonial setting. They were to encourage new mothers to breast-feed their babies and "generally . . . [preach] cleanliness in the homes of the people," ensuring that the "environment of the infant [was] made as sanitary as possible."[79] Wishart was certain that when this "ignorance disappear[ed], so [would] infantile mortality such as we know it to-day."[80] The health visitors were also responsible for monitoring the conditions in which newborns were raised, notably those regarded by contemporaries as detrimental to infant health. The reports provided to the health visitors included a variety of categories to be checked, including not only the manner in which infants were fed, but also the regularity with which the parents worked, the nature of the family's accommodation (whether they lived in cottages, tenement ranges, or tenement houses), and whether the newborns were illegitimate.[81]

Midwives were also to educate other women, but their responsibility was arguably even greater, given their much greater numbers.[82] I. M. Cowie, the superintendent of nurses at the Georgetown hospital, expected trained midwives to "work on their own responsibility" and "in some measure educate the people in modern ideas of asepsis and hygiene."[83] Similarly, Godfrey anticipated that the midwives placed in Georgetown would advise mothers about infant care and feeding.[84] League officials saw their midwives as the rural counterparts of the Georgetown health visitors, charged with "visiting, advising, and encouraging mothers in the rearing of their children."[85] But they worried that midwives might not be capable of carrying out their responsibilities and that without sufficient oversight, they would regress. As one official fretted, when "'planted out' in country districts where no conveniences [were] to hand, it [was] difficult for them, without help and encouragement, to keep themselves up to a high standard of cleanliness or care."[86]

The League's response indicates its concerns with overseeing the work of midwives. First, it attempted to transform the midwives into trained health visitors as a way to facilitate greater supervision of working-class mothers. The League's policies stated that its midwives should be replaced with health visitors in places where there were "sufficient" numbers of registered midwives. According to P. James Kelly, Surgeon General and President of the League, such a development would help "advance" the League's "activities" and ensure "more cordial co-operation between private midwives and the League." And, in the eyes of Nurse, the presence of more health visitors would ensure "watchful supervision" over infants and pregnant women.[87] Like the health visitors in Georgetown, those in the villages visited the homes of pregnant women and the mothers of infants under a year old. Their goal, according to Nurse's replacement, K. Wade, was to "gain the confidence of the people and then to educate, sympathetically and tactfully, with a view to bringing home to the mothers the vital necessity for a healthy generation." Such work, she believed, would establish "the foundation for a genuine change in the habits and customs of the people."[88] Thus, League midwives were encouraged to acquire a Health Visitors' certificate and a certificate of the English Royal Sanitary Institute. Doing so earned them a "promotion" to health visitor and a higher salary.[89] But relatively few took advantage of this. By 1932, the number of midwives significantly outnumbered health visitors by close to seven to one.[90]

The majority who remained midwives were subject to greater supervision. In 1920, the League created the positions of a medical officer and an inspector of midwives and health visitors.[91] The first medical officer, Ethel Minett, and the first inspector of midwives, Violet Nurse, were responsible for ensuring that the midwives did not backslide. Minett began to visit them regularly, inspecting their midwifery bags and equipment; she also had them keep weekly diaries of their work, with "full details" of each case.[92] To encourage excellence, she founded the "Minett medal," to be awarded to the two midwives with the "greatest number of satisfactory cases" in a six-month period. In a further effort to improve the "standard of midwifery," the length of the training program was extended to two years, and the number of deliveries students needed to perform increased from nine to twenty.[93]

League officials and supporters encouraged poor women to use formally trained and registered midwives. Its first female superintendent, Miss Cumming (no first name is given in the sources), visited "the homes of the people, settling difficulties and persuading wavers to employ" the midwife. A volunteer branch member helped out: Mrs. Manning attended the clinic in Ruimveldt and "visited the homes of the people" with the midwife, encouraging them to employ her.[94] The prenatal clinics which were established in 1923 were part of this effort; according to the League's medical officer, Fitzherbert Johnson, they facilitated a "close association" between the expectant mothers and the League midwife in "districts which were overrun with grannies."[95] The observation in one report that the "deaths and cripplings and hindrance to any progress" would continue until "untrained" midwives were prevented from practice indicates the powerfully felt reasons behind this concerted effort.[96]

Some members of the traditional elites supported this maternal education project. The governor and his wife were patrons and the Anglican bishop sat on the committee. But men and women from the Guianese middle and professional classes also played a role. Physicians employed as district medical officers volunteered at the clinics, but laypeople were active as well. They took out memberships in the local branches of the League, donated money and supplies, organized baby shows, and sat on district committees. Some even visited the clinics, offering advice to midwives and doubtless to new mothers as well.[97] The president of the Beterverwagting branch, for example, Mrs. L. Walker, was described as "always ready and willing to advise and assist the [midwife] . . . in all matters," and the honorary secretary of the East Coast branch, Mrs. Jemmott, attended its fortnightly clinic and gave "daily encouragement" to the midwife.[98]

As the examples of Walker and Jemmott suggest, women participated in League activities. They made up a large proportion of its committee members, comprising at least 50 percent, and often a much greater percentage, and some held executive positions as president, honorary secretary, or treasurer. One Colonial Office official suggested that, "perhaps the very fact that the men [were] too much occupied in business to undertake such public work [left] their wives with more time available than they would otherwise possess."[99] And indeed, although some of the female members were single, many were married to local physicians, clergymen, and politicians, some of whom served on the committees as well.[100] In 1914, the year the League was founded, the Georgetown branch included the bishop of British Guiana, the mayors of Georgetown and New Amsterdam, Georgetown's medical officer of health, and several Guianese and British-born physicians; the surgeon general, K. S. Wise, was the president.[101] The same mix of local religious and political luminaries, including government medical officers, made up the committees in the smaller regional branches.

Branch committees were multi-ethnic and multi-racial, including men and women of European, African, Indian, and Chinese ancestry, both Guianese and foreign-born. In this respect, they reflected the changing nature of British Guiana's professional class in the early twentieth century, particularly that of the medical profession, whose members represented all of the colony's major population groups.[102] Some of the male committee members were British, including several physicians, but a number—including those who served in executive roles—were not. For example, the Afro-Ceole Congregationalist minister, Revd T. B. Glasgow, joined the committee of the Den Amstel branch in 1916, the year it formed, and served as its vice president in 1917, and president between 1919 and 1924. His wife, "Mrs. T.B. Glasgow," was also part of the committee, acting as honorary secretary in the years he was president.[103]

These non-white Guianese men and women who were active in the League belonged to the colony's "respectable" middle class. Throughout the British Caribbean, this group expanded in the post-emancipation period, as black and mixed-race men and women gained education and advanced socially. Some of its male members entered the professions, such as law, medicine, and teaching, whereas others found "respectable" "white collar" employment as civil servants and clerks. There were fewer employment opportunities available for educated women, but the expansion of government services meant some could find work as teachers and health-care workers. Much of the scholarship on the political activities of the Caribbean middle classes in the nineteenth and early twentieth centuries has concentrated on men. Historians have argued that discrimination on the grounds of race and class limited their access to some occupations and political power, despite their education and cultural achievements.[104] These men, though, believed that these attributes "qualified them for participation in political life" and that they had a "'natural' claim to the leadership of the non-white population."[105] It can be argued that participating in philanthropic activities allowed them to exercise this kind of leadership. But the same can be said for women in the British Caribbean. Social welfare work gave them an opportunity to play a similar role and to oversee and "improve" the behaviour of the masses.[106] But, as in other English-speaking territories in this period, this work of "racial uplift" was closely linked to women's "traditional" tasks of nurturing children and caring for domestic life.[107]

Despite the participation of non-white men and women in the League, race and nationality figured in the administrative hierarchy of the colonial infant welfare system much as it did in other colonial institutions. For example, in the case of British Guiana's Government Medical Service, officials preferred British-born and -educated physicians, and the sources suggest that a similar bias operated in the nursing profession, at least for nursing supervisors.[108] Similar policies seemed to have governed hiring decisions for infant welfare work. Surgeon General K. S. Wise, in identifying the most important components of a successful infant welfare system, emphasized the necessity of appointing a "well qualified Lady Superintendent" with English qualifications, notably certificates from the English Central Midwives Board and the Royal Sanitary Institute as a health visitor and school nurse, and some prior English work experience.[109] Although Wise was not explicitly advocating that only white women be hired, their monopoly of supervisory positions suggests that such was his intent. White, English women supervised the day-to-day operation of the League. The League's first "lady superintendent" was Miss Cummings, an Englishwoman who had worked as a health visitor in London before going to British Guiana, and its first medical officer was the British-born Ethel Minett.[110] An "English divisional nurse" supervised the work of the outdoor midwives in Georgetown.[111]

Given the prevailing racial and social hierarchies in the colony, it is conceivable that government and League officials might have preferred to employ white British women as health visitors. Leone Manderson found this pattern in Malaya where, "ideally," health visitors were to be European. But the sources uncovered so far do not allow such a definitive statement to be made for British Guiana.[112] As the first health visitors were trained in Britain, they were likely British. Once health visitor training was available in British Guiana, Guianese women from the "respectable" middle classes may well have found work in this area. The racial and ethnic diversity of this group by the early twentieth century means that, in theory at any rate, health visitors could have been of British, Portuguese, or African descent. The small size of the female Chinese population and the relatively small number of educated, professional South Asian women in the early twentieth century make it unlikely that the health visitors were of Asian heritage.[113] But the availability of health-visitor training to midwives allowed for the possibility that some may have been promoted to these better-paying positions.

Detailed biographical information is even more elusive for midwives, with the result that their race and ethnicity cannot be identified conclusively.[114] But the fact that officials emphasized training "local, respectable" women who were practicing in their home communities implies that these women likely reflected the ethnic and racial background of their regions, as was the case in other British colonies.[115] Some tantalizing evidence hints that such was the case. In his report for 1906, the Surgeon General, Godfrey, noted that a "Spanish Arawak Indian woman" from one of the interior districts entered the training program. He believed that she would be a "great assistance to her own people amongst whom she [would] practice."[116] Although names are an uncertain indicator of ethnicity, the name of one midwife working in an area with a large South Asian population is suggestive. Miss Jaundoo was based in the League's Den Amstel branch, which was located on the West Coast, in the county of Demerara, the population of which was close to 50 percent South Asian in 1921.[117]

LOCAL RESPONSES AND OFFICIAL ACCOMODATIONS

Uncovering the response of poor Guianese women to the midwives and health visitors, and indeed to the larger maternal educational project, is difficult. For the most part, their views were not explicitly recorded in the sources. In the few instances where they were, they may have been distorted by the biases of the individuals recording their perspectives. Despite these uncertainties, evidence suggests that women slowly came to accept the midwives while continuing to rely on traditional sources of help during childbirth.

Historians have argued that the attitudes of working-class women toward health visitors often changed over time. This was the case in Britain, according to Porter. But the sources used by British historians are not available for British Guiana. Dwork, for example, has shown that mothers' letters about infant welfare work expressed not only a "widespread desire for and appreciation of education, maternity centres, and 'baby welcomes'," but also repeated some of its ideological underpinnings, namely the importance of the mother and the "rhetoric of the future of the Empire to emphasize their needs."[118] For British Guiana, one must rely on accounts produced by government and League officials and health visitors. But the race and gender biases that informed these sources mean that scholars must exercise caution in their use.[119] The Guianese material identifies the kind of change in popular attitudes seen in Britain. The Georgetown health visitors and Medical Officer of Health maintained that the visits of the first two health visitors appointed in 1913 were "looked upon with a certain amount of suspicion by mothers, and in some cases regarded as of an inquisitorial nature."[120] But relations became friendlier over time. One visitor, E. Fennens, noted that the "mothers listen[ed] very attentively and tr[ied] to carry out instructions"; her colleague, Josephine Legall observed that they "cheerfully" remedied any failings in their housekeeping that she pointed out. [121] Since the visits began, they claimed, the "standard of motherhood ha[d] been steadily improving."[122] The sources are problematic, of course, as they consist of anecdotal accounts produced by the health visitors on which Wishart seemed to have based his own reports. Whether these representations of grateful and obedient poor women were accurate or the result of misperception or self-justification is unclear. And, the speed with which Wishart reached his conclusions also gives one pause. Barely seven months after the first health visitors were hired in the city of Georgetown, he concluded that they were "received with greater courtesy."[123] Clearly, more detailed information about the race and ethnic background of the health visitors would help in drawing more certain conclusions about their relations with working-class women. Other factors may also have influenced these interactions, namely the middle-class "respectable" status of the health visitors. Perhaps their marital status did as well: the first Georgetown health visitors were not married, in accordance with the city's policy to hire only single or widowed women.[124] One can imagine that child-rearing advice offered by single and childless women might not have been welcomed enthusiastically, regardless of the visitor's skin colour.

Working-class women's reactions to midwives are also difficult to decipher with complete certainty, but they seem to have become more accepting over time. Soon after the League began its work in Georgetown, a Georgetown-based medical officer, Andrew Craigen, observed that the "poorer classes" continued to employ the "Sarah Gamp and their vile methods" rather than "better trained and more educated women."[125] His comment points to the opposition that registered midwives, including those employed by the League, initially encountered, both from the population as a whole and from traditional midwives. A League report from the early 1920s noted that few communities invited League midwives to practice among them, and that those appointed without local interest or support had to cope with "passive, and often active resistance" and with pregnant women's preference for employing "untrained women."[126] Class differences between formally trained midwives and poor women, hinted at by the official emphasis on training "respectable" women, may have contributed to this reluctance. Perhaps their advocacy of "elite" birthing and child-rearing techniques also made them unacceptable. Indeed, their government-supplied sign plates, uniforms, and "midwife bags" all helped mark them as "foreign."[127]

Over time, more women seemed to have turned to the formally trained and registered midwives. The League's reports point to an increasing proportion of women using its midwives for their births, up from 7 percent of live births in 1918 to close to a quarter in 1927. The growing number of registered, government-trained midwives in British Guiana, both employed by the League and working on their own, certainly made it easier for pregnant women to find such midwives. By the early 1930s, the number of League midwives and health visitors combined had risen to close to fifty.[128] They were part of the much larger group of trained, registered midwives being produced by the government midwifery programs; by 1920, 288 midwives had graduated from these programs.[129] The presence of antenatal and infant clinics may also have brought women into the orbit of the League and hence of its midwives. Although their growth was at times sporadic—new clinics opened, but others closed—the numbers grew overall. There were eighteen in 1917 and approximately sixty by the early 1930s, along with twelve clinics on sugar estates.[130] The number of women visiting the antenatal clinics was considerably smaller than those seeing midwives and fewer than attended the infant clinics. Also, the infrequency with which some clinics were held—once a month in some places—clearly limited their impact.[131] But perhaps these services reinforced each other: a woman turning to a League midwife for the birth of her child may have been convinced to become a regular at the infant clinic and to use the antenatal clinic for her next pregnancy. The clinics themselves were places of health care and instruction. There, mothers and their infants could see a medical officer and be educated in the finer points of mothercraft.[132] Although cost doubtless played a role in women's decisions about the services they would use, the extent of its influence is uncertain. Mothers were charged one shilling a year for membership in their local League branch; in exchange, they could attend its antenatal and infant clinics and receive free medicine for their babies. But this did not seem to include a midwife, whose fees appeared to have been separate.[133]

The sources examined do not permit a comparison of the fees charged by formally trained and registered midwives and the "grannies." But Ethel Minett's suggestion that those imposed by the latter were lower is intriguing and directs scholars to think about the reasons working-class women still saw them, as they clearly did.[134] Familiarity with the traditional remedies they offered, as noted earlier in this chapter, may have played a role, as did their ongoing presence in the villages, where they were doubtless well known to their neighbours.[135] Perhaps the patronage they continued to enjoy was responsible for the official decision not to prosecute those practicing in areas experiencing a dearth of midwives unless they actually did "harmful work," a kind of de facto compromise in the face of local realities.[136] This policy seemed to have been encouraged, at least initially, by Colonial Office officials who advised the Guianese government against prosecuting unregistered midwives until the new registration system was well known.[137] The small number of prosecutions some twenty years after the Colonial Office offered its advice suggests that principle had to give way to more practical considerations.

A similar imperative was at work in the attempts to incorporate "traditional" midwives into the formal government system. Legislation providing for the registration of midwives restricted inclusion on the Midwife Register to those women holding "certificates of competency," either granted by British Guiana's physician-dominated Medical Board or institutions in the United Kingdom, and threatened fines for unregistered midwives who refused to stop practicing. But the legislation allowed for exemptions: specifically, the Medical Board had the right to allow "granny" midwives to practice as long as they could convince physicians of their "knowledge of simple labour and of their fitness to continue," even though they had not passed a formal midwifery course.[138] Likewise, the League attempted to integrate these midwives into its own infant welfare network with varying degrees of success. It encouraged them to leave the practice of midwifery and become "home-helps" for post-partum women, an offer which not many women seemed to have taken up, "reluctant to give up the position they formerly held."[139] The League also tried to extend its influence over registered but untrained midwives by subjecting them to its oversight. By the mid-1920s, they were inspected and encouraged to acquire "a very few necessary articles to work with, in order to ensure their efficiency and cleanliness in the practice of midwifery." They were encouraged to send their patients to the League clinics, an effort which Nurse believed had been "fairly" successful. This, Nurse noted, was the most that could be done "until such time as they [were] replaced by trained nurses."[140] The number of informally trained but registered midwives is uncertain; a 1920 report put them at 700, whereas a report eight years later identified just 42, a precipitous and somewhat implausible drop that may have reflected poor record-keeping as much as anything else. This same report described most of them as "elderly," a fact which comforted the Surgeon General, P. James Kelly. He anticipated their eventual demise and replacement by trained midwives. Although conceding that they deserved "pity" rather than "any unforgivable condemnation" and that they had "lived their day and no doubt done their little best," he observed with some satisfaction that the "Colony [was] within measurable distance of a happy release as a result of senile decay."[141]

Through the 1920s and 1930s, infant mortality rates fell in the British Caribbean, a development that elsewhere has been linked to improved public health and medical infrastructure, vaccination campaigns, and maternal education.[142] In exploring this topic in Britain's Caribbean colonies, this chapter has concentrated on the emergence of state-driven infant welfare organizations in the late nineteenth and early twentieth centuries, emphasizing the significance of colonial ideas about race and gender and perceptions of emancipation's "failure." Its focus on the evolution of infant welfare work in one colony, British Guiana, highlights the influence of racial attitudes on the shape of public health institutions in the region. But the example of British Guiana also indicates the kinds of practical accommodations and compromises that marked the daily existence of these projects and emphasizes the role of mothers and "granny" midwives in this respect. Although the available source material prevents an easy and detailed reconstruction of the identities of the men and women charged with day-to-day operation of British Guiana's Baby Saving League, it reveals the participation of members of the multi-ethnic and multi-racial middle and professional classes, both male and female. Much more research is required to see whether these Guianese patterns were manifested in other British Caribbean colonies, and to identify the influence that they exerted over the public health policies and institutions of each other. The sources used in this chapter show the impact of British models on British Caribbean social welfare institutions, but they also hint that influences were more diverse than this, originating in territories outside the British Empire. Thus, they point to the necessity of an Atlantic-wide perspective in understanding the history of public health in the Caribbean.

NOTES

1. Research for this paper was conducted with the assistance of a fellowship at the University of Michigan, an Arts Research Board research grant from McMaster University, and a grant from the Social Sciences and Humanities Research Council of Canada. Earlier versions have been presented at the Association of Caribbean Historians, the Southern Historical Association, the American Historical Association, and at the University of Toronto, McMaster University, and York University. This paper has benefited from informal conversations with Woodville Marshall, Jacques Dumont, and Nancy Christie, and insightful readings by David Trotman, Michele Johnson, and Anne Macpherson. Any errors remain my responsibility.
2. My thinking about the incomplete nature of colonial states and their policies is indebted to Antoinette Burton, "Introduction: "The Unfinished Business of Colonial Modernities," in *Gender, Sexuality, and Colonial Modernities*, ed. Antoinette Burton (New York: Routledge, 1999), 1–16.
3. See, for example, Nancy Leys Stepan, *"The Hour of Eugenics": Race, Gender, and Nation in Latin America* (Ithaca, NY: Cornell University Press, 1991); *Degeneration: The Dark Side of Progress*, eds., J. Edward Chamberlain and Sander L. Gilman (New York: Columbia University Press, 1985); Richard Soloway, *Demography and Degeneration: Eugenics and the Declining Birthrate in Twentieth-century Britain* (1990; repr., Chapel Hill: University of North Carolina Press, 1995), 39, 41, 139. Citations here refer to the 1995 edition.
4. Margaret Jolly, "Other Mothers: Maternal 'Insouciance' and the Depopulation Debate in Fiji and Vanuatu, 1890–1930," in *Maternities and Modernities: Colonial and Postcolonial Experiences in Asia and the Pacific*, eds. Kalpana Ram and Jolly (Cambridge: Cambridge University Press, 1998), 180, 177–212.
5. See, for example, Dorothy Porter, *Health, Civilization and the State: A History of Public Health from Ancient to Modern Times* (London: Routledge University Press, 1999), 179; Deborah Dwork, *War is Good for Babies and Other Young Children: A History of the Infant and Child Welfare Movement in England, 1898–1918* (London: Tavistock Publishers, 1987), 155; Catherine Rollet, "The Fight against Infant Mortality in the Past: An International Comparison," in *Infant and Child Mortality in the Past*, eds. Alain Bideau, Bertrand Besjardins, and Héctor Pérez Brignoli (Oxford: Clarendon Press, 1997), 38–60. See also Anna Devin, "Imperialism and Motherhood: Population and Power," *History Workshop Journal* 5 (1975): 7–65.
6. Dwork, *War is Good for Babies and Other Young Children*, 155; see also Devin, "Imperialism and Motherhood," 24.

7. See Susanne Klausen, "'For the Sake of the Race': Eugenic Discourses of Feeblemindedness and Motherhood in the South African Medical Record, 1903–1926," *Journal of Southern African Studies* 23, no. 1 (1997): 43, 44.

8. See Lenore Manderson, "Shaping Reproduction: Maternity in Early Twentieth-Century Malaya," 26–49; and Jolly, "Other Mothers," in *Maternities and Modernities* (see footnote 4).

9. Richard Steckel, "Women, Work, and Health under Plantation Slavery in the United States," in *More than Chattel: Black Women and Slavery in the Americas*, eds. David Barry Gaspar and Darlene Clark Hine (Bloomington: Indiana University Press, 1996), 52–53. In the same collection, the following essays address this point: Wilma King, "'Suffer with Them Till Death': Slave Women and Their Children in Nineteenth Century America," 147–168; and Bernard Moitt, "Slave Women and Resistance in the French Caribbean," 239–258.

10. See Barbara Bush, "Hard Labor: Women, Childbirth, and Resistance in British Caribbean Slave Societies," in *More than Chattel*, 207; see also Sheena Boa, "Experiences of Women Estate Workers during the Apprenticeship Period in St. Vincent," *Women's History Review* 10, no. 3 (2001): 389–391.

11. Earl Grey to (governor) Sir Charles Grey, 15 Feb. 1851, in *Copies or Extracts of Despatches and other Documents relating to the Outbreak of the Cholera in the island of Jamaica, and respecting any Applications made to Her Majesty's Government for the adoption of Measures to meet the Difficulties thus brought upon the Colony* (1851), in Bound Pamphlets, v. 879, New York Academy of Medicine 31, 32.

12. Longden to Earl of Carnarvon, 1 Feb. 1877, Colonial Office (CO) 111/410, no. 22, National Archives (NA).

13. J. G. Pearson, "The Negro in the West Indies," *Timehri* 8 (1894): 250.

14. *Report of the Commission Appointed to Enquire into and Report upon the General and Infantile Mortality* (Georgetown, British Guiana: The 'Argosy,' Company, 1906), iv (hereafter *Report of the Mortality Commission*). It has not been possible to locate detailed information about Pearson and Ritchie. But "Revd Ritchie" was likely W. B. Ritchie, the president of British Guiana's School Managers' Union (1890s) and a local educator. Norman Cameron, *150 Years of Education in Guyana (1808–1957), with Special Reference to Post-Primary Education* - Georgetown, Guyana: Labour Advocate Printery of the author, 1968, 9.

15. See, for example, James Ogilvie, *Annual Report on the Health of and Sanitation of the City [Kingston], for the Year Ending 31th December 1909*, London School of Tropical Medicine (LSTM), p. 6.

16. These attitudes about the consequences of "improper" feeding appeared in many sources. See, for example, [no author] "The Transactions of the British Guiana Branch of the British Medical Association for 1898," *British Guiana Medical Annual* 10 (1898): vi, xxi, xxii, xxiii (hereafter "Transactions, 1898"). And see also J. R. Dickson, "Medical. Annual Report of the Surgeon General for 1903–4," *Council Paper No. 75* (1904), National Archives of Trinidad and Tobago (NATT), p. 13; W. de Weaver Wishart, *Annual Report of the Public Health Department of the City of Georgetown for the Year 1913* (Georgetown, British Guiana: 1914), 13. Discussions about efforts to obtain clean milk supplies and the importance of milk for infant health occurred in a number of jurisdictions. Deborah Dwork, "The Milk Option: An Aspect of the History of the Infant Welfare Movement in England 1898–1908," *Medical History* 31 (1987): 51–69; Angus H. Ferguson, et al, "The Glasgow Corporation Milk Depot 1904–1910 and its Role in Infant Welfare: An End or a Means?" *Social History of Medicine* 19, no. 3 (2006): 443–460; P. J. Atkins, "White Poison?

The Social Consequences of Milk Consumption, 1850–1930," *Social History of Medicine* 5, no. 2 (1992): 207–227; Milton Lewis, "Milk, Mothers, and Infant Welfare," in *Twentieth Century Sydney: Studies in Urban & Social History*, ed. Jill Roe (Sydney: The Sydney History Group, 1980), 194–207; De Barros, "'To Milk or Not to Milk: Regulation of the Milk Industry in Colonial Georgetown,'" *The Journal of Caribbean History* 31 (1997): 36–53.

17. See De Barros, "'Spreading Sanitary Enlightenment.'"

18. Wishart, *Annual Report of the Public Health Department of the City of Georgetown for the Year 1930* (Georgetown, British Guiana: "The Argosy" Company, Ltd., 1931), 7.

19. "Transactions of the British Guiana Branch of the British Medical Association, for 1913 and 1914," *British Guiana Medical Annual for 1913* 20 (1913): 131, 132 (hereafter, "Transactions, 1913 and 1914"). CO correspondence described Craigen as Guianese-born and as "appear[ing] to have dark blood in him." See confidential correspondence in British Guiana no. 37072, CO 111/546, NA.

20. J.W. Hawkins and A.J. Hanschell, "Minority Report B," encl. in *Report of the Public Health Commission, 1925–1926* (Barbados), in CO 28/306/6, no. 37510, NA.

21. See, for example, *Report of the Mortality Commission*; H. A. A. Nicholls to Harcourt, under-secretary of state for the colonies, 5 June 1914, CO 323/649, no. 20820, NA, pp. 83, 84. See also medical reports from the early 1900s and 1910s produced by Trinidad's J. R. Dickson, British Guiana's W. De W. Wishart, Barbados' John Hutson, and Jamaica's James Ogilvie. Dickson's observations are included in the Trinidad Surgeon General's reports, at the NATT; Wishart's are in the Georgetown public health reports (LSTM), but see also "The Transactions of the British Guiana Branch of the British Medical Association for 1898," *The British Guiana Medical Annual* 10 (1898); Hutson's are in the Barbados Poor Law Inspector's reports and, after 1913, in that colony's public health reports at the Barbados Archives (BA); finally, Ogilvie's are in the health and sanitation reports for Kingston, Jamaica (LSTM).

22. Scholars, such as Bonham Richardson, Michele Johnson, and Brian Moore, have discussed elite perceptions of a link between marriage and illegitimacy in the post-emancipation British Caribbean. See Richardson, *Panama Money in Barbados, 1900–1920* (Knoxville: University of Tennessee Press, 1985), 79; and Johnson and Moore, *Neither Led nor Driven: Contesting British Cultural Imperialism in Jamaica, 1865–1920* (Kingston, Jamaica: University of the West Indies Press, 2004), esp. chapter 4. Contemporary attitudes about the purported relationship between infant mortality and illegitimacy were also expressed in testimony before British Guiana's commission of inquiry into mortality rates, and in the public health reports of Barbados' John Hutson. See the *Report of the Mortality Commission*, especially i, ii, 14; and see Hutson's reports in BA.

23. Angus Macdonald, *Health Department Report on the Health of the City and Parish of Kingston, Jamaica, during the Year 1911* (Kingston, Jamaica: 1912), 90.

24. For example, see the editorial, "Some Facts of the Case," in *The Gleaner*, 11 January 1909, n.p.

25. See Enid Fox, "Powers of Life and Death: Aspects of Maternal Welfare in England and Wales between the Wars," *Medical History* 35 (1991): 339.

26. Harriet Deacon, "Midwives and Medical Men in the Cape Colony before 1860," *Journal of African History* 39 (1998): 274. Forbes discusses attacks on traditional midwives (*dais*) in colonial India; they too were seen as contributing to high rates of infant mortality. See Geraldine Forbes, "Managing

Midwifery in India," in *Contesting Colonial Hegemony: State and Society in Africa and India*, eds. Dagmar Engels and Shula Marks (London: British Academic Press, 1994), 154. See also Sean Lang, "Drop the Demon *Dai*: Maternal Mortality and the State in Colonial Madras, 1840–1875," *Social History of Medicine* 18, no. 3 (2005): 357–378.

27. For example, see Peter A. Espent, custos, St. Thomas, to Henry Irving, Colonial Secretary, 20 Aug. 1867, in Governor to secretary of state for the colonies, 23 Mar. 1868, CO 137/432, no. 62, NA, pp. 328, 329. See also Patrick Bryan, *The Jamaican People 1880–1902: Race, Class and Social Control* (London: Macmillan Caribbean Ltd., 1991), 110, 111.

28. Henry Kirke, *Twenty-five Years in British Guiana* (1898; repr., Westport, U.S.A.: Negro Universities Press, 1970), 269. Citation here refers to 1970 edition. See also Charles Daniel Dance, *Chapters from a Guianese Log-Book* (Georgetown, British Guiana: The Royal Gazette Establishment, 1881), 77.

29. See, for example, "Transactions, 1898," xxii, xxiii.

30. "Transactions, 1898," v, vii.

31. See Mrs E. P. Minett, "Infant Mortality," in *Report of the Proceedings of the West Indian Medical Conference, 1921* (Georgetown, British Guiana: "The Argosy" Company, Ltd., 1921), ICS, 58. Most sources identify Ethel M. Minett by her married name (Mrs E. P. Minett); she was married to Dr Edward P. Minett, an English medical officer based in British Guiana. See also The British Guiana Infant Welfare and Maternity League (BGIWML), *The Eleventh Annual Report, 1924,* 8. For biographical information about Edward P. Minett, see CO 111/627, no. 18120, NA. The Baby Saving League was renamed the Infant Welfare and Maternity League in 1924, "[i]n conformity with the custom prevailing in other parts of the Empire,"BG IWML, *Eleventh Annual Report, 1924,* 7.

32. Minett, "Infant Mortality," 58. These points were repeated in a report of the Baby Saving League when Minett was League medical officer. Although she was not listed as the author of the report, she may well have been the source of the information, if not the author of the report. See Baby Saving League of British Guiana, *The Eighth Annual Report, 1921,* 7.

33. Minett, "Infant Mortality," 58.

34. E. D. Gideon, "Response to presentations," in *Report of the Proceedings of the West Indian Medical Conference, 1921* (Georgetown: "The Argosy" Company, Limited, 1921), ICS, 60.

35. BGIWML, *The Eleventh Annual Report, 1924,* 11.

36. BGIWML, *The Eleventh Annual Report, 1924,* 11. On the discursive relationship between obeah and bush medicine, see Juanita De Barros, "Dispensers, *Obeah*, and Quackery: Medical Rivalries in Post-Slavery British Guiana," *Social History of Medicine* 20, no. 2 (2007): 243–261.

37. Lang, "Drop the Demon *Dai*," 367.

38. James Ogilvie, *Annual Report on the Health and Sanitation of the City for the Year ending 30th December 1905* (Jamaica, 1905), LSTM, 7. Ogilvie made similar points in his reports for other years. See, for example, James Ogilvie, *Annual Report on the Public Health and Sanitation of the City of Kingston, Jamaica, for the year ending 31st December 1908* (Jamaica, 1909), 11, LSTM.

39. Wishart also quoted Newman in his 1914 report. See Wishart, *Annual Report of the Public Health Department of the City of Georgetown for the Year 1913* (Georgetown, British Guiana: 1914), 13–14; Wishart, *Annual Report of the Public Health Department of the City of Georgetown for the Year 1914,* Georgetown British Guiana, 1915-18; and Dwork, *War is Good*

for Babies and Other Young Children, 23. See also Davin on Newman, 30, 31.

40. G. B. Mason, "The British West Indian Medical Services," *United Empire* 13 (November 1922): 696.

41. BSLBG, *The Fifth Annual Report of the Baby Saving League of British Guiana, 1918*, 7.

42. Wishart, *Annual Report of the Public Health Department of the City of Georgetown for the year 1923* (British Guiana, "The Daily Chronicle," Limited), Georgetown, British Guiana, 1924: 7, Municipal Storage Building, Georgetown, British Guiana (MSB).

43. J. Hampden King, government secretary, to Georgetown Town Clerk, 22 Apr. 1905, 1003, Minutes of Town Council, Georgetown, British Guiana (MTC), 1003. Research conducted so far suggests that British Guiana was the only British Caribbean colony to hold such an inquiry, although Barbados organized two small gatherings of the colony's Poor Law officials (1911 and 1912) to investigate infant mortality rates. See "Second Annual Report of the Public Health Inspector, 1914," in *Minutes of Proceedings of the Honourable Board of Legislative Council and Honourable House of Assembly of 1914 and 1915* (Barbados: Advocate Co. Ltd., 1915), 3, BA. See also Richardson, *Panama Money*, 79. See Catherine Rollet on the response of states to the pressure of such demographic concerns (Rollet, "The Fight against Infant Mortality in the Past," 45).

44. See, for example, Minute by GG, 11 June 1915, CO 111/600, no. 259, NA; Minute by G. Grindle, 11 June 1914, CO 323/649, no. 259, NA; Ibid., no. 20820, NA, 78–80. See also the Wood Report. *Report by the Honourable E. F. L. Wood on his Visit to the West Indies and British Guiana. December, 1921–February, 1922*, in British Parliamentary Papers (BPP), 1922 Cmd. 1679, xvi: 355, 3, 57, 58.

45. The sources suggest that the inclusion of this information in the annual reports was due to CO encouragement. See CO 111/536, no. 3798, NA.

46. In Trinidad, the 1903–1904 Surgeon General's report noted the rate and likely causes of infant mortality in that colony. Although the author of the report, J. R. Dickson (an assistant medical officer), provided Trinidad's average rate of infant mortality for the years between 1892 and 1900 (160/1000), these figures do not seem to have been regularly included in the Surgeon General's reports before 1903. Similarly, in Barbados, such information does not seem to have been regularly recorded before 1903. For Trinidad, see J.R. Dickson, Annexure C. Infantile Mortality in Port-of-Spain, in "Annual Report of the Surgeon General for 1903–1904," in *Council Paper No. 75* (1904), 13, 14, NATT; for Barbados, see *The Half-yearly Report of the Poor Law Inspector July–December 1903*, BA, 802.

47. Charles O'Brien, Barbados governor, to the House of Assembly, 3 October, 1920, in *Minutes of Proceedings of the Honourable Board of Legislative Council and Honourable House of Assembly for Session of 1920–1921* (Barbados: T. E. King & Co., 1921), BA, 17.

48. Draft minute from Bonar Law, secretary of state to the colonies, 24 Sept. 1915, in CO 111/601, no. 285, NA. The minute was sent to the following colonies: Ceylon, Hong Kong, Mauritius, Seychelles, Trinidad, Barbados. Windwards, Leewards, Jamaica, Bahamas, British Honduras, and Bermuda. See also K. S. Wise, Surgeon General, to Governor Egerton, 31 July 1915, encl. in Egerton to Bonar Law, 7 Aug. 1915, CO 111/601, no. 285, NA.

49. CPL to Mr. Lucas, 7 July 1906, CO 111/551, no. 29159, NA; Minute, 16 Nov. 1915, BG no. 27782, CO 111/600, no. 259, NA.

50. Dr. Hutson, Response to "An Auxiliary Medical Service," in *Report of the Proceedings of the West Indian Medical Conference, 1921* (Georgetown, British Guiana: "The Argosy" Company, Ltd., 1921), ICS, 7.

51. Minute by G. Grindle, 11 June 1914, CO 323/649, no. 20820, NA, 78–80.

52. ERD, 27 Apr. 1918, CO 111/616, no. 19767, NA; J. Chancellor, governor, to H. Long, secretary of state for the colonies, 2 May 1918, CO 295/516, no. 143, NA, 445.

53. H. E. Sutherland Richards, "Response to Presentations," in *Report of the Proceedings of the West Indian Medical Conference, 1921* (Georgetown: "The Argosy" Company, Ltd., 1921), ICS 61.

54. The few exceptions include Clare Millington's unpublished paper, "Maternal Health Care in Barbados, 1880–1940" (seminar paper, Department of History and Philosophy, University of the West Indies, Cave Hill, November 1995) and Anne Macpherson's excellent work (the citation for Macpherson's articles are included in the following footnote). Tara Inniss has done work on the health of children during slavery. See her "'Fed with the Bread of Slavery': Children's Health in Barbados During Slavery and the Apprenticeship Period, 1790–1838" (PhD thesis, University of the West Indies, 2006). For Jamaica, see James C. Riley, *Poverty and Life Expectancy: The Jamaica Paradox* (Cambridge: Cambridge University Press, 2005), esp. chapters 2–4.

55. Information for this paragraph is drawn from a number of sources. For Grenada, see Minute by G. Grindle, 11 June 1914, CO 323/649, no. 20820, NA, pp. 78–80; for Belize, see Anne Macpherson, "Colonial Matriarchs: Garveyism, Maternalism, and Belize's Black Cross Nurses, 1920–1952," *Gender and History* 15, no. 3 (2003): 514, 515; Anne Macpherson, "Citizens v. Clients: Working Women and Colonial Reform in Puerto Rico and Belize, 1932–45," *Journal of Latin American Studies* 35 (2003): 294, 295; for St. Lucia, see Edith G. Floissac, *Ninth Annual Report of the Child Welfare Association*, St. Lucia, 1938, CO 950/417, 1, 2, NA; for Jamaica, see Mary Manning Carley, *Medical Services in Jamaica* (Kingston: Jamaica: The Institute of Jamaica, 1943), 17; see also "Report on the Health of the Parish of Kingston, Jamaica" for 1918, 1919, and 1920; and for Trinidad, see the following: E. A. Turpin, "Medical Administrative Report of the Acting Surgeon-General for Year 1918," in *Council Paper No. 99* (1919), NATT, p. 13; C. F. Lasalle, "Administration Reports of the Medical Inspector of Health, the Medical Officers of Health, and the Port Officer for the Year 1918," *Council Paper No. 101* (1919), NATT, 11, 12; J. Chancellor, governor, to H. Long, secretary of state for the colonies, 2 May 1918, CO 295/516, no. 143, NA, 445. See also R. Seheult, *A Survey of the Trinidad Medical Service 1814–1944* (Part of Spain, Trinidad and Tobago: The Government Printer, 1948), NATT, 50–53. The sources for developments in British Guiana are provided later in this chapter. In Barbados, the governor's wife, Lady O'Brien, founded a Healthy Baby Clinic in 1921; its establishment seems to have occurred in tandem with that of the Women's Social Welfare League. For these related developments, see the following sources: "The Eleventh Annual Report of the Public Health Inspector, 1923," in *Official Gazette*, 4 May 1923, BA, 587; "The Ninth Annual Report of the Public Health Inspector, 1921," in *Minutes of Proceedings of the Honourable Board of Legislative Council and Honourable House of Assembly for session of 1923–1924* (Barbados: Advocate Co. Ltd., 1924), BA, 8; "The Tenth Annual Report of the Public Health Inspector, 1922," in *Minutes of Proceedings Honourable Board of Legislative Council and Honourable House of Assembly for session of 1923–1924* (Barbados: Advocate Co. Ltd., 1924), BA, 2; see also Frank C. Ramsey, "Child Care in Barbados:

Past Achievements and Future Needs," *The Barbados Association of Medical Practitioners* 135 (1995), BA, 2–6.

56. Similar kinds of midwifery training schemes were established in other parts of the British Empire from the mid-nineteenth century on. See especially Lang, "Drop the Demon *Dai*"; Deacon, "Midwives and Medical Men in the Cape Colony before 1860"; and Carol Summers, "Intimate Colonialism: The Production of Reproduction in Uganda, 1907–1925," *Signs* 16, no. 4 (1991): 787–807.

57. Manderson, "Shaping Reproduction," 37.

58. BGIWML, *Eleventh Annual Report, 1924,* 11.

59. No. 5 of 1886, An Ordinance to Establish a Government Medical Service, and to enforce the Registration of Practitioners in Medicine or Surgery, in *The Laws of British Guiana (1884 to 1891)*(Oxford: 1895), 3: section 42. This section also made provision for the training of dispensers. In the (amended) 1895 version of no. 5 of 1886, section 42 was renumbered as section 52. See also D. Palmer Ross, *Report of the Surgeon General for the Year 1895–1896,* 7.

60. "Transactions, 1898," v, vii; *Report of the Surgeon General for the Year 1897–1898,* 6.

61. *Report of the Surgeon General for the Year 1897–1898,* 6, 7; and *Report of the Surgeon General for the Year 1903–1904,* 14.

62. The identity of these "intelligent" women will be discussed later in the chapter.

63. *Report of the Surgeon General's Office for the Year 1904–1905,* 14.

64. *Report of the Surgeon General for the Year 1906–1907,* 13, 15.

65. Its length was similar to that of midwifery-training programs in Britain and some of the colonies. For example, Enid Fox has pointed out that in early twentieth-century Britain, midwifery-training programs ran for three months, but were then lengthened to six months by 1916, and to twelve months by 1926. In nineteenth-century Madras, midwives trained for nine months. Fox, "Powers of Life and Death," 339; Lang, "Maternal Mortality in Colonial Madras, 1840–1875," 360. See also *Report of the Surgeon General for the Year 1895–6,* 7, 8; A. J. Craigen, "The Hospitals of British Guiana and Their Administration," in *Report of the Proceedings of the West Indian Medical Conference, 1921* (Georgetown, British Guiana: "The Argosy" Company, Ltd., 1921), ICS, p. 17. See also De Freitas, "A Retrospect of Medical Practice in British Guiana, 1900–1935," 151.

66. *The Report of the Surgeon General for the Year 1920,* 11; see *Report of the Surgeon General for the Year 1913–1914* (Georgetown, British Guiana: "The Argosy" Company, Ltd., 1914), 17; *Return of the Surgeon General for the Nine Months April–December 1915,* 20; *Report of the Surgeon General for the Year 1908–1909,* 40; *Report of the Surgeon General for the Year 1909–1910,* 16. For the names of the districts, see *Report of the Surgeon General for the Year 1907–1908,* 15, 16.

67. BGIWML, *The Eleventh Annual Report, 1924,* 8.

68. Female health visitors were employed in other British Caribbean territories, such as Jamaica, by the early 1910s. See *Proceedings of the First West Indian Intercolonial Tuberculosis Conference* (Trinidad, 1913), 90. Dwork, *War is Good for Babies and Other Young Children,* 105, 125–129, 155–156; The British Guiana Society for the Prevention and Treatment of Tuberculosis, *The Sixth Annual Report,* 1912, LSTM.

69. Female health visitors were employed in other British colonies, from around the same time. Manderson has noted the introduction of women health visi-

tors in urban areas of Malaya in 1911. See Manderson, "Shaping Reproduction," 39. See also *Daily Chronicle*, 7 Jul. 1921, p. 7.

70. BSLBG, *The Fourth Annual Report*, 10; Wishart, "Infant Welfare Work in Georgetown—Past, Present, and Future," 54.

71. Minutes, 13 Nov. 1928, MTC, Jan.—Dec. 1928, MSB, p. 593. Initially, poor Portuguese women were also the targets of this official concern. Portuguese immigrants had arrived in the post-slavery period as sugar estate workers, but many soon migrated to the towns and urban areas where they found employment in the petty retail sector. Although some Portuguese became wealthy and entered the middle and professional classes, many others remained poor, particularly in Georgetown.

72. Wishart, "Annual Report of the Public Health Department of the City of Georgetown for the year 1924," MTC, July–Dec. 1925, MSB, 633–8, 633–9; *Annual Report of the Public Health Department of the City of Georgetown for the Year 1933*, 13.

73. For information about the educational background of individual health visitors, see the following: Wishart, *Annual Report of the Public Health Department of the City of Georgetown for the Year 1914*, 23; Application from M. Earle to J. B. Woolford, town clerk, 1 Jan. 1923, 294, MTC, Jan.–Mar. 1923, MSB, 294; Application from Kathleen E. Wilson to J. B. Woolford, town clerk, 3 Jan. 1923, MTC, Jan.–Mar. 1923, MSB, 294; Department of Maternity and Child Welfare, *Annual Report of the Public Health Department of the City of Georgetown for the Year 1933*, 42; The British Guiana Society for the Prevention and Treatment of Tuberculosis, *The Seventh Annual Report, 1919*, 9, 10.

74. Dr. E. P. Minett, Response to "An Auxiliary Medical Service," in *Report of the Proceedings of the West Indian Medical Conference, 1921* (Georgetown, British Guiana: "The Argosy" Company, Ltd., 1921), ICS, p. 4.

75. Application from Uranie E. D. Goulding, 8 Jan. 1923, 285, MTC, Jan.–Mar. 1923, MSB; "The Report of the Public Health Committee," MTC, Jan.–Mar. 1923, MSB, 256.

76. The British Guiana Society for the Prevention and Treatment of Tuberculosis, *The Seventh Annual Report, 1913*, 6.

77. "The Report of the Public Health Committee," 12 Feb. 1923, MTC, Jan.–Mar. 1923, MSB, 256.

78. Wishart, "Annual Report of the Public Health Department of the City of Georgetown for the Year 1924," MTC, July–Dec. 1925, MSB; 633–6, 633–7, Wishart, "Annual Report of the Public Health Department of the city of Georgetown for the Year 1920," MTC, July–Dec. 1921, MSB, 508, 509.

79. Health visitors in Birmingham, England, were given similar instructions. See Rosetta E. Gardiner, "The Work of a Health Visitor," *Journal of The Sanitary Institute* 21 (1900): 174–175. See also Wishart, *Annual Report of the Public Health Department of the City of Georgetown for the Year 1914*, 18.

80. Wishart, "Annual Report of the Public Health Department of the City of Georgetown for the Year 1924," MTC, July–Dec. 1925, MSB 633–6, 633–7,; Wishart, "Annual Report of the Public Health Department of the City of Georgetown for the Year 1920," MTC, July–Dec. 1921, MSB; 508, 509, Wishart, "Infant Welfare Work in Georgetown," 53, 54.

81. See the reports completed by the health visitors between 1914 and the early 1920s, and Wishart's annual reports for the Public Health Department for the City of Georgetown in the same period.

82. League midwives outnumbered the health visitors by seven to one in the early 1930s, a proportion that would have been even greater in the 1920s. The num-

bers of midwives and health visitors will be discussed in more detail later in this chapter.

83. *Report of the Surgeon General for the Year 1908–1909*, 39.
84. *Report of the Surgeon General for the Year 1909–1910*, 16.
85. BSLBG, *The Fifth Annual Report*, 1918, 7; see also BSLBG, *The Seventh Annual Report, 1920*, 7. Between 1914 and 1922, the reports did not include an author's name, but from 1922 the League's medical officer was listed as author.
86. BSLBG, *The Seventh Annual Report, 1920*, 9.
87. BGIWML, *Seventeenth Annual Report, 1930*, 8, 11.
88. BGIWML, *Nineteenth Annual Report, 1932*, 14.
89. BSLBG, *The Seventh Annual Report, 1920*, 9, 10.
90. See reports of the BSLBG and the BGIWML for the years 1924, 1926, 1930, 1932, and 1936.
91. The supervisor of health visitors divided her services between the Baby Saving League and the Tuberculosis Society. See BGIWML, *The Eleventh Annual Report, 1924*, 8. A similar position was established considerably later in at least one other British Caribbean territory, Belize (British Honduras), though not until 1941. See Macpherson, "Colonial Matriarchs," 516.
92. BSLBG, *The Seventh Annual Report, 1920*, 8.
93. BSLBG, *The Eighth Annual Report, 1921*, 6, 7; BSLBG, *The Tenth Annual Report, 1923*, 7.
94. BSLBG, *The Second Annual Report, 1915*, 13.
95. Fitzherbert Johnson replaced Minett as the League medical officer. BSLBG, *The Tenth Annual Report, 1923*, 6.
96. BSLBG, *The Seventh Annual Report, 1920*, 12, 13.
97. See, for example, BSLBG, *The Fifth Annual Report, 1918*, 10; BSLBG, *The Fourth Annual Report, 1918*, 8.
98. See, for example, BSLBG, *The Fourth Annual Report, 1918*, 14; and BSLBG, *The Second Annual Report, 1915*, 13.
99. EDW to Sir G. Fiddes, 16 Nov. 1915, CO 111/600, no. 27782, NA.
100. See BSLBG, *The Second Annual Report, 1915*, 3, 12. The League's reports do not note the men to whom these women were married, but the fact that the married female committee members were invariably identified by their married names, including their husbands' initials and surname, allows some conclusions to be drawn.
101. The current Surgeon General was always the president of the League.
102. See De Barros, "'Spreading Sanitary Enlightenment.'"
103. See the reports of BSLBG for the years between 1916 and 1924. The League reports do not identify the race and ethnicity of the committee members, but occasionally other sources fill in the gaps. For information about Glasgow, see A. W. Wilson to Rev. George Cousins, LMS Joint Foreign Secretary, 24 May 1907, LMS Incoming Letters-West Indies (with British Guiana) 1900–1908, box 2, folder West Indies 1907, School of Oriental and African Studies, pp. 4, 5; see also Juanita De Barros, "Congregationalism and Afro-Guianese Autonomy," in *Nation Dance: Religion, Identity, and Cultural Difference in the Caribbean*, ed. Patrick Taylor (Bloomington: Indiana University Press, 2001), 89–103. At least two more of this branch's committee members may have been of African descent, P. A. Browne and his wife (identified only as "Mrs. P. A. Browne), if this was the same P. A. Browne identified in various sources as the "negro" Guianese barrister and representative for Georgetown in the colonial government. See Clementi to Long, confidential, 26 Mar. 1917, CO 111/611, no. 21957, NA.

104. Raymond T. Smith, *British Guiana* (London: Oxford University Press, 1962), 116.

105. Bridget Brereton, *A History of Modern Trinidad 1783–1962* (Kingston: Heinemann Educational [Caribbean]Books, Ltd., 1981), 127–129.

106. There is a considerable amount of scholarship on this subject in the US context. See, for example, Eileen Boris, "The Power of Motherhood: Black and White Activist Women Redefine the Political," in *Mothers of a New World: Maternalist Politics and the Origins of Welfare States*, eds. Seth Koven and Soyna Michel (New York: Routledge, 1993): 213–245. See also Linda Gordon, "Black and White Visions of Welfare: Women's Welfare Activism, 1890–1945," in *"We Specialize in the Wholly Impossible": A Reader in Black Women's History*, eds. Darlene Clark Hine, Wilma King, and Linda Reed (New York: Carlson Publishing, 1995): 449–485; Glenda Elizabeth Gilmore, *Women and the Politics of White Supremacy in North Carolina, 1896–1920* (Chapel Hill: University of North Carolina Press, 1996). For the British Caribbean, see Macpherson's work and Rhoda Reddock, *Women, Labour and Politics in Trinidad and Tobago: A History* (Kingston, Jamaica: Ian Randle Publishers, 1994), esp. chapter 6.

107. See, for example, Seth Koven and Sonya Michel, introduction to *Mothers of a New World*, ed. Koven and Michel, 1–42.

108. On the hiring of non-white physicians in British Guiana, see De Barros, "Spreading Sanitary Enlightenment." On the employment of nurses through the Overseas Nursing Association, see correspondence in Collet to Milner, no. 544, 13 Nov. 1920, CO 111/632, NA. See also H. C. Hawkins, Acting Honorary Secretary of the Overseas Nursing Association, to the Undersecretary of State, 16 Sept. 1920, no. 42072/1920, CO 111/634; see also Application for Employment as Divisional Nurse in the Colonies, CO 111/634, NA. Reports of British Guiana's surgeons general for the following years note the employment of (white) English and Scottish female nurses in supervisory positions in British Guiana's hospitals in the early twentieth century: 1904–1905; 1907–1908; 1911–1912; 1918.

109. K. S. Wise, surgeon general, to Governor Egerton, 31 July 1915, encl. in Egerton to Bonar Law, 7 Aug. 1915, CO 111/601, no. 285, NA.

110. This conclusion as to Minett's ethnicity is based on her account of her background. She described herself as having worked in England for eleven years before going to British Guiana. See Minett, "Infant Mortality," 56, 57. Also see BGIWML, *The Eleventh Report, 1924*, 9. For biographical information about Cumming, see BSLBG, *The First Annual Report, 1914*, 10

111. "Transactions, 1913 and 1914," 138–141.

112. Manderson, "Shaping Reproduction," 38.

113. According to Brereton, very few children of South Asian descent attended secondary school until after the Second World War. Bridget Brereton, "Society and Culture in the Caribbean: The British and French West Indies, 1870–1980," in *The Modern Caribbean*, eds. Franklin Knight and Colin Palmer (Chapel Hill: University of North Carolina Press, 1989), 85–110. See also Clem Seecharan, *'Tiger in the Stars': The Anatomy of Indian Achievement in British Guiana, 1919–1929* (London: Macmillan Education 1997), chapters 17 and 18.

114. As the League reports do not indicate the midwives' race/ethnicity and the census reports for 1911 and 1921 do not include midwives as an occupational category, it is impossible to identify their race and ethnicity with any certainty. But, as these reports note the number of South Asian dispensers, druggists, and midwives, and as most druggists and dispensers were male in this period, it is possible to estimate the number of South Asian midwives. In 1911, there were thirty-three, and in 1921, there were twenty-four. See *Report on the Results of the Census of the Population, 1911* (Georgetown,

British Guiana: The Argosy Company, Ltd., 1912), 71; *Report on the Results of the Census of the Population, 1921* (Georgetown, British Guiana: The Argosy Company, Ltd., 1921), 72, 74, 75.

115. See, for example, Carol Summers, "Intimate Colonialism: The Imperial Production of Reproduction in Uganda, 1907–1925," *Signs* 16, no. 4 (Summer 1991): 799, 803; Lang, "Drop the Demon *Dai*."

116. *Report of the Surgeon General for the Year 1906–1907*, 13, 15.

117. Jaundoo's ethnicity is suggested by her name. Unlike many League midwives, Jaundoo was identified in the sources because she won a medal for "best Infant Welfare and Maternity work" in 1924. For references to Jaundoo, see BSLBG, *The Eighth Annual Report, 1921*, 19; BGIWML, *The Eleventh Annual Report, 1924*, 11.

118. Porter, 179; see also Davin, 36, 37; Dwork, *War is Good for Babies and Other Young Children*, 164, 165. In the case of Belize, Anne Macpherson has noted some "popular aversion" to its Black Cross Nurses. Macpherson, "Garveyism, Maternalism, and Belize's Black Cross Nurses," 517.

119. Some of the reports of the Georgetown-based health visitors have survived, either in their original form or reproduced for inclusion in the city's public health reports. However, copies of the reports produced by League midwives have not been found.

120. Wishart, *Annual Report of the Public Health Department of the City of Georgetown for the Year 1913* (Georgetown, British Guiana: 1914), 15.

121. Josephine Legall, "Report for May, 1916," MTC, Jan.–Dec. 1916, MSB 626; E. Fennens, "Report on January, 1916," MTC, Jan.–Dec. 1916, MSB, 186.

122. Wishart, "Annual Report of the Public Health Department of the City of Georgetown for the Year 1920," MTC, July–Dec. 1921, MSB, 508. This observation was repeated a number of times. See, for example, *Daily Chronicle*, 7 July 1921, 7; Wishart repeated these observations in his report. See Wishart, *Annual Report of the Public Health Department of the City of Georgetown for the Year 1929*, 19; Wishart, *Annual Report of the Public Health Department of the City of Georgetown for the Year 1920*, 5; Wishart, *Annual Report of the Public Health Department of the City of Georgetown for the Year 1930* (Georgetown, British Guiana: "The Argosy" Company, 1931), 9, 13.

123. Wishart, *Annual Report of the Public Health Department of the City of Georgetown for the Year 1913* (Georgetown, British Guiana: 1914), 15.

124. See "The Report of the Public Health Committee," 12 Feb. 1923, MTC, Jan.–Mar. 1923, MSB 256.

125. "Transactions, 1913 and 1914," 138, 139, 140, 141. By "Sarah Gamp," Craigen was likely referring to unregistered, "traditional" midwives; this derogatory term was used in Britain to refer to such women. See Deacon, "Midwives and Medical Men in the Cape Colony before 1860, 272.

126. BSLBG, *The Eighth Annual Report, 1921*, 8; see, for example, BSLBG, *The Ninth Annual Report, 1922*, 6.

127. BSLBG, *The Eighth Annual Report, 1921*, 9.

128. See reports of the BSLBG and the BGIWML for the years 1924, 1926, 1930, 1932, 1936.

129. *Report of the Surgeon General for the Year 1920*, 11.

130. See BSLBG, *The Fourth Annual Report, 1917*, 8; BGIWML, *The Nineteenth Annual Report, 1932*, 11.

131. See, for example, BSLBG, *The Eighth Annual Report, 1921*, 7.

132. See BGIWML, *The Eleventh Report, 1924*, 9, 11.

133. See BGIWML, *The Eleventh Report, 1924*, 9, 11.

134. BSLBG, *The Eighth Annual Report, 1921*, 7.

135. BSBGL, *The Seventh Annual Report, 1920,* 12.
136. BSLBG, *The Ninth Annual Report, 1922,* 6. The number of those "prosecuted and fined" is uncertain. An examination of police reports between 1906 and 1920 indicates that "uncertified midwife" was rarely singled out as an offence under the 1886 Medical Act. For most years, the total number of violations of this ordinance was noted. The exceptions were in 1918 and 1919; for those years, six and seven individuals, respectively, were convicted as "uncertified midwives" under the 1886 Medical Act. In 1918, three were acquitted, and in 1919, three were reported to the police in Essequibo. See *Report of the Inspector General of Police for the Year 1918,* 517; *British Guiana Report of the Inspector General of Police for the Year 1919,* 545, 548.
137. Draft response to Cavednish Boyle, 22 Dec. 1900, British Guiana no. 429, CO 111/522, no. 39724, NA.
138. Such was the recommendation of the Surgeon General, David Palmer Ross; from a reading of the amended legislation, it seemed to have been carried out. See *Report of the Surgeon General for the Year 1897–1898,* 6, 7. This "exemption" was not included in the 1886 version of this ordinance, but was added when it was amended in 1900. See British Guiana, no. 5, 1886. An Ordinance to Establish a Government Medical Service, and to enforce the Registration of Practitioners in Medicine or Surgery, in *The Laws of British Guiana (1803 to 1921)* (London: Waterlow & Sons Limited, 1923), 3: sectios 40, 41, 43, 44. This is the (1900) amended version of this ordinance.
139. BGIWML, *The Eleventh Annual Report, 1924,* 11, 12.
140. BGIWML, *The Thirteenth Annual Report, 1926,* 10; BGIWML, *The Twelfth Annual Report, 1925,* 10.
141. BGIWML, *The Eleventh Annual Report, 1924,* 9.
142. "Medical Services" (Submission and testimony at the West India Royal Commission), CO 950/47, 1–3, 72–3, NA.

9 Health in the French Antilles

The Impact of the First World War[1]

Jacques Dumont

The era of the First World War seems to represent to the Antilles and French Guiana—the 'old colonies'[2] tied to France since the beginning of the seventeenth century—a real watershed in sanitary policy. As Pierre Guillaume commented, "[although] outdated in 1900, the medical organization of the Antilles acted as a model for that which occurred later [in France], by experimenting with solutions which prefigured those that were ultimately adopted in the Metropolis."[3] Without necessarily subscribing to quite the same optimistic tone, one could argue that there was indeed a major transformation, one which coincided with two considerable events in colonial life: the enactment of conscription and the First World War. Primary sources on sanitation and public health from the beginning of the twentieth century, are fragmentary and untrustworthy. With the extension of military service to Guadeloupe, Martinique, and Guiana, however, comprehensive health statistics for young male populations finally became available.

This period highlights all of the ambiguities of health policy of 'old colony' nationals. In order to better comprehend the chain of events that resulted locally in the enactment of public health policy, this chapter attempts, in the first section, to explore the sanitary repercussions of the first experiences of conscription in 1913, before examining what followed during the first global conflict. The themes that emerge from these discussions permit us to address the extent of hygiene policy put in place from the end of the War onward. This chapter is based principally on unpublished military archives,[4] keeping in mind that colonial medicine remained, until the first half the twentieth century, largely a military responsibility, only yielding slowly and progressively over time to civilian control. It will demonstrate how medical examination of Creole conscripts provided scientific justifications for social exclusion, whereby morbidity was ascribed not to the social conditions of the Antilles, but to the innate inferiority of coloured troops bound for the European conflict.

THE EXTENSION OF MILITARY SERVICE

The abolition of slavery in 1848 granted citizenship to all of the inhabitants of the Antilles and French Guiana. It remained, however, an ambiguous situation, since the people of these places were given the same rights and responsibilities as other Frenchmen, but remained colonized. This situation generated a drive for equality, for full recognition of the rights of citizenship on the same level as other Frenchmen. The demands for conscription in the Antilles and French Guiana lie within this larger political context. It was the subject of repeated requests by the deputies from the beginning of the Third Republic.[5] But the right of military service was constantly rebuffed. Several factors account for this rejection, but above all, there was a fundamental judicial question: To what extent should metropolitan laws apply to the colonies, to people with a very different legal status? The law of 21 March, which imposed military service in France, did not explicitly discuss its applicability to the *outre-mer*. The symbolic meaning of the measure, highlighted by the demands of the Antillean politicians, was not sufficient to accelerate its application.[6] To these difficulties, of which there is abundant evidence in commissions and reports, one can add the reticence, on behalf of the French government, to extend conscription. The anxiety lay principally in the additional expenditure that local implementation of conscription might entail. For many politicians, this 'unjustified' expense did not seem to "correspond to any practical increase in the capabilities of colonial defence."[7] But concerns were also voiced about the value of creole soldiers.[8] Creole soldiers included a population that was principally of colour. The voluntary enlistment reinforced a prejudice against blacks:[9] "the Creole soldier appears to be very mediocre during times of peace as well as war."[10] Such value judgments were based on a racialized perception: "the Creole soldier is not very conscientious, and is whiny, lazy, slow, clumsy and not very careful (. . .) it is very difficult to inculcate in him the military habits of order and exactitude due to his inherent indolence."[11] Voluntary enlistment in the army was thus informed by an explicit and important racial balance between "Europeans and non-Europeans."[12] Military enlistment was coordinated according to this principle: "by way of respecting the proportions between white and Creole elements, we ensure a satisfactory military spirit in the troops stationed in the colonies."[13] All this together merely strengthened the distrust toward Creoles. The reports indicated that the candidates for enlistment did so less out of a sense of vocation than from miserable social circumstances. Moreover, "the recruitment of creoles continued to attract a good number of illiterates"[14] and the Creole non-commissioned officers were very few in number: "experience has shown that it has been difficult to form, in this cohort of troops, corporals and sergeants of suitable valour."[15]

The *physical* state of the enlisted also appeared to be problematic. The assertion of a general weakness referred back to an alarming sanitary situation, one caused in great part by colonial exploitation:

> in Martinique and Guadeloupe, of the numerous young men who seek to be enlisted, no less than 50% are not accepted on account of their poor constitutions (weakness, insufficient chest size) . . . [moreover] tuberculosis and syphilis exist in large numbers of them.[16]

The idea of a strong proportion of recruits being unable, for medical reasons, to perform standard duties was taken as axiomatic by the military authorities: "If the law of conscription becomes applied to the colonies [. . .] it will be wise to only count on 50% of the youth as listed in the census."[17]

The persistence of Antillean politicians succeeded in extending, in 1910, the (French) law of 1905 to the "old colonies";[18] it was, however, "limited to the operations of enumeration and of the medical examining board, to the exclusion of bringing recruits to their regiments."[19] The first medical examining boards were formal operations, where the great majority of conscripts were declared able if they did not present a medical certificate to the contrary,[20] as stipulated by the ministerial telegram of 19 April 1910. The directives were clear: "the designation of good men for service was made in a very large number since these men were not, until present, destined to be either incorporated into regiments or, above all, to be transported to the Metropolis."[21] The percentages of rejects on the grounds of physical deficiency, though noteworthy for enlisted men, did not reach the same level that one saw in the conscripts. As evidence, in 1912, of 3,795 enumerated men, the medical examiners in the Antilles declared 3,184 able.[22] This small number of rejects was immediately seized upon by the Antillean politicians and compared proudly to the other colonial territories, where the proportion of the men refused on medical grounds occasionally surpassed 50 percent.[23]

In 1912, following the decision of the Minister of Colonies, and despite military opposition, the decision to extend military service was made. The percentage of conscripts integrated on the spot was not able "to surpass the total contingent of recruits, who had already been well recognized for their service to the Metropolis."[24] The effective fighting force was evaluated at approximately 1,000 conscripts for both Martinique and Guadeloupe, and 100 for French Guiana. The departures in autumn—the first trip away from their home islands for the most of these individuals—constituted an unprecedented event in the colonies. Enthusiastic crowds saluted the embarkations. The conscripts were welcomed in France by Antilles notables. But the season of departure rapidly confronted the conscripts with problems of climate, food, and cold—essentially, of environmental adaptation. The military doctors in France were called upon to react to an unexpected problem of some significance.

SANITARY PROBLEMS OF THE FIRST CONTINGENTS[25]

From the moment of their arrival in France, the conscripts were subjected to a series of anthropometric measurements. Morphological files permitted the authorities to draw up a rudimentary taxonomy of health, following Pignet's index, in use by the Army, which was based on the relationship between the soldiers' height, his weight and his thoracic circumference. The index indicated whether or not the person was 'fit'. Thus, in Bordeaux, of 264 Antillean

Table 9.1 An Assessment of the Creole Contingent of Bordeaux, Following the Military Index for Fitness.

Classification	Index	Total
Very strong	5 to 15	26
Strong	15 to 25	92
Weak	26 to 35	122
Poor	36 +	24

soldiers examined, 118 were deemed very strong or strong, and 146 weak or poor, according to the index.

The physician major did not hesitate to conclude that "more than half of the contingent presents with mediocre physical attributes." These conclusions were repeated elsewhere, most particularly in the regular troop postings.

The report of the *général commandant* for the 16th Army Corps to the Minister of War spoke of "a physical state for the group that was below the average. These men are skeletal, with skinny chests, stooping shoulders, frail limbs, and narrow pelvises". It singled out a Guadeloupean of almost 2 m, who weighed only 61 kg and had a thoracic circumference of 82 cm, which gave him a disastrous coefficient of 52. As for the 22nd Colonial Infantry in Marseille, the recruits were judged to be "of mediocre rigour, too young, not at all tough, and, for the most part, insufficiently [physically] developed".[26]

The supposed weaknesses indicated by these indices seemed to be quickly confirmed by the unavailability for service of many troops, and the number of admissions to the infirmary and the hospital. In Montpellier, on 8 December, of the eighty-one soldiers unavailable for service on account of being in the infirmary, seventy-five were Creoles. Of the forty-four soldiers who had been hospitalized, forty-one were there due to flu or generalized complications from bronchitis, pulmonary congestion, or bronchial pneumonia. A death was reported on the 17th. The number of Creoles exempt from service reached 42 percent of the total force, with a "constant deterioration of the situation" from November to December.[27]

Table 9.2 Creole Fitness (Robusticité créole), the 24th Colonial Infantry Regiment (Montpellier).

Index	Total
1 to 10	18
10 to 20	95
20 to 30	118
30 to 40	26

THE RESPONSE OF MILITARY DOCTORS

Having arrived in France during the autumn, the new conscripts rapidly presented with health problems that were exacerbated by the difficult atmospheric conditions, unusual to the Antillean soldiers freshly arrived from a tropical environment they had never left before. The military doctors quickly found that they were confronted with health problems that were visited upon the Creole contingents sent to France. How does one construct diagnostics and therapeutics in these circumstances? How does one address sickness that arises in others who are different in their origin, their colour, and their customs?

In the first instance, the military doctors expressed their befuddlement in the face of such situations. They spoke of a double fatigue (*double fatigue*) due to the difficult climate and a problematic adaptation to different circumstances. The colonial military authorities were sensitized to the question of climatic adaptation. Since 1908, the interest in a "black force" (*la force noire*)[28] in Africa questioned the physical resistance of the soldiers of colour,[29] and the problems of health lay in the change of climate.[30] The strategic interest seemed to sweep aside the realities of the difficulties, inasmuch as the black soldiers had only been destined to serve in North Africa in order to replace the European contingents.[31] For the French Antilles soldiers transplanted into France itself, although the unfavourable atmospheric conditions were evoked—"they only had 8 days of sunshine since they arrived"—the authorities opposed giving them specific provisions, such as heating (*chauffage*), wool jumpers (*tricot de laine*), or special hot and spicy food, maintaining: "We approached these people cautiously."[32]

Quickly, the medical authorities insisted on the origins of these problems, signaling that the Creoles had "arrived in defective conditions of hygiene." When three deaths were recorded by military medical inspectors, all of whom were cognizant of the fact that the complications were due to the climate, they eagerly concluded that there were two cases of typhoid which had been contracted *prior* to the arrival of the soldiers in France. Elevated levels of amoebic dysentery were attributed to chronic infections, which corresponded well to the problems regularly cited by the health service in the Antilles and attributed to water-borne illnesses (*maladies hydriques*) and to the recurrent problems of nutrition and drinkable water, in the cities in particular.[33] Likewise, from the moment of the Creoles' arrival, numerous medical visits revealed venereal infections, which reinforced rumours to the effect that the sexually transmitted diseases had been previously contracted.[34] A report of 18 December 1915 indicated that, of the 328 Creoles enlisted in the Antilles, 88 were suffering from syphilis, 32 from gonorrhoea, with a further 28 already under treatment for syphilis, the total of infected men therefore was close to half of all the soldiers.[35] The situation seemed to affect other groups in the (French) army. A later medical thesis acknowledged:

"few of the [French] soldiers escaped the contagion [of venereal disease] during their colonial posting."[36] In the 3rd and 7th colonial infantry regiments, of 115 Creoles in the hospital, 35 had been admitted for venereal or coetaneous diseases,[37] but 56 were admitted for the flu and other respiratory problems. The illnesses, however, without being completely ignored, were far from predominant in the Antilles. For the Antillean conscripts in France, respiratory diseases[38] came to represent typical medical cases.

The first reports evoked many conditions concurrent to this vulnerability:

> in summary, the indigenous contingent of the 16th army corps is of mediocre physical condition, weakened by conditions of defective hygiene, exacerbated by a long and exhausting voyage, transplanted into a frigid climate . . . which turned out to be admirably prepared for the reception and development of morbid germs.

The report of the medical inspector, Pauzat, Director of health services for the 18th Army Corps, to the Minister of War, on "the sanitary state of the indigenous contingent arriving from the colonies on the 28 December 1913", underlined a "good general state" at the time of incorporation. He added, to emphasize the seriousness of the situation that "the sickness of the créoles had been three times that of the European contingent."

The report on the sanitary situation of the Creole contingent, dated 30 December 1913, enumerated 429 hospitalizations in two months, that being 25 percent of the 1,691 Creole soldiers. The escalation of sanitary problems for the contingents from the Antilles was sufficiently preoccupying to necessitate more inquests and a special envoy.[40] The medical inspector, General Charasse, was dispatched in turn on 20 December 1913 to visit the different regiments where conscripted Creoles had been incorporated.[41] A summary survey of "sickness and death in the Creole contingent since its arrival in France," dated 31 December, counted 9 deaths, 2 recoveries, and 7,626 cumulative days of unavailability for duty[42] for a contingent of 1,296 Creoles.

But this report no longer contented itself with listing "unavailability", of enumerating sicknesses; it slid insidiously into a moral indictment of the

Table 9.3 Creoles Hospitalized by Location.[39]

Place	Total	Hospitalized
Rochefort	257	28
Bordeaux	309	119
Cette	310	122
Marseille	385	128
Toulon	394	32

Table 9.4 Summary of the Days Unavailable for Service and of Medical Treatment.[43]

Confined to Bed?	Days unavailable for service	Having recovered	Entered the infirmary	Days treated in the infirmary	Hospital admissions
2058	2686	1892	2711	1260	234
Sick Sent to the Infirmary	Days of treatment	Cures	Entered the hospital	Dead	Remaining in the infirmary
274	1260	143	86	1	44
Sick Sent to the Hospital	Days of treatment	Discharged	Improved	Dead	Remaining in the hospital
305	3680	133	2	8	162

soldiers' valour. When the arguments of the preceding reports were reiterated, they emphasized the lack of physical and moral qualities of these soldiers. Was it the inspector general who reasoned more in terms of statistics than individuals? Or was it simply an expression of prejudice? Either way, it was always the deficiencies of the soldiers that garnered the most attention. Creoles presented "a vigorous bearing but they are lazy and fatigue easily." Proof was found in their feeble constitution: "there is a notable increase in the number of sicknesses the days before military marches of short duration". The sanitary realities were often marginalized in the discussion of the alleged lesser valour, which cemented conceptualizations of racial hierarchies: "the summary information collected by the chiefs of the army corps and the commandants of the company converge in agreement on this innate inferiority." The climatic conditions of the voyage and of the posting, and the transplantation into a radically different environment, were both blurred by the certainty of these soldiers' innate incapacity.

THE STIGMATIZATION OF CREOLE UNFITNESS

From that time onward, symptoms were no longer read as indices of sickness, but rather as signifiers of chronic unfitness: "[they have] no resistance to the cold or bad weather, [they are] extremely susceptible to respiratory viruses". Worse still, this deficiency seemed irredeemable: "the sanitary situation is thus very disquieting due to the number of sick, and the nature and the seriousness of the pulmonary infections observed, which denote a veritable inability to acclimatize even though the bad season has scarcely started." It did not matter that the situation became worse still in the south of France with the arrival of winter, where "an elevated number of pneumonias were reported starting on the 18th of December". It didn't matter that, in Rochefort, where the reports of the preceding months did not seem to indicate an unusual situation, 74 Creoles out of 257 (28.9 percent) were henceforth totally unavailable for service. At the heart of the problem lay the perception of the (in)abilities of Creoles.

The conclusions of the various commissioned reports shifted away from the effects of climate to a condemnation of a 'natural' fragility: "the cold and the sickness have, amongst them, a more depressing effect which exaggerates their innate laziness . . . it is necessary to watch them like children". A detailed report emanating from the 18th Army Corps reported: "the sick permit themselves to be rapidly discouraged and don't put up any type of fight (*résistance morale*)". Even if the document evoked an "inevitable nostalgia amongst the uprooted", the racist clichés found a pretext for their development, questioning the military usefulness of these soldiers that had already been suggested before the advent of conscription. The conclusion was incontrovertible: "their aptitude to wage battle appears to us to be pretty close to zero. The slightest scratch, the tiniest contusion reduces them to a state of infancy."[44] A report from Bordeaux, dated 30 December 1913, insisted that "of the 30 créoles actually in service in our regiment, I do not believe that we will have even 20 after 8 days at the front."

Medical and military reports thus moved rather swiftly from statistics on the sanitary situation to a "report on the capacity of the créole contingent to serve [in battle]"; the morbidity and mortality only henceforth ever came second,[45] as a way of confirming the self-evident inaptitude. Pathologies shifted from a neutral list of medical illnesses to proofs of weakness. A conclusion seemed to present itself: "The creoles are not able to handle the life of a soldier in France; the facts demonstrate that. They are plants of a warm greenhouse and our country's climate, even the southern climes, do not agree with them."[46] With more neutral terms and without negating the impact of the transplantation (of the soldiers), General Vautier, commandant of the Army Corps of colonial troops, nonetheless arrived at the same conclusions.[47]

From this moment onward, solutions largely escaped the grasp of the military doctors. What were they to do with these soldiers who did not seem able to adapt to European conditions? What were they to do with "useless and cumbersome" Creole soldiers? The law of 7 August 1913, which dealt with recruitment, prohibited a return home of the Creole soldiers. Nevertheless, measures were proposed which looked to postpone recruitment in the old colonies.[48] Whilst waiting for a decision, alternatives were envisaged: "We ought to wait until the springtime for the arrival of the special contingents."[49] Several reports suggested sending the Creoles to a nicer climate and closer to their country of origin. The Minister of War decided on 10 January 1914 that "the young soldiers of the class of 1912, of Creole origin, will be moved to Algeria and Tunisia". The result of the first contingent's posting in France had been catastrophic: "More than half of the contingent was relieved of duties [due to inaptitude]; the other half were transferred to Algeria and Tunisia."[50]

A SELECTION PROCESS IN FLUX

The most efficient solution, according to the military hierarchy, lay in better filtering the recruits at the outset. The principle of a "very rigorous selection [process]" in order to "eliminate the unfit [*non-valeurs*]"[51] became the leitmotif of the directives concerning Créole recruitment. The necessity of a very strict medical inspection was constantly identified, always in reference to the dramatic experience of the recruitment of the class of 1912. In this way, the fitness of the first conscripts enumerated on the spot was quickly questioned:

> The review council [*conseil de revision*] charged with examining the conscripts of the class of 1914 ought to have rejected, for unfitness, 80% of the young men presented to them. This proportion exceeded that of those deferred and exempted from the class of 1913, who themselves have notably exceeded that of the class of 1912.[52]

The intention of this work is not to judge the real sanitary state of the population subjected to colonial exploitation, to verify the statistics themselves, or to contest the indices as did Antilles politicians from 1915 and military doctors in 1930s Africa;[53] rather, the aim is to acknowledge the ebb and flow of estimations, and point out that observations were due less to real issues of physical aptitude than to the apprehension of the observers. The perspective had changed with the first, disastrous experiences. In Martinique, the Catholic journal, *La Paix*, published by the Bishop's diocese, went along with the point of view that a rigorous selection process necessitated a "very strict medical visit, as much in the interest of the créoles as in the general interest to avoid the cost of repatriation."[54] This opinion agreed with, while not explicitly echoing, the persistent opposition of the estate owners, who were fearful of being deprived of manpower by the extension of conscription. The machinations of the large landowners is clearly pointed out, however, in an intervention in the National Assembly by the deputies Lagrosillère of Martinique and Boisneuf of Guadeloupe, on 23 March 1916: "the physician-majors involved in the recruitment board have deliberately, under the pretext of local economic necessity, placed the interest of property owners before that of national defense."[55]

The declaration of war in 1914 changed very little. The leaders of colonial troops found it "opportune, in the interest of utility and humanity, to keep in their location, until ordered otherwise, the contingents of our old colonies who participate in the auxiliary service, of the territorial army and of the reserve."[56] In this way, until April 1915, "the two Antilles companies functioned in many ways as reserve companies [*compagnies de depot*] (until April 1915)."[57] Not only did the review councils continue to reject a significant proportion of potential soldiers, but the majority of (successful) conscripts were consigned to the Antilles. The reticence seemed suddenly to disappear in April 1915: there were no longer enough soldiers, regardless of their origins, their colour, or their health. An incorporation plan of non-reviewed classes[58] and previously deferred soldiers was established. All the classes from 1889 to 1916 were to be examined, wrote the newspaper *La France coloniale*: "The order of general mobilisation of the créoles is in the course of being executed and will involve progressively all legitimate men of the colony from aged 19 to 45."[59] Measures were even taken in Guadeloupe: "for the class of 1917 back to the class of 1890, all legitimate men were called forth". The possible exemptions were curtailed to include only "those men who presented with serious illnesses, such as the loss of a foot or a hand, paralyzed, obese beyond 100 kilos, etc."[60]

However, even if the call to arms was generalized, the effective incorporation of troops and the departures to the front were still very selective. Despite the War, resistance persisted "due to difficulties, confirmed by the experience of those suffering from acclimatization."[61] What were the criteria by which aptitude was determined? What norms were applied? The rejection of a good proportion of the Creoles continued to depend on the morphological index of Pignet, which served the goals of justifying exclusion orders and reinforcing the sanitary and civilizing mission of the Army: "what is lacking in these young men is weight and thoracic circumference, a consequence of insufficient and insubstantial nutrition, but after several weeks in the barracks, their weight and their circumference augment nicely."[62]

The change was ultimately less in the rate of recruitment[63] than in the urgency of its operationalization. The three months of initiation and training, previously presented as indispensable and carried out on the spot,[64] were now rapidly judged as no longer necessary, and the number of departures accelerated. The questions of a change of location, the difficulties of climactic adaptation, or physical unfitness were no longer germane.

REPERCUSSIONS IN THE ANTILLES

These health restrictions had great repercussions in the old colonies. The delays in the application of conscription and the strict medical measures toward recruitment were understood as forms of discrimination, aimed at tarnishing Creole patriotism and the possibility of full civil integration.[65] They would ultimately accelerate the establishment of public health policy.

The declaration of war, on 3 August 1914, exacerbated the feeling of being taken for granted: "Is it not, however, a cruel irony that, just as our compatriots spontaneously came to offer their lives for the defense of the homeland, they were rejected from this supreme sacrifice on account of unfitness?"[66] When the official publication of 2 April 1915 left no doubt about the generalization of recruitment, this announcement was welcomed favourably in the Antilles. The newspaper *La France coloniale* saw in it proof of:

a denial of the evidence of history, the trenchant proponents of the in-equality of races who describe us as unqualified for military services. Less than three years ago, at the moment when the uninterrupted efforts of the colonial representation resulted finally in the application of the military law on the young generation, créole recruitment has been sabotaged with pleasure in France by the opponents of our participation.[67]

From the first rumours of the extension of the mobilization of troops, the Catholic press was explicit as to the meaning attributed to Martinique: "We have suffered from prejudices against the state of our health; the exaggerated belief that the rigours of the winter will not be able to be endured by the créoles have postponed for too long ministerial decisions."[68] The defence of the homeland was associated with recognition. It offered an opportunity to bypass the question of colour:

> this cursed war, which costs so much in blood, so much in tears in France, will have at least this one unexpected result: it will dissipate the prohibitions and prejudices that we have in Europe against blacks and their descendants (. . .) After the war, what will persist in the stories spread against us in all of the Metropolitan circles? Just a little mud lying submerged in the blood shed by créoles on the battlefields of France. Yesterday one could consider us as intruders within the great French household; today, France can count us amongst the finest of their children.[69]

Nevertheless, the restrictions on recruitment also raised bitter recriminations about the deficient physical condition, seen as "physiological decadence analogous to that recorded in certain savage peoples"—in other words, referred to as an unacceptable step down on the ladder of civilization:

> The humiliation will be certainly huge for the entire country, if it comes to be demonstrated that, owing to a gradual weakening of the annual contingent, we were incapable of this military services so long demanded by us (more as an honour than an obligation) because it completed our assimilation as sons of the Metropolis.[70]

Faced with a substantial percentage of rejects, the local press did not hesitate to evoke the theme of a problematic waste (*un fort déchet*)[71].

From thence onward, recruitment became the symbol of good citizen health, and an occasion to periodically stigmatize "neurasthenic youth"[72] and to champion the virtues of physical education and military preparation. The *Union des Sociétés Martiniquaises de Sports Athlétiques*, founded in 1912, strengthened training in the sports associations.[73] *La Française*, a gymnastics and military preparedness association, authorized by the Minister of War, took the opportunity to justify its requests for grants, approved unanimously by the General Council of Martinique. In Guadeloupe, the person responsible for health care, Doctor-Major Pichon, founding president of the Guadeloupian Society, formed a *"Union sacrée"*[74] for the recovery and the radiance of the island. He was named responsible for military preparedness and promoted a "physical education *œuvre*" which would elicit the post-war congratulations of Clémenceau, the "father of the victory".[75]

For Dr Pichon, the population continued to lack not only the most elementary conditions of health, but also 'physical valour':

> In effect, here as in many other countries, it is urgent to combat the causes of the degeneration of the population, the scourges which influence little by little physical, intellectual, and moral deterioration: inebriety, tuberculosis, syphilis [*l'avarie*][76] (the last of which has made considerable advances since the war) and hereditary degeneration. For this fight, it behooves us to establish a first line of hygienic defense at the schools; they must be a centre of action and education, where we prepare healthy, energetic, passionate generations for an active life and for exercise or fortifying sports.[77]

A political maxim was recalled by the Head of Antilles health care, Dr Arnould, in Martinique: "Hygiene is a creature of habit and of education: It is a pleat to be ironed [*C'est un pli à prendre*]"[78] A new association appeared in the colonies: 'Hygiene and Physical Culture'.[79] Now, the real problem was to transform this dream into reality. Sanitary conditions remained rudimentary, and malnutrition rampant. Anticipating the compulsory law voted on by the Senate in 1920, Dr Pichon prepared a program for physical education in the schools. He published a small manual of practical hygiene and insisted on the need for creating a medical inspectorate. Pichon was an archetypal doctor of this time: his preoccupations revolved around what could be systematically measured.[80] Data cards, calibrations, grades, scales, norms, and statistics, all part of a medical arsenal needed to evaluate the physical state of the population, its progress, and its corporeal manifestations. This hygienic education also had as its goal the prevention of 'moral deviancies.'[81] The sanitary apprenticeship was the first step on the ladder to a 'civilized' life.

The dramatic experience of the War justified to the colonies the redeployment of the idiom of 'human capital'[82]:

> after such proof of courage, of bravery, of devotion, of loyalty displayed by the colonials, the Government conceived that it was no longer sufficient to pursue the economic development of its overseas colonies, but that it ought, in particular, to dedicate itself to the conversation and addition of its colonial human capital.[83]

Bills concerning the protection of hygiene and public health in the colonies were tabled by deputies from different parties. A medical school in the Antilles was envisaged.[84] Private medical practice developed, but was largely inaccessible to the great majority of the population. Certainly, civic hospitals and sanatoria welcomed indigents, but a true politics of public health remained unrealized. Thus, the law of 15 July 1920—rendering applicable, in theory, the arrangements of the law of 15 July 1893 on the organization of free medical assistance—left "to the authorities responsible the practicalities of adapting to the local conditions"[85]. And it was necessary to wait until the end of the 1930s to see the beginnings of a recognizable infrastructure. If the newspaper *La Paix* was able to write, "If we consider the actual state of Martinique, we are struck by the distance we have covered in several years",[86] we must not forget the especially high rate of infant morbidity that existed before the War, and the weak and sporadic attention paid to a deprived population. Although a real sanitary debate emerged at the beginning of the twentieth century, amplified by conscription and the First World War, public health reform remained marginal in the Antilles.

NOTES

1. This chapter was translated from the French by David Wright, with the assistance of the author.
2. The term also designates the island department of *La Réunion*. Although situated in a different geographical location—the Indian Ocean—the historical problems there were similar.
3. P. Guillaume, "Pathologies antillaises et politiques de santé publique au début du XXᵉ siècle," in *Identités caraïbes*, ed. P. Guillaume (Paris: Editions du CTHS, 2001), 161–169.
4. The main primary sources for this article are housed in the archives of the former historical service of the armed forces, *Service Historique de l'Armée de Terre* (SHAT), thereafter the *Service Historique de la Défense* (SHD) in Vincennes (France).
5. J. Corzani, "Conscription," in *Dictionnaire encyclopédique des Antilles* (Fort de France: Désormaux, 1993).
6. *Rapport au conseil supérieur de la Défense nationale*, 10 Oct. 1906, labeled 'secret', 7N78.
7. The bill modified articles 89 and 90 of the law of 21 March 1905, (n.d.), 7N78.
8. SHD Supplementary series: Créole contingent, 9N1147. This appellation was in accord with the republican idea that did not differentiate by place of birth and designated, in a neutral way, "the French citizens of the colonies".
9. For a comparison in the Caribbean, see G. Howe, *Race, War and Nationalism: A Social History of West Indians in the First World War* (Kingstown/Oxford : Ian Randle/James Curey, 2002).
10. *Rapport général de l'infanterie*, 1 Oct. 1906, 13H1/d1.
11. *Rapport du commandant supérieur des troupes des Antilles*, 1905, 13H1/d1.
12. Medical Statistics, French Guiana, 1906, 13H3.

13. *Letter from the Minister of Colonies*, 6 Oct/ 1914, 7N78.
14. 1906 Report, Antilles Group, 13H3. The report indicated that one-quarter seemed to be unable to read or write. This problem was more pronounced according to other military sources, such as the first conscription registers.
15. *Rapport au conseil supérieur de la Défense nationale*, 10 Oct. 1906, 13H3.
16. Information on Recruitment, 1906, 13H3. A report from 1906 indicated that nineteen out of fifty-seven Martiniques and thirty-four out of ninety-two Guadeloupians were accepted, that being about one-third of each group.
17. Information on Recruitment, 1906, 13H3.
18. The laws were not automatically applied to Antilles colonials, and sometimes required additional clauses.
19. *Journal Officiel de la Martinique* (JOM), local ordnance (*arrêté*) of 2 September 1910.
20. The ruling of 30 January 1911 specified the qualifications of doctors responsible for the medical inspections, 1911, JOM, 51.
21. Letter from the Minister of War to the Minister of Colonies, 6 June 1912, no. 131 1/8, 7N78.
22. One thousand four hundred seventy-four for Martinique, 1,469 for Guadeloupe, and 156 for Guiana. Numbers determined according to articles in the press.
23. *La Vérité* (political, commercial, literary, sports organ), Fort de France, Wednesday, 3 September and Thursday, 5 September 1912.
24. Letter of 6 June 1912, op. cit.
25. The principal data of this section comes from the supplementary series 9N692; in particular, *Documents d'ordre statistique et rapports médicaux au sujet de l'état sanitaire des militaires du contingent créole*. The other sources will be indicated later.
26. Report of Gl Mercier, 15th army corps, to the Minister of War, Marseille, 28 Dec. 1913.
27. Report of the medical inspector, director of health services for the 16th army corps, Montpellier, 19 Dec. 1913.
28. Mangin (général), *La Force noire* (Paris: Hachette, 1911).
29. Dr. Major Cazanove, *Rapport sur l'endurance et la résistance physique au climat du tirailleur sénégalais*, 31 Aug. 1910, 7N81, SHD.
30. For example, the report of one Colonel Bulleux, commandant of the 5th mixed colonial regiment of Morocco, noted on 25 October 1913: "the Senegalese soldiers are very sensitive to the cold which causes severe, and rapidly progressive bronchitis and pneumonia in them. Out of 700 men in the 2nd Senegalese battalion, from the first of January 1913, 315 were suffering/ill, 40 had been hospitalized, and 6 had died," 7N81, SHD.
31. *Historique sur la question des troupes noires*, 7N81, SHD.
32. *Etat sanitaire du contingent indigène*, Bordeaux, 21 December 1913.
33. Information on Health Provision/Services, 1905, 13H1/d2.
34. See 13H1/d1. Information on Health Provision/Services, *Défense Martinique: journaux de mobilisation*, 13H3; and for an introduction, see P. Guillaume, op. cit.
35. Information on Health Provision/Services, 13H1/d2.
36. J. Lutrot, "Les maladies sociales aux Antilles françaises" (thèse de médecine, 1932).
37. *Report on the Sanitary State of the Indigenous contingents coming from the colonies*, 28 Dec. 1913.
38. *Rapport du médecin principal,* Lafage, Paris, 31 Dec. 1913.
39. *Rapport sur la situation sanitaire du contingent créole*, 30 December 1913.

40. *Rapport du médecin inspecteur général sur la situation sanitaire du contingent créole incorporé en France*, Paris, 30 Dec. 1913.
41. The 22nd colonial infantry in Marseille, the 8th in Toulon, and also the 3rd colonial artillery in Rochefort, the 7th infantry in Bordeaux, and the 24th in Cette (Sète 1926), Perpignan.
42. 13h1/d2, SHD.
43. *Report of the Organization of Health Services for the Colonial Troops*, 31 Dec. 1913.
44. General Mercier, Director of Health Services for the 15th Army Corps (Marseille) to the Minister of War, 28 Dec. 1913.
45. *Rapport sur l'aptitude à servir du contingent créole, sa morbidité et sa mortalité,* by the principal doctor, Lafage, Paris, 31 Dec. 1913.
46. *Rapport du médecin inspecteur general*, Charasse, 30 Dec. 1913.
47. Letter of 5 January 1914, *état sanitaire des contingents créoles*, addressed to the Minister of War.
48. *Note historique au sujet de l'incorporation des contingents créoles*, manuscript, *Direction des troupes coloniales*, Minister of War, n. d. .
49. *Rapport sur l'état sanitaire du contingent indigène provenant des colonies*, Medical Inspector Pauzat, Director of Health Services for the 18th Army Corps to the Minister of War, Bordeaux, 28 Dec. 1913.
50. *Note de la direction des troupes colonials*, [date indecipherable], 9N1147.
51. *Lettre du ministre des colonies au ministre de la guerre*, 5 Mar. 1915.
52. *Conseil général de la Martinique, session ordinaire*, Nov. 1914.
53. J. Dumont, "Santé et conscription créole: le tournant de la première guerre mondiale," *Outre-mers* (revue du SFHOM), June 2007.
54. *La Paix*, 26 May 1915.
55. Cited by G.B. Mauvois, *Louis Des Etages (1873–1925) Itinéraire d'un homme politique martiniquais* (Paris: Karthala, 1990), 44–45, 142.
56. *Projet de rapport au Président de la République au sujet de la mobilisation des creoles*, n. d., 9N1147.
57. Letter of 15 January 1915, *Direction des troupes coloniales*.
58. *Courrier* of 21 April 1915, Lieutenant-colonel Mauger, Superior Commandant of the Antilles Troops.
59. *La France coloniale*, 17 April 1915.
60. *La Paix*, 31 April 1915.
61. Dispatch no. 6590 1/8, 17 July 1915.
62. Letter of 6 October 1915 to the Minister of War, Superior Commandant of the Antilles Troops.
63. In total, an estimated 18 percent of the male population of the Antilles was sent to the European front.
64. *La Paix*, 3 February 1915.
65. J. Dumont, "Conscription antillaise et citoyenneté revendiquée," *Vingtième siècle Revue d'histoire* 92 (2006): 101–116.
66. *Conseil général de la Martinique*, regular session, November 1914.
67. *La France coloniale*, 17 April 1915, paper founded by Victor Sévère, Mayor of Fort de France.
68. *La Paix*, 13 January 1915.
69. *L'Union sociale*, 12 February 1915.
70. *Conseil général de la Martinique*, regular session, November 1914.
71. *La Paix*, 22 May 1915.
72. *La Paix*, 2 August 1913.
73. J. Dumont, *Sport et formation de la jeunesse à la Martinique, le temps des pionniers (fin XIXe-années 1960)* (Paris: L'Harmattan, 2006).

74. One finds in the leaders of this society owners, industrialists, politicians of all stripes including socialists, masons, a bishop, and several priests.

75. On this period and the role of Dr Pichon, see J. Dumont, *Sport et assimilation à la Guadeloupe* (Paris: L'Harmattan, 2002), esp. chapter 3.

76. The former, and then largely obsolete, name for syphilis.

77. *La Guadeloupéenne*, Nov–Dec 1918, 160.

78. Dr Arnould, "Hygiène et éducation physique," *Discours de distribution des prix du pensionnat colonial*, Fort de France, 1921. Reported in *La Guadeloupéenne*, March–April 1922.

79. *La Paix*, no. 897, 26 July 1922.

80. S. Fauché, "Hygiène de l'enfance et de l'éducation physique," *Revue STAPS* 40 (May 1996): 39–52.

81. *La Guadeloupéenne*, May–June 1919, 85.

82. M. Spivak, "Un concept mythologique de la Troisième République : le renforcement du capital humain," *Journal of International History* 4, no. 2 (1987).

83. *La Paix*, "La salubrité publique,". no. 901, 9 August 1922.

84. *La Paix*, "Une école de médicine à Fort de France," 19 August 1925.

85. Second draft bill [*avant-projet*] for the reorganization of public medical insurance in Martinique, February 1936, D 164, Archives Départementales de la Martinique.

86. *La Paix*, "L'essor médical de la Martinique," 17 May 1922.

10 The Difficulty of Unhooking the Hookworm

The Rockefeller Foundation, Grace Schneiders-Howard, and Public Health Care in Suriname in the Early Twentieth Century

Rosemarijn Hoefte

In 1915, the governor of Suriname informed the International Health Commission (IHC) of the Rockefeller Foundation that he "gladly accepted" its offer to eradicate ankylostomiasis, or hookworm disease, in the Dutch colony. The Foundation took a two-pronged approach: first, it wanted to eradicate the disease; and second, to engage in public health education and establish a permanent basis for public health work.[1] It soon emerged, however, that the governor had not spoken for all the colony's inhabitants, as the relief and control program encountered resistance from different sides: from agricultural workers, planters, and local dignitaries. After less than a decade in Suriname, the Rockefeller Foundation closed its operation there in 1923.[2] Local sanitation workers, trained by the Foundation, were left to continue the campaign.

The leader of this local effort was Grace Schneiders-Howard (1869–1968), who, as the daughter of a British planter and an upper-class Dutch–Surinamese–Jewish mother, became a social activist, taking up the cause of the poor and the powerless, including prisoners, British Indian indentured labourers, deportees from French Guiana, and Amerindians.[3] In the second and third decades of the twentieth century she became involved in sanitation programs, starting as a casual labourer and finally becoming the colony's chief sanitary inspector. She was a champion of the poor, but, according to her, changes in their conditions had to be initiated by the elite and not by the masses themselves. She firmly believed in the American foundation's modernist and technical approach.

This chapter focuses on the efforts of both the Rockefeller Foundation and Schneiders-Howard in the fight against hookworm in Suriname in particular, and their efforts to improve the public health system on the plantations and in the capital city of Paramaribo in general. It will be shown that the Foundation and the local public health and sanitation officials encountered not only enthusiasm and admiration, but also indifference, cynicism, and hostility. Groups of labourers, planters, and officials all showed their hostility to the Foundation's approach, intrusiveness, and superior attitude. Negative sentiments prevailed, thus eroding the first impressive results obtained by the Americans. The lack of local cooperation and financial support, a *sine qua non* for the Rockefeller Foundation, and inattention to the importance of sanitation, undermined the efforts to permanently improve public health in the colony, whether by the Americans or local health workers. The energy and enthusiasm of a few individuals did make a difference, but without broad support, most of their work ultimately was in vain.

INTRODUCTION

In the first decades of the twentieth century, Suriname was a colonial society in flux and in decline. Large-scale agriculture was still considered the backbone of the economy, even though the number of sugar plantations had declined dramatically in the nineteenth century. On the other hand, the total area under cultivation grew from 2,113 hectares in 1890 to 2,878 in 1930. Through this increase in scale and modernization, production was kept at the pre-abolition level of eight to nine million kilograms per year, but the rapidly declining price of sugar posed severe problems.[4]

The workers on these plantations were mostly Asian indentured migrants. After the abolition of slavery in 1863, a ten-year "apprentice" period was established to ease the transition to free labour, in which the former slaves were to work for employers of their own choice under the supervision of the state. Cheap and docile workers were of utmost importance to the plantation owners, who wanted to continue their economic activities in the post-slavery era. They found the source of this type of malleable labour outside the region—from indentured immigrants from British India. Three weeks before the period of state supervision ended on 1 July 1873, the first indentured labourers arrived in Suriname from British India. During the period 1873–1916, more than 34,000 British Indians entered Suriname.[5] In 1890, a second group of Asian immigrants were moved to Suriname. Almost 33,000 migrants from Java, the largest island in the Netherlands East Indies, were shipped to the Dutch colony in the West. World War II ended this flow of labourers from Asia. The great majority of these immigrants from British India and the Dutch East Indies settled in the Caribbean.[6] At present, more than half of the population of the Republic of Suriname is of Asian descent.

The movement of a large number of people from one continent to another with a different disease environment brought with it an increased chance of malaise and ill health. Moreover, these Asian migrants had to adapt to a new life, diet, and work rhythm. It is therefore not remarkable that many different afflictions plagued the new plantation inhabitants.

THE ROCKEFELLER FOUNDATION

The Rockefeller Foundation started its activities in public health care in the US South,[7] but convinced of the excellence of its approach, soon adopted the goal of promoting "public sanitation and the knowledge of scientific medicine" throughout the world in the hope of furthering peace and harmony.[8] Until the founding of the World Health Organization in 1948, the Foundation's international branch was the world's most important public health organization.[9] The international division, organized in 1913, was engaged in research to cure disease and promoted the institutionalization of public health care in countries that wanted to advance the fight against curable diseases such as hookworm.[10] Hookworm was one of the main foci of the Foundation's health-care campaigns; other diseases it took on were malaria and yellow fever. Tellingly, the Foundation called hookworm "the germ of laziness", as it sapped the energy of workers.[11] The Foundation identified an equatorial "hookworm belt" from 36° north to 30° south, and stated that labour immigration in particular facilitated the spreading of the disease. The Caribbean was one of the first places that attracted the attention of the Foundation's international division. The region's proximity to the United States and the small size of its countries' populations made it an ideal testing ground for an international experiment. In small-scale societies, the impact would be great, while the operational costs were limited. According to Marcos Cueto, this careful start in a quiet corner of the world was characteristic of the cautiousness of the Foundation's advisers.[12]

Hookworm caused a considerable loss of labour productivity, which, for example, Surinamese employers generally did not understand.[13] This debilitating but rarely fatal disease led to unauthorized absences from work, which according to the labour contract, could result in fines or even jail sentences. In could also lead to an inability to complete tasks, which led to lower wages, since most plantation workers in Suriname were paid per task. This reduced income in turn affected the standards of nutrition, and thus created a vicious circle.

On some plantations in Suriname, everybody was infected.[14] Several factors contributed to the spread of hookworm in the colony; the main problems were the improper disposal of human waste—causing pollution of the soil and drinking water pools—and inadequate drainage. Climatic factors, such as regular heavy rainfalls and heat, as well as the abundant vegetation that created shade, provided favourable conditions for the hatching and development of worms. Although planters and labourers often did not recognize the threat of ankylostomiasis, it was the only disease leading to the organization of a full-scale eradication program in the colony, if only because it was simple to diagnose and easy and inexpensive to treat.

In March of 1915, the IHC of the Rockefeller Foundation received official permission to start a campaign to eradicate ankylostomiasis in Suriname.[15] A year earlier, the IHC had moved into British Guiana to combat hookworm and to set the standard for the rest of the region.[16] Other British Caribbean colonies and Central America were the Foundation's next targets.[17] The first hookworm campaign in South America started in Brazil in 1916.[18]

In Suriname, the IHC inaugurated its ambitious so-called relief and control program at the largest plantation, Mariënburg. In 1915, this plantation employed almost 2,000 Asian indentured servants. The number of British Indians declined rapidly during that period, while the number of Javanese continued to grow. In the period of 1912–1916, approximately 62 percent of the indentured labourers came from Java, and in the years from 1917 to 1921, this percentage had grown to 88.[19]

As elsewhere in the Caribbean and Latin America, the Rockefeller Foundation had selected a number of areas in which it conducted field investigations, demonstrations, and laboratory research. In these selected areas, the Foundation set out to register and examine every person and to treat all individuals who were infected until these patients were cured. The development of public health education was an essential element in the campaign. Modern ideas and methods had to displace traditional folk practices and medicine. One physician, Dr W.H. Kibler, and a staff of three clerks, a dozen nurses, and four microscopists, started the process by informing the inhabitants of the capital and the plantations in the surrounding areas about the effect, cause, and prevention of hookworm disease. To this end, the Foundation toured the colony with lectures and slide shows, and later the silent film "Unhooking the Hookworm."[20] In addition, the Foundation's representatives handed out 72,000 circulars written in Dutch, Sranantongo, Hindi, Urdu, and Malay.[21] Sometimes the microscopists also gave demonstrations to show eggs and young worms that had been hatched from eggs: "Seeing the young worms alive under the microscope proves very interesting to the people and makes about as much impression [. . .] as anything that is done to inform them about Ancylostomiasis."[22] These microscope demonstrations are a good example of how the population was instructed about the (almost) invisible organism that caused disease, and also about the way modern medicine could eradicate the disease.

Kibler combined this public spectacle with an almost military operation to inform and biomedically register, examine, and treat as many individuals as possible. The nurse who was in charge of a selected area visited each house to record the names of all inhabitants, while explaining the symptoms, effects, and prevention of hookworm disease. Each person received a box to be filled with his or her faeces. The nurse then collected these boxes and locally trained microscopists examined their contents. A first indication of the prevalence of the disease occurred when 95 percent of a group of 2,380 persons were infected. Treatment consisted of the administration of the potentially dangerous poison, thymol, and the purgative, Epsom salts. The regime prescribed a dose of salts at 6 p.m. the first day, two doses of thymol the next morning at 6 and 8 a.m., and then another dose of salts two hours after the last dose of thymol. The belief was that locally trained practitioners would soon be capable of continuing this work.

The first quarterly report by Kibler was almost brimming over with enthusiasm about the results and the local cooperation. On New Year's Day 1916, the Rockefeller staff had treated 1,800 patients. In 1917, the Foundation examined more than 13,000 people and concluded that 91.5 percent suffered from the disease. The recovery rate was close to 83 percent.[23] Yet, despite these apparent successes, the Rockefeller Foundation was fighting a losing battle. The tone changed in the following reports, when its representatives identified problems that they considered insurmountable: the lack of cooperation by groups of Javanese labourers, some planters and local officials, and the government administrations in both Paramaribo and The Hague made it impossible to attain the Foundation's goals.

The first antagonists were the Javanese—not only the most numerous but also the most heavily infected population group, that, according to the Foundation's Suriname staff, objected to treatment by refusing to heed instructions and even using force against the medical staff. Their opposition seems to have been based largely on religious grounds. Many Javanese were suspicious of Kibler and viewed him as a disguised missionary who would force them to convert to Christianity through the use of secret potions; it was believed that the use of thymol would lead to conversion. On the other hand, some of the non-Javanese nurses were afraid of the Javanese because the latter were said to use secret poison on individuals they mistrusted.[24]

In addition, Javanese workers argued that they would lose their pay while being treated. Yet, to the obvious annoyance of Kibler, they would not take treatment during their free time. Kibler's successors employed Javanese nurses and educated Javanese to convince their compatriots to participate in the eradication program. This strategy had some success, despite the fact that Kibler previously concluded that:

> [t]hey seem to have no natural or religious leaders such as the *Maharaj* among the British Indians and they have little or no respect for their better educated country men. If they fear their immediate superior they will follow his instructions without trouble, if they do not fear him, they will resist treatment.

Free Javanese, who could not be coerced by managers or overseers, were even more difficult to handle. Kibler chided the "superstitiousness" and "fatalism" of the Javanese, their suspicious minds and reticence made it impossible for him to approach the Javanese.[25] Kibler obviously had difficulty communicating with the largest population group on the plantations. He did not have the knack of some of his colleagues in Trinidad and British Guiana, who displayed a sympathetic stance towards people/cultures from the East, developing "a particular fascination with the East Indian populations," and thus managed to build a rapport with the masses.[26] Unlike

Kibler, the white Grace Schneiders-Howard made it clear that she had indeed been able to convince free Javanese to build latrines; unfortunately, she never revealed how she really did this.

According to the Foundation, the problems with Javanese labourers did not arise on plantations, where the manager demonstrated his power and authority. Although some planters fully supported the hookworm campaign, and even wrote enthusiastic letters to the Foundation, others refused to back the program, possibly because they did not perceive the negative impact of ankylostomiasis. In a carefully worded letter to the Surgeon General in Suriname, who was formally in charge of the campaign, the Rockefeller Foundation's representative in the United States argued that the doctor was unable to secure from the managers a sufficient number of workers each day in order for treatment to be useful, and in some instances, promises were not kept. Plantation Mariënburg was a case in point: the managers wanted to stop the health campaign during the harvesting season. Mariënburg's director told Dr Kibler that he thought him to be a "typical American" who wanted to achieve maximum results in no time.[27]

The negative attitude of a number of local officials probably fostered the lack of cooperation on the side of the planters. To be sure, there was ambiguity in administration circles as the government officially embraced the hookworm eradication program, yet it was not forthcoming with either financial contributions or with the promised implementation of public health legislation. Next to curing the disease and public health education, the construction of a permanent basis for public health work was an essential element of the Foundation's mission. However, neither the Netherlands nor Suriname were forthcoming in providing the necessary funds. The colonial government needed extra capital to finance such new projects, but The Hague was not willing to provide the money required. The colonial minister bluntly stated that he refused to subsidize the Rockefeller Foundation, which he thought to be rich enough.[28] Such a remark was not uncommon, given that the British also viewed the Rockefeller Foundation first and foremost as an unlimited source of money.[29] It showed that governments did not (want to) understand the mission of the Rockefeller Foundation: it was not a charitable but a philanthropic organization that encouraged self-help, not dependence.[30] The host nations would gradually have to self-finance public health care and education after the Foundation had demonstrated the benefits of treating hookworm and the importance of hygiene.

Even though some public officials expressed doubts about the Foundation's program, there also existed a genuine enthusiasm for Kibler's efforts among the population and in the press. Already in 1916, the legislature adopted a motion of appreciation to thank the Foundation for its work in the colony. The conservative paper *De West* called for continued government support for Kibler's efforts.[31] *De Surinaamsche Bode* praised Kibler for his zeal and dedication, and the short-lived weekly, *Op den Uitkijk*, suggested that Kibler receive a royal medal.[32] In July 1917, Kibler gave a lecture on hookworm for colonial government officials and prominent members of the community. The director of the Suriname Bank chaired the session. Kibler emphasized the importance of the building and use of latrines and pleaded for the appointment of sanitary inspectors to enforce observance of the ordinance for combating the disease. *The New Paramaribo Times* expressed the hope that the Rockefeller Foundation "represented here by the genial doctor, may find the co-operation it deserves."[33] The well-known Dutch journalist, M. van Blankenstein, who visited Suriname in 1922, also praised the work of the Rockefeller Foundation and criticized the lack of financial support from, and the inertia of, the administration.[34]

Experts agreed with Kibler that only the improvement of hygiene, and the correct disposal of human waste in particular, would lead to the eradication of hookworm. The Foundation regularly urged the government to take more aggressive action on this issue:

> The original agreement made it quite clear that the government was to secure such sanitary conditions as would reduce the dangers of reinfection to the minimum, and we have the right to expect, and insist on the fulfilment of this agreement as far as is practicable.[35]

The Surgeon General objected to the Foundation's proposal to build latrines, arguing that it was a ridiculous idea, since the "Javanese, Creoles [Afro-Surinamese], and British Indians were known to be dirty and unhygienic."[36] The promotion of the construction and use of latrines turned out to be the most challenging part of the campaign.[37] Many planters embraced the Surgeon General's opinion, as it bolstered their resistance to building and maintaining latrines which they had to pay for. According to the Foundation, this lack of active official support resulted in a low percentage of cures after several treatments, and a high percentage of reinfections.

What the Rockefeller Foundation in all likelihood did not take into account was that its founding notion that US-trained physicians and paramedical personnel, and American organizational and research skills, were superior could cause resentment and even resistance among individuals who were trained in Suriname or in Europe. In other words, the Rockefeller Foundation's technical-elitist, almost triumphalist approach not only created allies, but also provoked challenges and conflict.[38] In addition, Kibler had no success in reaching across the cultural divide to convince the Asian population of the importance of treatment and hygiene.

In 1917, Dr Kibler went on leave in the United States and chose not to return to the colony where he had met such obstruction. The US participation in World War I frustrated plans to dispatch a new physician. Only in 1921 did the executive committee of the International Health Board, the former IHC, vote for funds to resume the work in Suriname. The Foundation's representatives continued to praise the positive response of the population, yet the campaign's results were discouraging. In 1921, the Foundation examined more than 900 individuals: 88 percent were infected. Of these patients, 91 percent were treated, and the recovery rate was 77 percent. In 1922, almost 12,000 persons were examined; the infection rate was 97 percent, treatment was given to 93 percent, and the recovery rate declined to 59 percent.[39] However, the reinfection rate remained unacceptably high because of the lack of progress in the government sanitation program. According to the new man in charge, the physician W. Hausheer, "I think it will be a case of their [government officials] doing the least they think they can possibly get away with in order to receive the most."[40] Despite the fact that the most important officials in Suriname for this program often refused to cooperate with the Americans, the popular endorsement had not waned now that Hausheer was in office. Several high officials, including the governor and some social organizations, remained loyal to the educational, eradication, and sanitation campaigns, but were unable to make a decisive difference. It seems that, in the end, the fact that the Foundation could not implement a culture of hygiene was more important than the fact that cure and recovery rates were disappointing, even though hygiene and finding a cure were, of course, closely intertwined. The Rockefeller Foundation's representative in New York advised Hausheer to close his "eyes and fail to see, as far as is possible, all slights, inuendoes etc. [and forget] the people and the conditions which have been so disagreeable and difficult."

The Rockefeller Foundation decided to withdraw from Suriname, citing the "official ingratitude with which we have had contact in Dutch Guiana [. . .] We may console ourselves with the thought that since our work in Dutch Guiana will close near the end of the present year [1923] we will not be subjected to this injustice again."[41] The Netherlands refused to financially support the necessary sanitary measures because it was more concerned with its short-term policy of reducing the colony's deficit than with such long-term goals as public health care. By 1930, the Foundation had terminated its hookworm campaigns in the rest of the region, yet other programs combating yellow fever and malaria continued there.

In 1927, the Suriname-born Dr P. C. Flu confirmed the Rockefeller Foundation's assessment and its expectations about the future of the hookworm campaign in Suriname. During a visit to Plantation Mariënburg, he concluded that the hygienic conditions there were the worst in the colony and that the medical staff did nothing to suppress hookworm disease: "The physician, head of the hospital, very proudly showed me eight patients, all suffering from an advanced [ankylostomiasis]".[42] In other words, the results of the Rockefeller Foundation were not lasting, as its representatives already expected.

THE ROCKEFELLER FOUNDATION'S EXPERIENCES ELSEWHERE IN THE CARIBBEAN AND LATIN AMERICA

Was the experience of the Rockefeller Foundation in Suriname exceptional? By the early 1920s, hookworm campaigns had been carried out in Latin

America and the Caribbean, as well as in Asia and the United States. A comparison with other countries in the region shows that the Foundation's record, as well as the assessments thereof, is mixed. For example, Christopher Abel argues that, based on the Foundation's reports, the ankylostomiasis campaign in Colombia was successful in broadening support to actively control "filth" diseases by properly disposing of human waste and enacting sanitation measures.[43] Efforts in Mexico, however, show that it was not easy to change the habits of the population there.[44] Steven Palmer points out sharp contrasts in the Central American situation. The hookworm campaign's success in Costa Rica was based on the establishment of an extensive public education system. It is important to underline that, in Costa Rica, the principal departments in the public health organization and the government had gained substantial knowledge about the disease and its treatment well before the arrival of the Foundation. The Costa Ricans were very aware of what the Foundation could offer and used the mission to strengthen its existing public health apparatus. Other Central American countries were not able to do so. There were no strategic alliances between local elites and the Foundation to expand the public health departments in Panama, Nicaragua, or Guatemala. Interestingly, Palmer notes that a comparison between the experiences in Central America "suggests that there was no positive correlation between direct U.S. geopolitical influence and the realization of the Rockefeller Foundation's imperial public health mission."[45]

Also complicated is the evaluation of the Foundation's success in the British colonies. John Farley judges the hookworm campaigns as failures,[46] yet James Riley disagrees and points out successes in Jamaica, where the use of latrines controlled the spread of diseases associated with human waste.[47] Both the number of people who tested positive for hookworm and levels of infestations had dropped sharply. Furthermore, a School for Sanitary Inspectors opened in 1927. In that way, US ideas about health and health inspection became internalized in Jamaica. This level of success in both eradicating the disease and prevention and education was never achieved in Suriname.

GRACE SCHNEIDERS-HOWARD'S ROLE IN THE SANITATION MOVEMENT

Even though the Rockefeller Foundation left Suriname on a sour note, it certainly did not mean that the fight against hookworm was doomed. The Foundation's banner was held aloft by Grace Schneiders-Howard. She was trained by the Foundation and was probably the greatest, and definitely the most strident, supporter of its work and its policy to promote the building and use of latrines. First, she served as a sanitary inspector without pay. According to the Foundation, her great enthusiasm did not really catch on in Suriname.[48] For decades she lobbied in both Paramaribo and The Hague for the return of the Foundation, financial means to implement the Foundation's policy, and more staff, but generally could not convince the authorities, which clearly frustrated her. In effect, she accused the Dutch of callousness.[49] Her own goals were set high: "Suriname is one infection, all infection [. . .] This Suriname shall become parasite free."[50] And according to her, Suriname was poor and powerless in the fight against hookworm, malaria, and filariasis.[51] It was not that the Rockefeller Foundation had awakened her: by 1914—a year before the Foundation came to Suriname— Schneiders-Howard had written a ten-page letter to the colonial minister in the Netherlands:

> The town is dirty, terribly dirty [. . .] I wish they would make me chief inspector for 3 months (without a salary) to clean up this mess. The living conditions are very sad [. . .] I know the town and out- skirts and see everywhere how miserable everything is because of in- difference.[52]

Grace Ruth Howard was born in Paramaribo in 1869 in an upper-class family. She spent most of her youth in Europe and returned to Suriname in 1902 with her husband and children. Despite her background and upbring- ing, she had not chosen a partner from the Dutch or Surinamese upper class, and instead married Wilhelm Schneiders, a German headmaster. Soon, Schneiders-Howard made plans to become active in the social life of the colony, but not like many white women in charitable or philantrophic organizations. This may be explained by the fact that Grace Howard had married below her social status, and her participation in such organiza- tions would not enhance her husband's standing. She became a social activ- ist, taking up many causes, including those of prisoners, British Indian labourers, deportees from French Guiana, Amerindians, and the poor and indigent in general. In the second and third decades of the twentieth cen- tury, Schneiders-Howard became involved in various sanitation and public health projects, including the building of a sewage-and-drainage system and a water supply system. She openly called for more financial support for public health care and less for education.[53]

In 1919, Grace Schneiders-Howard started at the sanitation depart- ment as a casual employee. Two years later, she was made a temporary sanitation inspector. In 1923, the governor finally decreed a special hook- worm ordinance and appointed sanitary inspectors trained by the Rocke- feller Foundation, but it was too late to keep the Foundation in the colony. A year later, in 1924, Schneiders-Howard was promoted to chief sanitary inspector; her official title was "head of inspection of latrines, refuse and weed in Paramaribo and latrines elsewere." She was responsible for the sanitation in town, but also for the surrounding plantations and settle- ments of smallholders.

In her letters, she contradicts Dr Kibler's statements about the unwillingness of Javanese to listen to "the white man" or to sanitize. In her first year as chief inspector, she enthusiastically reports on the progress made in sanitation among the Javanese at Plantation Mariënburg: "If you gain their confidence and convince them that it is in their own interest, he'll sanitize outstandingly. I proved it." She challenges colonial politicians who argued that all efforts had come to naught by pointing at the success of the Javanese settlement of Lelydorp, some 15 km outside of Paramaribo, with its "pleasant little houses" and "cheap, practical latrines."[54] How she gained the immigrants' confidence is less clear: in all likelihood, she did not speak any of the languages of Suriname except for the official Dutch.[55] Nor was she the maternal type who advised women how to take care of their children. It seems that she acted more as a stern teacher who explicitly told people what to do. In that respect she probably did not differ much from Kibler, but somehow she was more successful than the American doctor. The fact that she repeatedly visited the people living on the plantations and settlements may have reinforced her message on the importance of sanitation.

The career path of Schneiders-Howard is remarkable. It was not uncommon for women from the upper classes to become involved in public health and social welfare projects, but the great majority of these women concentrated their efforts on reproductive health and infant welfare, and (compulsory) education. Schneiders-Howard is exceptional because of the trajectory of her career, starting as a casual employee cleaning yards. Later, as an inspector, she was not a woman to sit at a desk in an office or clinic, but she actually did go out and biked and walked along smallholdings in tropical temperatures to check the latrines of the Asians. This was not considered to be a proper activity for a white woman. She certainly had her admirers, but she also had many detractors who openly doubted her mental stability.[56] Her influence depended, therefore, largely on her personal relations with the authorities: some officials valued her opinions and suggestions, while others tried to stay away from her as far as possible.

Needless to say, the degree of recognition she earned affected her work. According to one official, she was an enthusiastic and hard worker, in charge of some twenty men. Another official praised Schneiders-Howard's "excellent work," "great enthusiasm," "courage, " and physical power.[57] At the age of 68 she still worked ten hours per day inspecting urban yards and smallholder settlements. The abovementioned Dr Flu wrote that she was "diligent and enthusiastic."[58] These three men lauded Schneiders-Howard's enthusiasm, as did the representative of the Rockefeller Foundation, but her spirits were dampened by the lack of cooperation from other authorities. The police's inertia especially frustrated her. She would fine people 10 Dutch guilders for not building a latrine, and 6 for not cleaning it.[59] As one informant stated, "we were deadly afraid of her, because she would give fines."[60] One can imagine that people would not only be afraid of the financial consequences, but also resented someone inspecting their yards or houses. Matters became even more complicated when Dr P. H. J. Lampe, who had become Surgeon General in 1929, terminated his activities as head of the Sanitation Department in 1933 and was not replaced.[61] Simultaneously, financial cutbacks in government spending on public health had their effects on inspection and prevention.

In 1930, the extremely outspoken Schneiders-Howard was fired for defamation of her superiors and other high-ranking officials. All these changes led within months to the neglect of the latrine system. In 1933, Schneiders-Howard reported that the smell in Paramaribo was unbearable because public health was being neglected and fines were no longer being given. According to her, Paramaribo was becoming "a danger."[62] Schneiders-Howard was without a job at that time, and this statement was self-serving, but other people must have concurred, because in that year, Schneiders-Howard was reinstated as a sanitary inspector. Another aspect that probably played a role in this decision was that Schneiders-Howard was becoming increasingly politically active, and it was hoped that her sanitation work would reduce her political activity. She retired in 1937 at age 68. In reality, she had been fired once again because of insubordination, but was ultimately given an honourable discharge.

CONCLUSION

The activities of the Rockefeller Foundation show the potential, as well as the limitations, of what a well-funded, foreign philanthropic organization could achieve in a poor colony like Suriname. The combination of assistance and notions of supremacy, also known as the white man's burden, were prevalent in the West in the late nineteenth and early twentieth centuries, but not necessarily appreciated at the receiving end. Thus, knowledge, technology, skills, and ideas—in short "civilization," in the eyes of the Foundation—were transferred, but did not always find fertile ground. The immediate effects of the hookworm campaigns, as measured in treatments and recovery rates, were impressive but not lasting. It turned out to be difficult to convince workers, local doctors, officials, and planters of the value of modern public health and medicine. The open racism of a man like Kibler could not have helped to enhance the cause of the IHC. Even if the environment was receptive, officials were unwilling or unable to allocate resources to sustain public health efforts.

The work of the active, and sometimes imprudent Schneiders-Howard— her temperament and actions both helped and hindered the progress of the sanitation movement in Suriname—showed the importance of the efforts of some individuals in the colony, but on the other hand, the limited interest of the colonial authorities in improving health conditions in town, and on the plantations for that matter. The sanitary evangelism of Schneiders-Howard was the driving force behind the hygienic movement once the Rockefeller

Foundation left Suriname. The technical-elitist approach of the Rockefeller Foundation fit her like a glove. She was convinced that change should occur from above. She firmly believed in American and European superiority, and her own class background reinforced her eagerness to teach the, in her eyes, backward, population. Schneiders-Howard is remembered in Suriname as the first female politician. I would argue, however, that the legacy of Schneiders-Howard should be based more on her work in the field of sanitation and public health.

The experience of the Rockefeller Foundation in Suriname is rather unique in the history of the Foundation. It must have been one of the few times that the American Foundation decided to pull out of a country because of a lack of cooperation. Thus, both the Rockefeller Foundation and Grace Schneiders-Howard could only temporarily make Suriname a healthier colony. Ultimately, most failures to act decisively were to be blamed on the constantly deteriorating economic and financial situation in the colony, the lack of public awareness regarding the disabling effects of diseases like hookworm, and the lack of trust in the population's ability to understand the importance of sanitation. In 1948, an international report concluded that Suriname had a bad reputation for sanitation and public health care because of lack of planning, manpower, and enthusiasm. The damning final conclusion was that Suriname was thirty years behind British Guiana.[63]

NOTES

1. This is also known as the "American Method" or "Intensive Method."
2. As this chapter will show, the Rockefeller Foundation de facto worked less than five years in Suriname.
3. For more on Grace Schneiders-Howard, see Rosemarijn Hoefte, "The Lonely Pioneer: Suriname's First Female Politician and Social Activist, Grace Schneiders-Howard," *Wadabagei* 10, no. 3 (2007): 84–103.
4. Rosemarijn Hoefte, *In Place of Slavery: A Social History of British Indian and Javanese Laborers in Suriname* (Gainesville: University Press of Florida, 1998), 15–16.
5. In total, more than 530,000 British Indians migrated to the Caribbean, representing approximately one-fourth of the total British Indian emigration numbers. The major destinations in the Caribbean were British Guiana, Trinidad, Guadeloupe, Jamaica, and Martinique.
6. For more details on the British Indian and Javanese contract migration to Suriname, see Hoefte, *In Place of Slavery*, 25–60.
7. On this campaign in the US South, see, for example, John Ettling, *The Germ of Laziness: Rockefeller Philanthropy and Public Health in the New South* (Cambridge, MA: Harvard University Press, 1981).
8. Christopher Abel, "External Philanthropy and Domestic Change in Colombian Health Care: The Role of the Rockefeller Foundation, ca. 1920–1950," *Hispanic American Historical Review* 75, no. 3 (1995): 342.
9. John Farley, *To Cast Out Disease: A History of the International Health Division of the Rockefeller Foundation (1913–1951)* (Oxford: Oxford University Press, 2004), 2.

10. For a history of the International Health Division of the Rockefeller Foundation, see Farley, *To Cast Out Disease*.
11. See, for example, Ettling, *The Germ of Laziness*. Ankylostomiasis is an infection caused by 7- to 13-mm-long worms that attach themselves to the mucous membrane of the intestines and damage the blood vessels, ultimately leading to anaemia. Walking barefoot exposed the workers to the parasites which burrow through the foot soles and eventually gestate in the small intestines. The worms reproduce, and their eggs leave the body with the faeces. After approximately two weeks, new infections will occur.
12. Marcos Cueto, "Visions of Science and Development: The Rockefeller's Foundation's Latin American Surveys of the 1920s" in *Missionaries of Science: The Rockefeller Foundation and Latin America,* ed. Marcus Cueto (Bloomington: Indiana University Press, 1994), 2.
13. H. Baron van Asbeck, "Rockefeller's bestrijding van de mijnwormziekte in Suriname," *West-Indische Gids* 1, no. 2 (1919–1920): 506; C. Bonne, "De maatschappelijke beteekenis der Surinaamsche ziekten," *West-Indische Gids* 1, no. 1 (1919): 304; P. C. Flu, "Sanitaire verhoudingen in Suriname," *West-Indische Gids* 4 (1922–1923): 590; P. H. J. Lampe, *Suriname: Sociaal-hygiënische beschouwingen* (Amsterdam: Koninklijke Vereeniging Koloniaal Instituut, 1927), 140.
14. Bonne, "De maatschappelijke beteekenis," 304; Flu, "Sanitaire verhoudingen," 590.
15. The Surgeon General of Suriname at that time, H. A. Hovenkamp, convinced H. H. Howard of the Rockefeller Foundation to start a hookworm campaign in Suriname. Hovenkamp, however, left his job in the very year the Foundation arrived in the colony (Geert-Jaap Hallewas, *De gezondheidszorg in Suriname* [Meppel, The Netherlands: Krips, 1981]), 158.
16. On the campaign in British Guiana and the other Anglophone Caribbean colonies, see Rita Pemberton, "A Different Intervention: The International Health Commission/Board, Health, Sanitation in the British Caribbean, 1914–1930," *Caribbean Quarterly* 49, no. 4 (2003): 87–103; and Steven Palmer "'O Demônio que se transformou em vermes': a tradução da saúde pública no Caribe Britânico, 1914–1920," *História Ciências, Saúde-Maguinhos* 13, no. 3 (2006): 571–589. (For an English translation, see http://www.scielo.br/hcsm.) For information on sanitation and living conditions in Georgetown, the capital of British Guiana, see Juanita de Barros, "Sanitation and Civilization in Georgetown, British Guiana," *Caribbean Quarterly* 49, no. 4 (2003): 65–86.
17. In 1914, Costa Rica was the first Latin American state to host the Rockefeller Foundation. In the next two years, hookworm campaigns were started in Panama, Guatemala, Nicaragua, and El Salvador. Steven Palmer, "Central American Encounters with Rockefeller Public Health, 1914–1921," in *Close Encounters of Empire: Writing the Cultural History of U.S.-Latin American Relation*, eds. Gilbert M. Joseph, Catherine C. LeGrand, and Ricardo D. Salvatore (Durham, NC: Duke University Press, 1998), 311–332.
18. Additional surveys and campaigns were initiated in Colombia (1920), Paraguay (1922), Argentina (1923), and Venezuela (1927). In total, the Rockefeller Foundation started its health care activities in fifteen Latin American countries. Marcos Cueto, introduction to *Missionaries of Science*, x; and Cueto, "Visions of Science and Development: The Rockefeller Foundation's Latin American Surveys of the 1920s," in *Missionaries of Science*, 1.
19. Hoefte, *In Place of Slavery*, 72.
20. "Unhooking the Hookworm" was the first feature-length public health motion picture made by the Rockefeller Foundation. It was first used in 1921.

According to Fedunkiw, the scenes in the film were "distinctly American." Marianne Fedunkiw, "The Rockefeller Foundation's 1925 *Malaria* Film: A Case Study in Early Public Health Filmmaking," in *Philanthropic Foundations and the Globalization of Scientific Medicine,* eds. Benjamin B. Page and David A. Valone (Lanham, MD: University Press of America, 2007), 17.

21. On the difficulty of addressing a muti-ethnic public, see Palmer, "'O Demônio que se transformou em vermes.'"

22. "Report on work for the relief and control of Ankylostomiasis in Dutch Guiana from Dec. 31, 1915 to March 1916," and "Report on work for the relief and control of Ankylostomiasis in Dutch Guiana quarter ending June 30, 1916," series 2, RG 5, Rockefeller Archive Center (RAC).

23. Hoefte, *In Place of Slavery,* 147–150. This high cure rate may be explained by the failure to locate eggs in light infections; see Farley, *To Cast Out Disease,* 75.

24. Hausheer to Howard, 14 Jul. 1921, series 1, box 124, file 1666 RG 5, RAC; Annual Report 1921, series 3, box 229, RG 5, RAC; and Annual Report 1922, series 3, box 230, RG 5, RAC.

25. Report on work for the relief and control of uncinariasis in Dutch Guiana from Oct. 15, 1915 to Dec. 31, 1915, series 2, box 57, file 366, RG 5, RAC. What the Rockefeller Foundation's report did not mention was that fear might have played a role as well. Rumours circulated on the plantations that some children had died from the prescribed treatment. Others claimed that thymol had unwelcome side effects: a Javanese accused of theft claimed that the pills had caused such hunger that he was forced to steal food—a defence the judge did not consider believable, *De West,* 18 May 1917, Royal Library, The Hague.

26. Palmer, "O Demônio que se transformou em vermes," 23.

27. Report on work for the relief and control of Hookworm Disease in Dutch Guiana 1915–1916, series 3, box 229, RG 5, RAC; Mariënburg (Mb), 30 May 1916, Stichting Surinaams Museum (SSM) 10, 1229; Mb, 24 Sept. 1917, SSM 8, 651; Mb, 28 Aug. 1918, SSM 12, 1279.

28. Staten-Generaal, Voorlopig Verslag II, 1916 Nationaal Archief, The Hague, the Netherlands (NA); see also M. van Blankenstein, *Suriname* (Rotterdam: Nijgh en Van Ditmar's, 1923), 25–26.

29. Farley, *To Cast Out Disease,* 62.

30. Farley, *To Cast Out Disease,* 4; Palmer, "'O Demônio que se transformou em vermes'," 22.

31. *De West,* 25 May 1917, Royal Library, The Hague.

32. *De Surinaamsche Bode,* 14 March 1917 and 20 June 1917; *Op den Uitkijk,* 28 July 1917, National Archives in Paramaribo, Suriname.

33. *The New Paramaribo Times,* 28 July 1917.

34. van Blankenstein, *Suriname,* 292–301.

35. Howard to Kibler 10 Sept. 1917, series 1, box 55, RG 5, RAC.

36. Mb, 28 Aug. 1918, SSM 12, 1279; Mb, 5 Sept. 1915, SSM 10, 1209; P. C Flu, "Sanitaire verhoudingen in Suriname," *West-Indische Gids* 4 (1922–1923): 590.

37. See also Anne-Emanuelle Birn, "Revolution, the Scatological Way: The Rockefeller Foundation's Hookworm Campaign in 1920s Mexico," in *Disease in the History of Modern Latin America: From Malaria to Aids,* ed. Diego Armus (Durham, NC: Duke University Press, 2003), 165–166.

38. See also Diego Armus, "Disease in the Historiography of Modern Latin America," in *Disease in the History of Modern Latin America: From Malaria to Aids,* ed. Diego Armus (Durham, NC: Duke University Press, 2003), 8–10.

39. Hallewas, *De gezondheidszorg in Suriname*, 159.
40. Hausheer to Howard, 24 May 1922, series 1, box 146, folder 1936, RG 5, RAC.
41. Hausheer to Howard, 24 May 1922, series 1, box 146, folder 1936, RG 5, RAC; and Howard to Hausheer, 27 Jul. 1922; Howard to Hausheer, 7 Nov. 1922, box 147, folder 1937, RG 5 RAC series 1, box 146, folder 1936, RG 5 RAC; Howard to Andrews, 9 Mar. 1923, box 168, folder 2169, RG 5, RAC.
42. P. C. Flu, *Verslag van een studiereis naar Suriname (Nederlandsch Guyana) Sept. 1927–Dec. 1927 en beschouwingen dienaangaande* (Utrecht, The Netherlands: Kemink, 1928), 149–150.
43. Abel, "External Philanthropy," 370.
44. Birn, "Revolution, the Scatological Way," 165–174.
45. Palmer, "Central American Encounters with Rockefeller Public Health, 1914–1921," 327.
46. Farley, *To Cast Out Disease*, 61–87.
47. James C. Riley, *Poverty and Life Expectancy: The Jamaica Paradox* (Cambridge: Cambridge University Press, 2005), esp. 82–90, 104, 113.
48. Series 1.2, box 55, folder 812, RG 5, RAC—note by Howard, attached to a letter by Schneiders-Howard (1917).
49. Letter, 10 Apr. 1917, series 1.2, box 17, folder 251,RG 5, RAC.
50. Letter, 1 Mar. 1917, Ibid.
51. Letter, 29 Sept. 1928, Collection Rollin Couquerque (RC) 2.21.142, inv. no. 20, NA.
52. Letter, 21 Nov. 1914, RC 2.21.142, inv. no. 19, NA.
53. Letter, 10 Nov. 1924, RC 2.21.142, inv. no. 19, NA.
54. Letter, 30 Nov. 1924, RC 2.21.142, inv. no. 19, NA.
55. Schneiders-Howard claimed to speak Javanese (letter, 29 Jul. 1928, RC 2.21.142, inv. no. 20, NA), but I have found no evidence of this.
56. Schneiders-Howard undoubtedly was the most visible woman in the colony, and considered herself the best-informed individual in Suriname, candidly advising governors and colonial ministers, as well as high-ranking officials and parliamentarians in The Hague. She was the first woman to be elected to the Colonial States (legislature) in the late 1930s. This self-proclaimed Social Democrat was benevolent, but never a radical, and she had full confidence in Dutch colonial rule. For more on the life and work of Grace Schneiders-Howard, see Hoefte, "The Lonely Pioneer."
57. Letter, district commissioner to governor, 6 Apr. 1937, Kabinet Geheim (KG) 2.10.18, inv. no. 66, NA.
58. Flu, *Verslag van een studiereis naar Suriname*, 2.
59. Letter, 4 Nov. 1924, RC 2.21.142, inv. no. 19, NA. In the years 1924–1925, $1 US was equivalent to 2.5 Dutch guilders. 'How Much is That?', EH.net/ hmit/ (Exchange rates between the United States Dollar and Forty-One Currencies).
60. Personal communication, Dr. Johan Ferrier, May 2004.
61. Hallewas, *De gezondheidszorg in Suriname*, 157.
62. Letter, 18 Mar. 1933, RC 2.21.142, inv. no. 22, NA.
63. 2.10.18, no. 850, NA. Report Assistant Military Surgeon of the USA, 11–13 November 1948.

11 World War II to Independence
Health, Services, and Women in Trinidad and Tobago, 1939–1962

Debbie McCollin

INTRODUCTION

This chapter investigates the system of public health care in the colony of Trinidad and Tobago in the pre-independence era, beginning from the Second World War. It focuses specifically on the traditional role of women as health-care providers and their subsequent role in the formal health structure of the colony. The chapter first gives an overview of the health system and the concerns of the time. Its investigation into the impact of the Second World War demonstrates that the conflict played a dual role, creating grave problems for women but also encouraging their empowerment through health-care work. Women's services, particularly in the area of nursing and maternity activities, will be examined to highlight the rate of progress for women as patients and as employees in the health sector. This chapter also aims to place the unofficial female health-care provider—the mothers and grandmothers within the home—in their rightful place as important contributors to the local health-care system. It begins with a brief look at the general state of health, the existing services, and the changes that took place in health care and sanitation between 1939–1962, particularly in areas which directly touched women, as it is important in any assessment of this type to understand women within the context of their time and determine the conditions under which they existed.

OVERVIEW OF HEALTH

By 1939, the western region of Trinidad was the most densely populated, with the urban areas of Port of Spain (the northern capital) and San Fernando (located in the south) possessing the highest concentration of people (over one-fifth of the total population in the 1940s)[1]. By the 1960s, this pattern had changed little, despite expansion into certain rural areas in the north and southeast and a redistribution of some of the urban population to adjacent communities, particularly after the Second World War. The continued decline in the death rate (from 16 percent in 1939 to 8 percent in 1962), coupled with the steady rise of the birth rate, saw the population grow to over 870,000 by 1962,[2] an increase much greater than that of other islands like Jamaica and Barbados.[3] This growth outpaced the development of medical facilities and challenged the already problematic health-care system of the islands.

Most West Indian territories had, by 1939, established a fairly diverse medical system based on at least one government/colonial hospital, a district hospital, and special facilities to house those with leprosy and mentally disabled patients.[4] However, Trinidad and Tobago, like Jamaica and British Guiana, had developed a more extensive network of medical facilities with three colonial hospitals in the urban centres of Port of Spain, San Fernando, and Scarborough (on the southern coast of Tobago), seven district hospitals, and health offices scattered throughout the colony.[5] Similarly, the specialized facilities were larger than average, and included a Leper Settlement on an island off the northwest coast of Trinidad called Chacachacare, that could accommodate 400 persons by 1939, and the St Ann's Mental Hospital in the north.[6] Criticism was rife about the conditions, service, and care provided in these establishments, and it was obvious that facilities were insufficient to service the rising population. The bed ratio of 1:458 persons (in the colonial and district hospitals), while not as poor as other islands, was still a clear indication of the importance of increasing accommodations.[7] However, Trinidad did possess small, specialized services in the form of tuberculosis, venereal disease (VD), and maternity wards, and these would continue to expand and diversify during the next two decades.

As such, and in accordance with the trend in Britain[8], the capacity for health-care provision improved in the 1940s with the establishment of new specialized hospitals, such as the Caribbean Medical Centre for Venereal Diseases, established with the assistance of the United States military during the Second World War, and the Masson Tuberculosis Hospital in 1948.[9] Efforts to expand the facilities at the colonial hospitals, which culminated in the 1950s with the rebuilding of the San Fernando and Scarborough hospitals—completed in 1954 and 1957, respectively—opened more avenues for services to women through new female wards and improved spaces for obstetrics and gynaecology.[10] Nonetheless, medical facilities in the colony were constantly overcrowded, demonstrating the inadequacy of the colony's medical services. There were persistent difficulties in the administration of health care, especially in rural communities, as problems with getting the inhabitants to these facilities, due largely to the lack of a proper ambulance service and the inconsistent maintenance of district services, continued unabated. Yet, there is no doubt that by 1962, health-care provision had improved in the colony, as the medical services had expanded and diversified, and mortality rates, including those specific to women—such as maternal mortality rates (see Table 11.1.)—continued to decline.

The 1940s and 1950s were decades characterized by movements (slow at times) toward the mechanization of basic services that would enhance the living conditions of all, but would lower the susceptibility of women to disease and ease their roles as caregivers in particular. The transition to a mechanized water system—the Central Water Supply Scheme, established in the early part of century—was slow, despite supplying an ever-increasing area in the west and north of Trinidad (the most populated areas) and improving the treatment of water supplies, both official and natural.[11] But by the late 1950s, the Trinidad and Tobago Health Department was still in the process of expanding this system to the southern and eastern parts of Trinidad, and southwest Tobago, and had only just begun to conduct surveys to establish an island-wide sewage system in Trinidad.[12] These advances could not keep pace with the growing population. Most households continued to use easily contaminated water sources (rain, shallow ponds, rivers, and wells). Women, because of their responsibility for washing, cooking, cleaning, and other domestic chores, were in frequent contact with these tainted water sources and sewage areas.[13] Thus, they were vulnerable to contamination diseases such as dysentery, which saw serious outbreaks as late as 1961, when 1,104 cases were reported.[14]

The twenty-four years under study, however, saw an epidemiological shift from infectious to degenerative diseases, such as cardiac diseases and cancers more associated with affluent countries. Improvements in the standard of living and health education, and the establishment of control and eradication programs during the 1940s and 1950s, saw the almost total eradication of malaria and a reduction of tuberculosis deaths to an estimated five per year.[15] Among the communicable diseases, these had been the two main causes of death, with tuberculosis notoriously being one of the main killers of the 15- to 34-year-old female cohort.[16] There was also a decline in the incidence of hookworm from an 80- to 60-percent infestation rate in the two decades.[17] The main causes of mortality gradually shifted from these illnesses to heart disease, cerebrovascular disease, cancers, and diabetes—which, by the 1970s, constituted the four main causes of death.[18] This shift did not, however, improve the plight of women, as they seemed to be more severely affected by these diseases. The 1962 statistics for cancer deaths (the fourth major cause of death in the colony) revealed that the capital city, Port of Spain, for instance, reflected the country-wide trend, as female cancer mortality was shown to far outnumber that of males (forty-nine male deaths compared to seventy-nine female).[19] This notable steady increase of degenerative diseases, this epidemiological shift, conversely reflected the improvements made in controlling communicable diseases and the rising standard of living. The shift slowly began to change the face of disease control in the post-independence era to one focused on individuals and lifestyle changes and less on enhancing the living environment. These diseases, even more so than communicable ones, required an expansion of the health education program, the main targets of which, throughout the two decades, were women.

WORLD WAR II, HEALTH, AND WOMEN

The conditions created by the Second World War in the colony emphasized the extent to which women were more vulnerable to the public health interventions, which were at their most acute during the conflict. An analysis of this period also gives insight into the involvement of women in health outside of the official system, the means by which the common woman with little training was able to infiltrate the system, though only in a semi-official capacity. Through an examination of the Trinidadian and Tobagonian female experience during the Second World War, the role of women as both objects and agents of health care in the period is easily discernable.

From the onset of the War in September 1939, Britain's participation in this global conflict involved the support of all of her colonies, including the British West Indies. Pledges of support were immediately sent to the imperial government from the colonies upon the declaration of war, and locally, support activities blossomed and would continue during the period. Female involvement in these local activities was enormous and sustained throughout the War. However, challenges created by the War particularly exacerbated female health issues.

Migration into the cities as a result of jobs created by American bases worsened the colony's already poor social conditions.[20] The influx of people from rural areas and from other West Indian islands, particularly Grenada, put pressure on housing, sanitation, and the water supply, which in turn affected the spread of disease and the functioning of the health services.[21] Death rates, which had been in decline throughout the 1930s, leveled off during the War, and actually rose in 1942 and 1943 to over 16 per 1,000.[22] The compromised standard of living placed women—especially those involved in high-risk professions (such as prostitution)—at greater risk of disease.

Water shortages across the country occurred frequently from 1940 to the end of the War, exacerbated by a severe dry season in 1941 that dried up reservoirs (such as in Maraval, in the northern part of Trinidad) and the shortage of materials preventing maintenance of the existing piping system. There were even reports of operations being postponed in Port of Spain Colonial Hospital due to shortages of water and medical supplies.[23] Water schedules were implemented, and water in Port of Spain was generally shut off daily from 2 to 5 p.m.[24] As the War intensified, with German U-Boat infiltration into the Caribbean Sea in 1942–1943, shortages of food and medical supplies became acute, as cargo and merchant vessels found it difficult to traverse these waters. The resulting shortages of goods, such as milk and certain staples, specifically affected the health of new mothers, as these products made up a large part of the nursing mother's and infant's diet. Milk was further rationed in 1942.[25] The negative impact of reduced consumption of specific foods for priority groups, which included new and expectant mothers in Trinidad (and Jamaica and Barbados), was itemized in a survey on nutrition conducted by B.S. Platt of McGill University in 1944.[26] He pointed out that their special needs were not being included in the estimates of food requirements for the community as a whole, and in those dire times, they suffered from a wide variety of nutritional issues.[27]

The overall trend of the declining death rates was marred by these wartime challenges, reflected in the increase in maternal deaths between 1939–1945, and especially in infant mortality rates, which had previously been in decline but escalated at the beginning of the War to a peak of 119 by 1942.[28] Infant mortality rates were generally used as indicators of the standard of living of a colony and, in particular, of mothers' and infants' health.[29] Thus, this rise during the War was an indication of the decline of social conditions and, as a consequence, a woman's ability to effectively care for herself and her child.

In addition, the loss of personnel to American bases and construction sites also hindered the operation of medical services, as it provided opportunities for the movement of women out of the health divisions into alternative employment with US forces which made it difficult to maintain general medical services, including women's programs.[30] By 1944, complaints of loss of personnel, which had been rife throughout the War, reached a peak, with eighty-nine vacant nursing positions in the colony's hospital and district service.[31] The work of the Child Welfare League and the District Nursing Service, which provided the basis of most of the structured maternity work in areas not served by the colonial hospitals, was greatly hindered by these staff shortages by 1944.

Despite its negative effects, the Second World War generated opportunities for women to participate in health care outside of the official health field through the formation and expansion of volunteer women's organizations. The Red Cross Women's Brigade, for instance, established in 1939 under the aegis of the British Red Cross, worked tirelessly from the nascent stages of the War to help organize the Medical Defence Organisation of the colony.[32] By 1944, this organization was responsible for assisting in the establishment of fourteen First Aid Posts (including one at Maracas, on Trinidad's north coast), seven Casualty Clearing Stations in the north, and seven First Aid Posts and four Clearing Stations in the south. They were also responsible for staffing two annexes at the San Fernando Colonial Hospital. In addition, they helped supply materials and equipment to overseas troops and facilities, such as The Allied Merchant Seamen Convalescent Home and hospitals and sick bays of both British and American troops, through work parties (in which they would congregate for one day and sew materials needed to treat patients). These women also visited the casualty patients at the various hospitals and gave first aid and home nursing classes to women throughout the colony.[33]

Another organization, The Women's Volunteer Service (WVS), was founded by the governor's wife, Lady Young, at the beginning of the War.[34] This organization mainly assisted in the care of the wounded, especially during the intensification of the War between 1942 and 1943 when, according to Admiral Hoover, Commander of the Caribbean Sea Frontier, "a 150-mile strip around Trinidad suffered the greatest concentration of shipping losses experienced anywhere during World War II."[35] Frequently, wounded men were reported to have washed up on the beaches of the island of Trinidad after these battles. The women of the WVS, like those of the Red Cross, organized clearing stations where the wounded were brought before being taken to hospitals.[36]

This organization was characterized by a more diverse recruitment process. Indian women were encouraged to enter service, as "many Indian seamen were brought in badly wounded from ships that had been sunk . . . and the Indian women were particularly good at providing curries and the kind of food the men liked to eat as they recovered."[37] These organizations provided supplementary service to the health-care system at a crucial time when personnel and materials were at their lowest. They also gave women typically confined to the home an alternative means of becoming involved in health care in the colony.

Although the Second World War generally increased women's vulnerability to diseases and decreased their ability to provide proper nutrition and care to their families, it also saw the beginnings of opportunities outside of maternity care for average and formally 'untrained' women to become involved in the administration of health care in a semi-official capacity.[38]

WOMEN'S SERVICES

After the early 1940s, the pregnant woman became a prime target for disease-control efforts. This could not be more obvious than in the area of VD. After a massive explosion of cases during the Second World War (already over 5,000 by 1939, this rate had risen to tens of thousands by the beginning of the next decade), the government instituted compulsory testing of certain groups of the society. Pregnant women attending clinics were targeted as a group that could be tracked and had been exposed to VD through sexual activity.[39] This group was particularly important to address, as diseases specifically associated with women—such as trichomonas vaginalis, vulvo-vaginitis (gonorrhoea), and congenital syphilis (passed from mother to child during fetal development)—were prolific, and in the late 1940s and early 1950s, continued to produce very high numbers.[40] These services contributed to the improvement of the treatment of VD among the female population by 1962, which is evident by the increase in attendance at clinics and in the steady reduction of diseases, such as diagnosed congenital cases of syphilis, by about 82 percent.

In addition to the increased targeting of pregnant women in specific disease-control efforts, the emphasis on the general care of the mother became acute after the 1930s. An investigation of maternal and infant mortality rates conducted by the Health Department in 1941, looking specifically at the difference between rural and urban rates, proved how crucial this attention would be to women's overall health. It was observed that the normal trend of lower rates in the rural areas of a country did not obtain in Trinidad, as both the rural and urban mortality rates tended to be very high and, at times, the rural rate was even higher than the urban (this was noted for at least two years of the study). The study attributed this to defective social conditions and its impact on mothers' ability to care for their children. Inadequate housing and food played a role, but so too did women's often speedy return to work (prompted by economic need) following the birth of the child. The shortage of child welfare organizations in rural areas merely aggravated this situation.[41]

By the 1930s, a government maternity service had been established, but it underwent considerable development between 1938 and 1962. At the beginning of the Second World War, maternity wards were already in place at the three Colonial Hospitals in Port of Spain and San Fernando in Trinidad, and Scarborough, Tobago. In addition, there were beds at four of the six district hospitals in Trinidad, St Joseph, and Arima in the north; Couva in the western central region; and Princes Town in the southwest. With the exception of Jamaica, whose Jubilee Maternity Hospital had 120 beds, the extent of hospital-based maternity services in Trinidad was roughly comparable to those in most British West Indian territories which had only small wards in their government hospitals.[42] But by the early 1960s, the number of beds used for maternity purposes had increased to 313, including district hospitals in Tacarigua, Cedros (in the southwestern tip of Trinidad), and Point Fortin, where a maternity hospital operated.[43] The preferential treatment given to Trinidadian facilities over those in Tobago was evident, as by 1961, the number of beds for maternity care in Tobago remained at a dismal fourteen, while a new maternity block was completed in Port of Spain Colonial Hospital.[44] Despite efforts to increase capacity for maternity cases, particularly in the capital, complaints of overcrowded wards and a shortage of nurses continued unabated throughout the period.

The early twentieth century saw an increase in the education and organization of women in the area of maternity care with the establishment of representative associations campaigning for improved services.[45] In Trinidad, the Child Welfare League, founded in 1918, fulfilled this purpose.[46] Other than at the facilities mentioned above, formal maternity work in the colony from this period was limited to the endeavours of district nurses and the nurses of the League. The Child Welfare League was an independent voluntary organization maintained by subscriptions of its members and contributions from private individuals, business firms, and other charities.[47] Activities included "assistance to expectant and nursing mothers in the way of advice, supplies of milk where necessary, either at a free or reduced rate, and helping suitable cases with layettes and garments."[48] This League maintained a hospital of four beds at Point Fortin in 1938, but by 1942, the initiative was taken to further organize the structure of the maternity services in the colony, and the nurses of the Child Welfare League were taken over by the government. It was at this point that efforts were made to coordinate a program of education in the area of maternity care in the colony.[49]

One of the main responsibilities of the district nurse in the area of maternity work was to organize and conduct antenatal clinics for women. In the beginning of the century, little thought was given to antenatal care. In most countries, antenatal care was absent from maternity services and only appeared as a late development of the infant welfare movement.[50] This pattern was clearly seen in Trinidad and Tobago through the work of the Child Welfare League, which took responsibility for these endeavours. Hilary Marland asserts that it was only after the 1940s that there was growth in global interest in antenatal clinics.[51] In Trinidad, however, the first organized clinic established to deal specifically with maternity needs, was opened as early as 1918 in an effort to reduce the high infant mortality rates of the time. The responsibility for this was later transferred to the Child Welfare League, which was operating twenty-three clinic centres throughout the colony by 1938.[52] Had it not been for the efforts of this League, however, Trinidad and Tobago would have followed this international trend closely, as it was only after the Second World War that there was an acceleration in the government's antenatal programs, not surprisingly led by the nurses formerly of the League. Clinics were conducted by the district nurse in charge of each area. In the clinic, this nurse had an opportunity to meet with expectant mothers and assist the medical officer in his routine examination. Her other duties, as laid out by the Health Department, included urine testing; providing advice on personal hygiene, diet, and preparation for delivery; and assisting in supervision of midwives.[53] These clinics became increasingly popular; attendance grew from around 4,000 women in 1939 to 120,000 by the early 1960s.[54] This steady increase over the period indicates the growing awareness of the importance of proper care during pregnancy, and reflected the success of the movement to educate women around the country in the post-war era.

In conjunction with the rise of clinics in the 1940s and 1950s, health education was increasingly used as a distinctive part of the maternal health program. As advances in technology, specialized training of personnel, and greater expenditure in this area allowed for the increased dissemination of information using mobile cinema units, health visitors, with the assistance of occasional experts and volunteers in the health field, moved into areas of Trinidad and Tobago to conduct educational sessions.[55] In 1941, a superintendent of Maternity and Child Welfare Services was appointed to institute a program of education throughout the colony.[56] During the 1940s, "mothercraft" classes and practical demonstrations were held in health offices and community centres across the two islands; district nurses and health visitors instructed senior secondary school girls throughout the colony, including Tobago, at the request of head teachers. These classes focused on the care of mothers and babies, preparation for delivery, outfitting the home with proper equipment for delivery, and ensuring that young women understood the responsibility of caring for a home and child. In the 1950s, breastfeeding was increasingly emphasized, in opposition to the global trend which saw artificial feeding promoted, a practice that many mothers in this area were probably unable to afford.[57] Health exhibitions, such as the one in 1948 in Port of Spain, Princes Town (southwest), and Sangre Grande (northeast), and a display in Tobago, were prime opportunities to spread the message of proper care and good health to women.[58] As a consequence of these improved practices, the extension of services, and no doubt the introduction of new drugs in the 1940s, the maternal mortality rate continued to decline from 6.1 per 1,000 to under 2 per 1,000 by the period of independence,[59] a rate that had sadly already been reached by more developed countries by 1940.[60]

THE CONTROL OF MIDWIVES

Midwives were the first and main group to be targeted in most societies in the battle against high infant mortality rates and maternal deaths, and the twentieth century saw the culmination of the controversies surrounding these health practitioners. The post-war period in Trinidad and Tobago saw an emphasis being placed on regulating midwives outside the official system. Government midwives or maternity nurses were typically trained at the colonial hospitals in a course undertaken in the fourth and last year of a nurse's training period. These nurses, particularly those sent to district hospitals, were the backbone of the official maternity service, and the only means of expanding the official system into rural areas. In addition to conducting clinics, they visited different communities to perform check-ups and evaluations on pregnant women (antenatal care), deliver newborns, and counsel new mothers. Therefore, as district facilities grew, there was a commensurate development of maternity services throughout the colony.

In various European countries after the 1930s, many unregistered midwives "sought to move into public health work themselves and were actively encouraged in this by legislators and medical reformers."[61] Similarly, by 1948, the government of Trinidad and Tobago, with an insufficient number of midwives to deal with the increasing number of births (birth rate at 40.25 per 1,000 women), opened its official doors to midwives involved in private practice.[62] Those who were licensed but not in the government service could attend to maternity cases referred to them from antenatal clinics across the country (initially in Success Village, Carenage, Gasparillo, and Fyzabad). These midwives were usually employed in areas not covered by the district nurses. By the early 1960s, the number had more than tripled (from seven in 1948 to twenty-three in 1960), and they dealt with 1,944 deliveries, as compared to 437 in 1950.[63] These nurses, contracted outside the official service, assisted greatly throughout the years in reducing the number of maternal and infant deaths by partially filling the need for qualified midwives in the communities.

Despite the yearly increases in nurses and the new schemes to train and contract midwives, a large proportion of expectant mothers within the colony, through necessity or refusal to abandon traditional ways, relied on midwives who had no formal training or qualifications to assist them during their pregnancy. These women, referred to at the time as 'handywomen', performed thousands of deliveries each year. These were average women who had taught themselves through experience or who had been instructed by former handywomen, usually a female relative. The medical officials of the time saw the operation of handywomen in communities as a grave problem not only because it resulted in inaccurate registration of births and mortality rates, but also because of the additional risk to mothers and infants through improper techniques and poor hygiene habits. Irvine Loudon suggests that the blanket dismissal of these types of midwives as "'relics of barbarism'" was unfair, as they often enjoyed success in their work; however, he insists that the training of the unofficial midwife was important.[64] It is vital to note that, even in the midst of the official controversies, nurses "on the district" in Trinidad and Tobago recognized the importance of the handywoman to the community and thus the need to work alongside her to gain the mother's trust and ensure the mother's health in an era when the handywoman was more trusted than the government nurse.[65] Nurse Sheila Proctor, assigned to the Maraval District in 1956, remarked that "you worked with them because you knew as soon as you left the mother would turn to these women and do whatever they wanted to do anyway."[66]

By 1953, despite the efforts of the health officials, the majority of births in the colony were still being delivered by handywomen (13,904, compared to 11,661 by official midwives).[67] The successful business of these women was a clear indication of a void within the official service and proved that in many poor, rural communities in the colony, birth and maternal survival continued to depend on the traditional village handywoman.

GOVERNMENT NURSES

In the first half of the twentieth century in Trinidad and Tobago, women within the official health service continued to hold mainly secondary positions. Female candidates for the position of medical doctor were unusual, and the roles for women were generally limited to the nursing service. The highest grade within the service was the post of matron, and there was typically one per hospital. These women were usually of European descent and acted as the heads of the nursing department and the nurse training school. Their subordinates were senior nursing sisters, and below them were ward sisters, who were in charge of different wards within the hospital. The staff nurses (district nurses were chosen from this group) made up the body of trained nurses, but by far, the largest group consisted of student nurses. In the Port of Spain Colonial Hospital in 1943, there were 11 senior nursing sisters, 21 ward sisters, 70 staff nurses, and 136 student nurses.[68] This compared favourably with other hospitals in the region, such as the Kingston Public Hospital in Jamaica and the Georgetown Public Hospital in British Guiana, where there were 150 and 105 student nurses, respectively.[69] So at any given time within a British West Indian hospital, there were by far more student nurses attending to patients than trained ones. Nurses, always at the core of the health-care system, may not have been principal players in the hospital hierarchy, but they made up the majority of the working staff and were the most involved with patient contact.

A 1957 commission, the Julian Commission set up by the Trinidad and Tobago Government to investigate the conditions at the Port of Spain Hospital "among doctors, nurses and all other grades of staff . . ." and conducted by Inskip Julian, reported that:

> the shortage of nursing staff is perhaps the most tremendous single problem of the medical and health service. The available staff is overworked. The long exhausting hours under depressing conditions necessarily lead to physical and mental fatigue with resultant loss of concentration and falling off in efficiency. The situation is aggravated by the chronic over-crowding of the wards and the lack of suitable nursing apparatus, supplies and equipment.[70]

This description encapsulates the experience of the nurses during the 1940s and 1950s. Difficulties in attracting and retaining nurses within the health system continued throughout the period because of these issues. At no point between the Second World War and independence was there a full complement of nurses in Trinidad and Tobago, and the medical reports of the time frequently expressed distress at the number of vacant nursing positions. Nonetheless, with the expansion of services throughout the period, especially the district service, the Health Department continued to increase the number of positions annually, for example, in the district system, where between 1951 and 1960, the number of positions more than doubled (from twenty-five to fifty-three).[71] However retention and attraction difficulties remained, and this expansion, though necessary, further emphasized the problems in the nursing service, notably inadequate conditions, poor accommodation, and little pay. By 1961, there were still twenty-five vacancies in the district service.[72]

Two commissions in the late 1930s and early 1940s brought official focus to the problem of salaries of government nurses. The Rushcliffe Committee report on the conditions of service for hospital nurses in England—which highlighted major discrepancies of salary scales—and the dissatisfaction of the nurses voiced during the West India Royal Commission (Moyne Commission) interviews of 1939, compelled the Health Department of Trinidad and Tobago to revise the emoluments of nurses.[73] It must be noted, however, that during the 1940s, compared to other West Indian colonies (in particular Jamaica, Antigua, and British Guiana), the pay scale of the local nurse was between 100 and 1000 British West Indian dollars, with salaries increasing along the scale depending on the rank of said nurse.[74] However, this did not reflect well on the Trinidadian pay scale, and simply underscored the awful plight of other West Indian nurses at that time. Beyond the period of independence, salary issues continued to be a major point of contention between nurses and health authorities in the colony of Trinidad and Tobago.

Not only was retention a problem, but the quality of young women entering the service was frequently questioned by health authorities; initiatives were taken to encourage better educated females to apply and to improve the training provided. Unlike their male superiors—medical doctors—nurses' training mainly took place locally. Young women between the ages of 18 and 25 were trained at the colonial hospitals in Port of Spain, San Fernando, and Tobago under the mentorship of a matron, usually a European sister. The student nurse had to undergo three years of general training and a fourth year for midwifery. After completion of this course of study (theoretical and practical), she would be required to take an exam to qualify for the Government Nursing Certificate. The nurses being trained at the Scarborough Colonial Hospital in Tobago spent their last two years of training at the Port of Spain Colonial Hospital, as it was felt that this hospital possessed the best equipment and training facilities and dealt with the largest population.

The quality of training was hampered by the insufficient number of sister tutors, which resulted in less time devoted to the training of student nurses who were usually thrown into practical work before being properly instructed. This is reflected in the 1957 Julian Report, which identified student nurses as the group most affected by the inadequacies in the provisions for nurses. The Report stated that "it seemed quite impossible for them to find time to devote to serious study under these conditions or to gain the fullest advantage of their theoretical instruction from practical demonstrations."[75]

Occasionally, there were opportunities for training at London institutions such as the four-year course offered to eighteen West Indian candidates in 1944 by the London County Council Hospitals, of which four girls were chosen from Trinidad.[76] But these opportunities were few and usually biased toward urban student nurses. A report by M. Houghton in 1953 further revealed that "many of the girls who had been given scholarships to undertake training in the United Kingdom either did not return to their own county on completion of training . . . [or] considered they should be given immediate promotion to a senior post" upon their return.[77]

The involvement of foreigners in the nursing service was also an area of contention for many local nurses, particularly with the issues of ethnic discrimination arising out of the post-World War I era, which also impacted the working class movements of the turbulent 1930s and coloured the movement toward independence in the 1940s and 1950s. As a result of drives by organizations such as the Overseas Nursing Association[78] in the early part of the century, hundreds of British-trained nurses entered into service in the colonies and were seen, according to Anne Marie Rafferty, as "crucial to the success of government hospitals throughout the 'Empire.'"[79] These European nurses held superior positions as sisters and matrons and were responsible for training the local student nurses. In 1939, while being interviewed by the Moyne Commission, Avis Metivier, a local nurse of some experience, revealed that "certain seniors posts were open only to overseas nurses," and that though local nurses were promoted to the position of nursing sisters (prior to the Medical Reorganisation Committee of 1933, this was uncommon), they were not allowed to wear the sister's uniform, carry out administrative work, or be referred to as "Sister," instead being called "Charge Nurse."[80] By the 1950s, this was slowly changing with the increasing incorporation of local nurses of experience to superior positions, including teaching posts. The account of Nurse Proctor, who entered the service in 1951, shows that the influence of foreign nurses remained strong, however, even in the run-up to independence:

> When I went in hospital the matron was from England, my sister tutor was from England. The eye ward departmental sister, that was a special thing, she was from England. And there was one other lady who I can't remember. So that our training . . . we had local tutors . . . but she (English) was the lady in charge of the training. They were beginning to train local tutors there (Port of Spain General Hospital). Valerie Foster, was one of the [local] tutors, she worked with us in the field but our main tutor was Mrs. Helen Middlecombe-Webb from England. So we were trained very much along de English system sometimes I think that we were more English than the English themselves.[81]

To alleviate the personnel problems in the nursing service, the health authorities at the time developed initiatives to entice foreign nurses or West Indian nurses living abroad to the colony to work. In 1960, for instance, two officers were sent to the United Kingdom to recruit West Indian nurses for service in the territory with satisfactory results.[82] Though efforts were made to incorporate more local women into higher grades of nursing, the ugly problem of preferential treatment of foreigners continued to plague the system. This struggle was reflective of the larger struggle taking place in the West Indies in the 1950s and 1960s between the colonies and their imperial masters, a battle that would be won in the political arena by Trinidad and Tobago in 1962.

A problem that continually beset the health authorities was inadequate housing for nurses, both for those stationed at government hospitals and district health facilities. Fortunately, the immediate post-war period saw improvements in this area, with nurses at the colonial hospitals being housed in hostels built by the government either on or near hospital premises. The Nurses Home at the Port of Spain Colonial Hospital, situated adjacent to the hospital, provided accommodation for approximately 250 residents. A nurses' hostel was also opened in March 1948 in San Fernando.[83] Accommodations for district nurses were dire when compared to those at the colonial hospitals, and the district nurses were usually also separated from their families and located in isolated areas. They were forced many times to find their own housing within their respective communities, but as the 1950s emerged, more attention was placed on providing proper housing for district nurses. New quarters, for instance, were constructed in areas such as in Moruga (in south Trinidad) in 1961,[84] and by 1961–1962, there were forty-six special quarters available around the colony for district nurses.[85] Inadequate nursing accommodations, however, remained a pressing issue for authorities throughout the 1940s and 1950s. Thus, for the district nurse, time and effort tended to be wasted on adjusting to a system that did not provide adequate "housing . . . clerical assistance . . . travelling allowances, telephones and other amenities," and this obviously affected their performance in their communities.[86]

Nonetheless, district nurses were usually well known in the district and respected. To be a good one, according to Enid Henry, a retired nurse who was stationed in Carenage and Sangre Grande—northwest and northeast Trinidad, respectively—and in Tobago in the 1940s and 1950s, one had to become part of the community to be trusted and welcomed into the homes of maternity cases and sick persons.[87] Another retired district nurse and matron of Port of Spain Colonial Hospital, Joycelyn Taitt, explained that, "nurses were highly regarded for their sense of duty both in the community and in the Hospital."[88] With inadequate numbers and poor accommodations, facilities, and equipment, the support of the community was extremely important to the effective functioning of the district nurse.

Despite the advances made for nurses in particular areas throughout the period, their progress was impeded time and again by administrative (personnel, salary, and accommodation) or ethnic issues. In the pre-independence period, the nurse remained an important part of the health-care scene, though she was treated in many ways with less dignity than her station deserved.

INFORMAL CAREGIVERS

As previously discussed, women's participation in health care outside of the official services was of paramount importance to the total well-being of the colony. If women within the service traditionally held secondary positions, those in the home were the primary caregivers to their families.

Lewis echoes this idea, as she itemized women's general function and significance in the home in the first half of the twentieth century as:

> informal health providers involving the provision of materially secure environment (including cleanliness and good diet), nursing the sick, teaching about health, mediating with outsiders (health visitors, social workers and doctors) and coping with health crises.[89]

Increasingly, throughout the British Empire in the first half of the twentieth century, the role of the female in the provision of health care in the home gained significance in official eyes. In Colonial Malaya, for instance, there was growing importance placed on preventive health programs, with an emphasis on health centres, nutrition, and "preventive health measures that could be undertaken domestically against disease such as malaria, tuberculosis and hookworm," and these campaigns focused on the education and instruction of women.[90] As seen through maternity work, this was also the reality of women in Trinidad and Tobago. However, it was not only these new methods of health care, but the persistence of traditional methods that kept the woman at the helm of health provision in the home and on the frontline of the unofficial system.

Throughout the West Indies, folk and herbal medicines have been traditionally used to deal with the prevention and cure of diseases. Rooted often in religious and cultural beliefs of the African, European, Indian, and indigenous Caribbean people, many of these practices evolved and were diluted by time and the more modern western medical traditions, making them easier to incorporate into the lives of the inhabitants of the colonies. In his work on Afro-Caribbean folk medicine, Michel Laguerre outlines the three ways in which this type of medical knowledge was passed on: "(1) collective or community practises, (2) family practices and (3) individual healer practices."[91] I propose here that the area of "family practises" was governed by women. Laguerre, using examples from Jamaica, Barbados, and urban dwellers in the Dominican Republic, explained that as traditions became more cemented in the family and "preserved recipes were handed on by parents," it became less necessary to call on folk healers.[92] Thus, in these areas it was left mainly to women, the 'recipe keepers' and healers in the home, to continue these traditional practices.

As such, herbal and alternative medicines, or bush medicines as they were locally known, were the first choice of most inhabitants of Trinidad and Tobago when attempting to cure an ailment; attending the hospital and visiting private doctors was typically the last resort. In the rural communities, where facilities and medical personnel were at a minimum or were totally absent, the females in the household—mothers, grandmothers and other female relatives—were well versed and practiced in the art of bush medicine, and used these methods to cure the sick and deal with maternity issues.[93] Edna Goodial of Cunupia in Central Trinidad, for instance, recalls her mother caring for her when she suffered from periodic outbreaks of sores (probably from yaws) and the common cold in her childhood in the 1950s:

> my mother used to boil fever grass, she used to put the yellow black sage leaf, and if you have cough, if coughing she boil a bush they call carpenter bush, she boil something they call chadon beni root, she pound it and she boil all this bush with the fever grass and whether you wanted to drink or not you had to drink it, you can't say no.[94]

Eileen Craig, resident of San Fernando, and Pearl Brereton of Port of Spain both describe the frequent use of other herbs, such as shining bush, chandelier, and, in particular, aloe vera, by their mothers for minor and severe illness, cuts, and bruises.[95]

The use of these types of medicines was common even in urban areas, where land was limited and 'bushes' were sold by bush sellers who cultivated them in Diego Martin and Maraval in the north, or grew them in an oil drum herbal garden.[96] The health authorities of Trinidad and Tobago recognized this and targeted women in their health education drives, encouraging them to attend workshops and film shows, as they believed that to educate the woman, the primary caregiver in the society, was to incalculably advance the health of the family and thus the colony.[97]

CONCLUSION

The poor social conditions—inadequate, untreated water supplies, problematic, primitive sewage disposal, and poor sanitation—all negatively affected women in particular because of their roles in society, professionally or personally (for instance, as cooks, washerwomen, and cleaners). The deterioration of their health due to war further emphasized their particular susceptibility to disease and general ill health under poor living conditions. At the beginning of World War II, health provisions for women, maternity programs in particular, were partially established and run mainly by a female volunteer organization. The developments in this area reflected the growing importance placed on female health care within the colony as the increase in the number of clinics and midwives contributed significantly to the reduction of the maternal mortality rate. Nonetheless, women, along with children and the elderly, were the most at risk in the society. Although this period could be considered one of the most progressive in the history of the colony, women remained vulnerable, further emphasising their plight as victims of poor health care.

Conversely, it has been demonstrated through this investigation that female workers were the backbone of health care within the local society. Nurses employed by the Health Department were involved in all aspects of public health, from working within formal medical institutions to personally administering to the sick in communities throughout the islands. And though there were general attempts at improvements in the 1940s and 1950s in terms of accommodation, salaries, and training, more needed to be accomplished before their working conditions could be deemed adequate. Under these circumstances, their accomplishments in the institutions and the community were even more impressive.

The impact of the informal sector on the operation of health care was diverse. The area of maternity care, more than any other, saw the results both negative and positive of the move toward professionalization that marked the pre-independence period. Handywomen (unlicensed midwives), through assisting in their communities, contributed to the high rate of maternal mortality and to problems in regulating medical care and births. The attempts by the authorities (often unsuccessful) to curb their influence saw the increasing professionalization of the midwife. However, the handywomen's work and the work of female organizations, such as the Red Cross Brigade during World War II and the Child Welfare League, which operated in conjunction with the established health service, were successful in bridging the gap between the colony's health services and the poor and rural communities.

Women in the home were the first line of care, and their initial command of herbal medicinal practices coupled with the increasing knowledge gained through health education contributed greatly to the lowering of infant and maternal mortality rates and improving the general standard of living. More than any other group in society, women contributed immensely to the development of health care in the colony and the improvement of services for themselves and the colony at large. Their issues reflected the challenges

Table 11.1 Death Rate, Maternal Mortality Rate, and Infant Mortality Rate, Trinidad and Tobago, c. 1928–1958.

Year	Population	Death rate (per 1,000)	Maternal mortality (per 1,000)	Infant mortality (per 1,000)
1928	379,093	19.4	8.0	127.0
1938	464,389	15.82	6.1	98.42
1948	586,700	12.26	3.2*	75.48
1958	788,600	9.2	2.1	62.6

*This was an unnaturally low rate in the 1940s, possibly due to improved efficiency at the Port of Spain hospital in this year. The maternal mortality rate rose again from 1949 to 1950, then continued its downward decline.
Sources: Director of Medical Services, Medical and Sanitary Report of Medical Services 1938 (Port of Spain, Trinidad and Tobago: Government Printing Office, 1939), 14. Director of Medical Services, Medical and Sanitary Report of Government Printing Office, 1949), 7. Director of Medical Services, Medical and Sanitary Report of Medical Services 1958 (Port of Spain, Trinidad and Tobago: Government Printing Office, 1959), 57.[98]

and problems faced by a colonial society in which the need for public health care outstripped the pace of its development. Thus, this study concludes that, in the public health system of Trinidad and Tobago, women occupied an ambiguous space as victims of contemporary diseases and the health-care workers empowered to fight endemic morbidity.

NOTES

1. Inskip Julian, *Julian Commission Report: Report Of The Commission Appointed To Enquire Into The Causes And Consequences Of Dissatisfaction With Conditions Obtaining At The Colonial Hospital Port Of Spain By Personnel Council Paper No. 14 (1957)* (London: Colonial Office [CO], 1958), 121.
2. Central Statistical Office, *Annual Statistical Digest of 1961* (Port of Spain, Trinidad and Tobago: Government Printing Office, 1962).
3. G.W. Roberts, "A Note on Mortality in Jamaica," *Population Studies* 4, no. 1 (Population Investigation Committee, June 1950): 83. Robert claims that during the years 1946–1947, Trinidad and Tobago showed a natural increase of 26.0 one, as compared to Jamaica with a rate of 17.9.
4. Colonial Office Reports, "Medical School" (London: CO, 1945), CO 318/464/6, British National Archives (NA), pp. 8–9.
5. Even by the early 1940s, islands such as Barbados and Antigua possessed one general hospital and no district hospitals.
6. Director of Medical Services of Trinidad and Tobago, *Medical and Sanitary Report of the Medical Services 1939* (Port of Spain, Trinidad and Tobago: Government Printing Office, 1940), 3. Trinidad had benefited from the movement in the mid- to late nineteenth century to establish leprosariums and mental asylums in the British West Indies. Barbados, Guiana, Jamaica, Antigua, Grenada, St Lucia, and St Vincent all possessed accommodations for lepers and mental patients. CO Reports, "Medical School," CO 318/464/6, NA, pp. 8–9.
7. *Medical and Sanitary Report of the Medical Services 1939*.
8. Roy Porter, ed., *Cambridge Illustrated History of Medicine* (Cambridge: Cambridge University Press, 1996), 330.
9. O.C. Wenger, *Caribbean Medical Center: The Organization, Development and Activities of the Caribbean Medical Center at Port of Spain, Trinidad, B.W.I. from February 9, 1943 to March 1, 1945* (Washington, DC: Caribbean Commission, 1946); and Director of Medical Services of Trinidad and Tobago, *Medical and Sanitary Report of the Medical Services 1948* (Port of Spain, Trinidad and Tobago: Government Printing Office, 1949), 11.
10. Peter Rostant, "A Story of the San Fernando Hospital From 1920/1958," *Caribbean Medical Journal* 41 (1980): 31.
11. The mandatory testing of water supplies began effectively in 1946, and chlorinated water, available in Port of Spain alone prior to the War, eventually spread to other areas under the Central Water Authority.
12. Director of Medical Services of Trinidad and Tobago, *Medical and Sanitary Report of the Medical Services 1957* (Port of Spain, Trinidad and Tobago: Government Printing Office, 1958), 24. By 1939, the country was virtually devoid of a proper sewage system except in part of Port of Spain, certain oilfields, and settlements.
13. Interviews conducted with Eileen Craig, 82-year-old female of African descent from San Fernando and Port of Spain (Interviewed at Mt. Hope, 15

June 2007); Edna Goodial, 73-year-old female of Indian descent who resided in Cunupia and St. Helena (Interviewed at St. Helena, 17 July 2007); and Pearl Brereton, 84-year-old female of African descent who resided in Mt. Hope (Interviewed at Mt. Hope, 15 June 2007).

14. Director of Medical Services of Trinidad and Tobago, *Medical and Sanitary Report of the Medical Services 1961* (Port of Spain, Trinidad and Tobago: Government Printing Office, 1962), 7.

15. Ibid.

16. William Santon Gilmour, *Tuberculosis in the West Indies: Interim Report on Sociological and Clinical Survey* (London: The National Association for the Prevention of TB, 1943), 15–16.

17. Director of Medical Services of Trinidad and Tobago, *Medical and Sanitary Report of the Medical Services 1961*, 12. Though this infestation rate remained high, it was an improvement worth highlighting since hookworm affected so many inhabitants of rural Trinidad and Tobago.

18. Ann Bissessar, et al., *The Historical Development of the Health System in Trinidad and Tobago,* Public Health and Policy Departmental Publication No. 34 (London: London School of Hygiene and Tropical Medicine, 2001), 8. It is important to note that degenerative diseases had been the causes of considerable morbidity throughout the early part of the twentieth century, but it was only during the 1950s that heart disease, for instance, overwhelmed the mortality statistics and claimed the position of the principal cause of death in the colony.

19. Medical Officer of Health, *Administrative Report of the Public Health Department of Port of Spain, 1962* (Port of Spain, Trinidad and Tobago: Government Printing Office, 1963), 47. The sites of highest frequency for cancer in women were the stomach, breast, and cervix uteri, in that order.

20. The American military set up bases in Chaguaramas and Wallerfield, Trinidad, in 1941–1942 and thus construction of these bases and access roads and the available civilian positions on bases caused a migration of workers to urban areas throughout the period.

21. Beverley A. Steele, *How Grenada Won World War II,* (Grenada: Grenada Centre, 2002), 9. There were reports of Grenadian citizens "gather[ing] outside shipping offices waiting for the opening hour when they could buy tickets" to travel to Trinidad.

22. Director of Medical Services of Trinidad and Tobago, *Medical and Sanitary Report of the Medical Services 1944* (Port of Spain, Trinidad and Tobago: Government Printing Office, 1945), 4.

23. Michael Anthony, *Port of Spain in a World at War,* vol. 2 (Port of Spain: Ministry of Sport and Culture, 1978), 210.

24. Staff Reporter, "Special Committee to Probe Water Shortage," *Trinidad Guardian,* 1 January 1942, 2.

25. Staff Reporter, "Food Controller Asked to Start Milk Ration Scheme," *Trinidad Guardian,* 23 July 1942, 3.

26. B.S. Platt, *Nutrition in the British West Indies* (Montreal: McGill University, 1944), 1–11.

27. Ibid, 11.

28. *Medical and Sanitary Report of the Medical Services 1946,* 49.

29. Bonham C. Richardson and Joseph L. Scarpaci, "The Quality of Life in the Twentieth Century Caribbean," *General History of the Caribbean Volume 5: The Caribbean in the Twentieth Century,* ed. Bridget Brereton (Paris: UNESCO Publishing, 2004), 659. They reasoned that "infants' health often depends upon among other factors, nutrition of both infants and mothers, family and community literacy and family income. Infant mortality rates

also indicate the quality of medical care, to include prenatal intervention and post delivery check ups."

30. In March 1941, the US military was officially granted permission to open bases in Trinidad, among other places, in an effort to secure the Western hemisphere from German infiltration. Construction had already begun on bases by this time, requiring the employment of hundreds of local workers.

31. *Medical and Sanitary Report of the Medical Services 1944*, 2.

32. "Red Cross Detachment to be Formed," *Trinidad Guardian*, 1 September 1939, 11. The Medical Defence Organisation was the name of the programme that coordinated the response of the official and voluntary organisations to the medical challenges that arose in the colony during the War.

33. "Red Cross Organized," *Trinidad Guardian*, 31 January 1943, 2A.

34. Molly Huggins, *Too Much To Tell, An Autobiography* (London: Heinemann, 1967), 54. Lady Young eventually turned the running of this organization over to Molly Huggins, wife of the Colonial Secretary.

35. Claus Füllberg-Stolberg, "The Caribbean in the Second World War," *General History of the Caribbean Volume 5: The Caribbean in the Twentieth Century*, ed. Bridget Brereton (Paris: UNESCO Publishing, 2004), 100.

36. Huggins, 54.

37. Ibid.

38. Women in the WVS underwent periods of basic first aid training, but no formal nursing training. The British Red Cross required their volunteers to be British-born and hold certificates in First Aid and Home Nursing.

39. *Medical and Sanitary Report of the Medical Services 1941*, 5.

40. *Medical and Sanitary Report of the Medical Services 1941–1961*. Thus, in the early 1940s, pregnant women attending antenatal clinics were required to attend the nearest VD clinic for blood tests. Often, antenatal clinics and VD clinics were not open on the same day, and women had to return on different days. This lowered attendances until 1956, when routine blood tests of all pregnant women were actually done at the antenatal clinic, and abnormal blood samples were referred to the Caribbean Medical Centre Clinics.

41. *Medical and Sanitary Report of the Medical Services 1941*, 11.

42. Colonial Office Reports "Medical School" 1944, 7–9.

43. *Medical and Sanitary Report of the Medical Services 1961*, 40.

44. Ibid.

45. Hilary Marland, "Childbirth and Maternity" in *Medicine in the 20th Century*, eds. Roger Cooter and John Pickstone (Amsterdam: Harwood Academic Press, 2000), 560. In Britain, professional, voluntary, and political organizations, such as the Women's Cooperative Guild, the National Council for Maternity and Child Welfare, and the Labour Party Women's Organisation all contributed to the movement to improve provisions and services in the area of maternity care.

46. R. Seheult, *A Survey of the Trinidad Medical Service, 1814–1944* (Port of Spain, Trinidad and Tobago: Government Printing Office, 1948), 13.

47. Sir Alexander Russell, *Russell Committee Report: A Review of the Medical and Health Policy of the Colony, Council Paper no. 65* (1944), CO 295/636/6, NA, 22.

48. *Medical and Sanitary Report of the Medical Services 1946*, 17. A layette was a complete outfit of clothing and equipment for a newborn.

49. *Medical and Sanitary Report of the Medical Services 1941*, 11.

50. Marland, "Childbirth and Maternity," 563.

51. Ibid.

52. *Medical and Sanitary Report of the Medical Services 1938*, 50.
53. *Medical and Sanitary Report of the Medical Services 1949*, 20.
54. *Medical and Sanitary Report of the Medical Services 1961*, 27.
55. The Mobile Cinema Unit operated throughout the 1940s and 1950s in Trinidad and Tobago.
56. *Medical and Sanitary Report of the Medical Services 1941*, 11.
57. Jacalyn Duffin, *History of Medicine: A Scandalously Short Introduction* (Toronto: University of Toronto Press, 1999), 325–326.
58. *Medical and Sanitary Report of the Medical Services 1948*, 21.
59. *Medical and Sanitary Report of the Medical Services 1928–1961*. Reference made to all reports between these years.
60. Anne Hardy, *Health and Medicine in Britain Since 1860* (New York: Pelgrave, 2001), 105.
61. Hilary Marland and Ann Marie Rafferty, eds., introduction to *Midwives, Society and Childbirth: Debates and Controversies in the Modern Period* (London: Routledge, 1997), 4. They refer to England, Sweden, and Denmark.
62. *Medical and Sanitary Report of the Medical Services 1948*, 7.
63. *Medical and Sanitary Report of the Medical Services 1940–1961*.
64. Irvine Loudon, "Midwives and the Quality of Maternal Care," *Midwives, Society and Childbirth: Debates and Controversies in the Modern Period*, eds. Hilary Marland and Anne Marie Rafferty (London: Routledge, 1997), 181, 196–197.
65. "On the district" was a local phrase used to describe being stationed at one of the district hospitals or health centres.
66. Interview with Nurse Sheila Proctor, 76 years old, from Diego Martin, Trinidad (Diego Martin, 13 August 2007). Nurse Proctor entered the system in 1951, and left as a staff nurse in 1958.
67. *Medical and Sanitary Report of the Medical Services 1953*, 27.
68. Seheult, 14.
69. Frank Stockdale, "Dispatch on Nursing Service in the B.W.I." (Barbados: Development And Welfare Organisation, 23 June 1943), CO 318/455/5, NA.
70. Julian, 21.
71. *Medical and Sanitary Report of the Medical Services 1951* and *1960*.
72. *Medical and Sanitary Report of the Medical Services 1961*, 26.
73. West India Royal Commission: Dr. and Mrs Vivian Metivier, Memorandum of Evidence, 1939 CO 950/769, NA. The West India Royal Commission of 1938–1939 assessed the social and economic conditions in the British West Indies and made recommendations to the Colonial and local governments which were published in full in 1945, after World War II.
74. Stockdale, "Dispatch on Nursing Service in the B.W.I."
75. Julian, 21.
76. *Medical and Sanitary Report of the Medical Services 1944*, 2.
77. Julian, 87. M. Houghton, Education Officer for the General Nursing Council for England and Wales, visited the British West Indies to assess the standards of nurse training in these territories.
78. Brigid Maxwell, "Colonial Nurse," *The American Journal of Nursing* 49, no. 7 (1949): 455.
79. Anne Marie Rafferty, "Nurses," *Medicine in the Twentieth Century*, eds. Roger Cooter and John Pickstone (Amsterdam: Harwood Academic Publishers, 2000), 521.
80. Staff Reporter "Mrs. Metivier Appeals for Equal Opportunities of Promotion For Local Nurses," *Trinidad Guardian*, 16 March 1939, 3.

81. Interview with Nurse Sheila Proctor.
82. *Medical and Sanitary Report of the Medical Services 1960,* 26.
83. Ibid., *1948,* 22.
84. Ibid., *1961,* 27.
85. Ibid.
86. Julian, 31.
87. Interview with Enid Henry, 88-year-old former nurse of African and indigenous Caribbean descent who entered the service in 1933 and was involved in both institutional and district nursing work in Port of Spain, Carenage, Sangre Grande, and Tobago (Interviewed at La Puerta, Diego Martin, Trinidad, October 2004).
88. James Damian Cummings, *Barrack Yard Dwellers* (St. Augustine, Trinidad and Tobago: The University of the West Indies, 2004), 184.
89. Jane Lewis, "Agents of Health Care: The Relationship between Family Professionals and the State in the Mixed Economy of Welfare in Twentieth-Century Britain," *Coping with Sickness: Perspectives on Health Care, Past and Present,* ed. John Woodward and Robert Jütte (Sheffield, UK: European Association for the History of Medicine and Health Publications, 1996), 166. Assessment taken from H. Graham, *Women, Health and the Family* (Brighton, UK: Wheatsheaf Books, 1984), 150–152.
90. Lenore Manderson, *Sickness and the State: Health and Illness in Colonial Malaya, 1970–1940* (Cambridge: Cambridge University Press, 1996), 218.
91. Michel LaGuerre, *Afro-Caribbean Folk Medicine* (South Hadley MA: Bergin and Garvey Publishers, Inc., 1987), 39.
92. Ibid., 42.
93. Julian, 28. The Julian Commission reported that, "in some country districts no nurse is provided and the doctor has to do his own dressing."
94. Interview with Edna Goodial. The bush medicines referred to Fever grass, *Cymbo pozan citrates*; Black Sage (bois noir), *Cordia curassavica Boraginaceae*; Carpenter Bush, *Justicia pectoralis*; Chadon Beni, *Eryngium foetidum*; all were used locally to treat malaria and other fevers.
95. Interview with Eileen Craig and Pearl Brereton. The bush medicines referred to here were Shining Bush, *Peperomia pellucida*; Chandelier Bush, *Leonotio nepetifolia*; Aloe vera, *A. Barbadensis.*
96. Cummings, 60.
97. This was not uncommon. In colonial Malaya, for instance, Lenore Manderson, author of *Health and Illness in Colonial Malaya, 1970–1940,* explains "the extent to which public health education that targeted women reflected their presumed primary role as nurturers and carers of their husband and children."
98. *Medical and Sanitary Report of the Medical Services, 1938,* 14. *Medical and Sanitary Report of the Medical Services, 1948,* 7. *Medical and Sanitary Report of the Medical Services, 1958,* 57.

12 Red Marly Soil

Medicine, Environment, and Bauxite Mining in Modern Jamaica, 1938 to Post-Independence

David McBride

During the early nineteenth century, one European visitor to Jamaica surveyed the land and used the term "red marly soil" to describe some of the mountainous areas. These landscapes turned out to be stretches of bauxite, a naturally occurring material composed of minerals. These minerals include alumina minerals, iron silicon, titanium, phosphorus, zinc, manganese, and quartz. Bauxite and its alumina derivative are used for production of aluminum. In 1942, bauxite mining commenced in Jamaica. Following World War II, the international demand for aluminum grew enormously. Consequently, Jamaica's bauxite production expanded rapidly and, by the 1970s, the nation's annual bauxite output was the largest in the world.[1]

This chapter will argue that bauxite mining produced significant transformations in the Jamaican population's health and environment. However, these far reaching environmental health changes were neither recognized nor confronted directly by the medical research of modern Western nations. In nations like United States and England, a strong tendency to attribute disease patterns in the Caribbean to racial traits and climate discouraged lines of research that would explore disease hazards associated with bauxite mining. Moreover, the foreign-owned mining firms erected highly efficient health centres to protect the health of employees and their families. Therefore, research questions about the larger health effects of mining in Jamaica were of little urgency to North American and European nations.

By contrast, Jamaica's sparse medical and geology community produced a small but significant stream of research and reports that broached the issue of unhealthy environmental exposures. This research suggested that more than racial determinants and tropical climate were behind disease occurrence in largely black, multi-ethnic-populated nations like Jamaica. To recreate critically the medical history of the Caribbean involving the health impact of bauxite mining, it was necessary to apply knowledge from several new subfields in the environmental sciences, especially geo-environmental research, toxicology, and occupational medicine.

BACKGROUND

Bauxite mining had a profound effect on Jamaica's economy and international prominence. One geographer studying Jamaica's mining industries in 1965 wrote that the bauxite industry had done for the nation "in little more than ten years what agricultural exports have been unable to achieve during a period of production for world markets stretching over three centuries".[2] This chapter begins with a brief overview of the origins and mechanics of the industry in Jamaica. Second, it explores the environmental impact of this industry. Third, it profiles Jamaica's medical institutions and health problems. In the fourth section, it demonstrates that, as the nation's bauxite industry expanded, medical studies were emerging by clinical researchers in Jamaica that cast doubt on the tendency to assume black populations were less susceptible to diseases linked to environment and pollution. These diseases included lung diseases and cancers. Finally, the chapter uses specific current-day medical and environmental science to raise issues for future investigation. Overall, this chapter suggests that the modern medical history of the impact of bauxite mining in the nations of the Caribbean region is just beginning to be written.

ORIGINS AND EXPANSION

The start of modern bauxite and alumina production in Jamaica can be traced to 1938. That year, a government agricultural chemist surveyed infertile red soils throughout Jamaica. The surveyor noticed that in the southern parishes of Manchester and St. Elizabeth, the soils had high contents of alumina. Subsequently, government and mining experts in London (at the Imperial Institute) and in Canada made a preliminary estimate that perhaps five to ten million tons of bauxite reserves lie in this region of Jamaica. By 1943, this estimate was raised to 100 million tons, and it rose again in 1953 to 315 million tons. In the late 1940s, US and Canadian companies began to acquire rights to bauxite lands throughout Jamaica from the Crown.[3]

Foreign companies were especially attracted to Jamaica's rich deposits of bauxite ore. Compared to deposits in other countries, Jamaican bauxite could be produced rapidly and on a grand scale. Its bauxite ore is found in karstified limestone and lies close to the surface. It could be found in pockets 10- to 30-feet deep at altitudes of 1,000 to 2,000 feet throughout the middle mountain range. Therefore, mine operators did not need to use any form of blasting or explosives. The mining sites selected by the bauxite–alumina companies depended not only on the ore bodies' richness and closeness to the surface. The sites needed proximity to ports that were to be constructed specifically for shipping the materials. Some of the sites that companies selected were in parishes with large deposits of bauxites:

Manchester, St Ann, St Elizabeth, and Trelawny. Other mining sites for bauxite deposits of lower grade or smaller size were placed in Clarendon, St Catherine, and St James.[4]

The production of aluminum is conducted in three stages. First, the ore must be mined and dried. The bulk of the bauxite industry in Jamaica focused on this stage and the subsequent shipping of the ore to processing centres, chiefly in Canada and the United States. Second, the bauxite is processed into alumina. One large Canadian company eventually built an alumina plant, Alcan's Kirkvine Works, in Manchester and Ewarton. In the final stage, this free-flowing, white powder substance is reduced to aluminum. The last two stages must be conducted in complex technical plants that necessitate large supplies of electrical power.[5]

Three large companies mined Jamaica's bauxite—Kaiser and Reynolds (both US companies) and Alcan. A fourth firm, the Aluminum Company (US), emerged in 1964. By 1972, there were six companies mining bauxite in Jamaica. In general, these companies headquartered the processing plants for alumina and aluminum in their countries. The US companies shipped their bauxite materials to refineries in Baton Rouge, Louisiana, and Corpus Christi, Texas, while Alcan refined some of their bauxite in Kirkvine, shipping the alumina to aluminum smelters in Canada, Scandinavia, and other foreign points.[6]

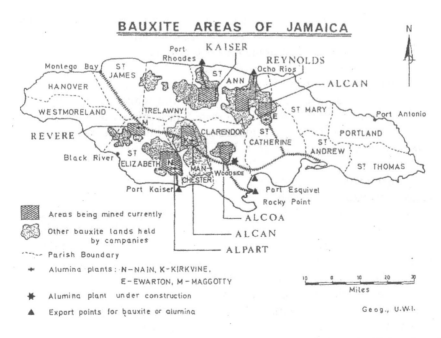

Figure 12.1 Jamaica's bauxite areas as depicted by researchers at the University of the West Indies (1987).

As aluminum gained wider use throughout the industrial nations, the expansion and concomitant domestic economic and social impact of bauxite mining in Jamaica became enormous. Before 1957, sugar, rum, and molasses were Jamaica's largest domestic exports. Within a decade, bauxite and alumina combined comprised 49 percent of the nation's domestic exports compared to the sugar, rum, and molasses that accounted for just 22 percent. Also, the government of Jamaica received nearly 14 percent of its revenues from royalties and taxes earned from bauxite and alumina.[7]

ENVIRONMENT AND LABOUR: THE INDUSTRIAL IMPACT

Bauxite and alumina mining and production brought fundamental changes to Jamaica's regional countrysides, cities, and ports. Dragline and shovel excavators were used to scoop up the ore from the surface. The rocky material was then loaded into various machinery, including tractor scrapers, bulldozers, rippers, and rear dump trucks. At some of the plants, in the early years of their operation, the ore was shunted onto railroad cars via canvas spout equipment. In later years, aerial ropeways conveyed ore-laden steel buckets. The railroads then brought the ore to ports, where workers unloaded it with forklift trucks, and stacked and stored it. Next, the materials were loaded onto ships by handlers using mechanical equipment.[8]

An additional chain of industrial processes occurred in the plants in Jamaica that converted the raw bauxite into alumina. These plants were complex arrangements of storage tanks, heavy machinery, and large buildings that, as one geologists stated, "cover . . . a very wide area, and are a dominant feature of the landscape for miles around". Most visible are precipitation tanks measuring 120 feet tall and with the capacity to hold 250,000 gallons of alumina in solution. These plants also have "stacks emitting vapour from [the] 270 foot long rotary oil-fired kilns" that operate at temperatures as high as 2,000 °F.[9]

Writing in the 1970s, a local geology professor, Barry Floyd, described the environmental changes bauxite–alumina caused to local environments adjacent to bauxite production sites. Floyd was the head of the Geology Department (from 1966 to 1972) at the University of the West Indies. "Visual evidence of bauxite mining, processing and shipping activities is all too obvious in those areas of Jamaica where the industry is established", he wrote. Describing the "environmental price" for the industry presence, Floyd stated: "Deep-red gashes on interior landscapes indicate the opencast mines, and provide a vivid contrast to the green, densely-wooded hills in surrounding limestone country . . .". The excavation and transportation of bauxite materials left behind "[c]llouds of red dust . . . and a fine layering of red covers much of the scene, spreading far downwind". Finally, there prevails "a distinct, acrid smell of bauxite dust in the air".[10]

The labour hierarchy performing the surface mining, processing, loading, and transporting of bauxite and alumina was a small, stable employee sector. The total number of workers at all plants combined in 1967 was an estimated 5,000–7,000 employees. These workers comprised only about 1 percent of Jamaica's total labour supply, and earned about 3 percent of the national wages and salaries.[11] Their occupations included process operators, drivers, mechanics, electricians, welders, plumbers, painters, heavy-duty equipment operators, and unskilled labour. Moreover, each company provided their employees with medical services at the company health centres. Bauxite mine workers in Jamaica benefited from union membership. The bauxite companies made agreements with unions that made wages for their employees among the highest in the nation. The bauxite companies found that working closely with certain unions in Jamaica's contentious political environment proved the best means to sustain high employee productivity. Unions also provided both management and employees in the bauxite companies an organized grievance mechanism.[12]

Jobs in the bauxite industry were highly paid and long-term for both the expatriate and local employees. The health facilities that the bauxite companies set up and operated assured a high level of worker satisfaction and health at the plants. The health centres served both employees and their families, and some developed supportive ties with Jamaican medical institutions. While the health conditions and medical care for company employees in the plants were carefully attended to throughout the bauxite companies' production sites, the island's general population and ecology encountered environmental impacts from the industry's expansion. Eventually, the human health effects of these industrial enclaves were not a priority for the nation's health-care institutions to track, much less to try to prevent. This indisposition to take own environmental and occupational health problems linked to the bauxite industry has two key explanatory factors. One has to do with the unsophisticated stage that medical specialties relating to occupational health and environmental epidemiology were in at the mid-twentieth century. The second concerns the organizational character of institutional medicine in Jamaica during the decades immediately preceding and following independence. Hospitals, physicians, and public health measures to promote colonial commerce were the major foci prior to independence, and medical modernization and primary health care were concerns after independence. We look at both of these factors in the subsequent section.

JAMAICAN MEDICAL INSTITUTIONS CONFRONT NATIONAL AND INDUSTRIAL GROWTH

From the beginning of the twentieth century through World War II, medical institutions in Jamaica were formed primarily as part of the tropical medicine movement that British authorities and operations initiated throughout Britain's colonies in Africa and Asia. During this era, Jamaica was an international trade centre vital to the British Commonwealth. As such, medical and public health affairs critical to the commercial production process on the island were a persistent concern to British authorities and its international business partners.

The relationship between British medical involvement in Jamaica and Britain's commercial expansionism is exemplified by events in 1908. That year, bubonic plague broke out in Kingston, a key port city for shipments to the Americas and Western European countries. The next year, the School of Tropical Medicine of Liverpool sent an expedition to conduct a survey of health in Jamaica.[13] In subsequent decades. numerous other diseases became the focus of special scientific research bodies organized by British research institutes or government commissions.[14] During the mid-twentieth century Britain devised a substantial network of colonial medical resources throughout its colonies that included a number of hospitals of high standards, staffed by well-trained physicians and nurses. Initially these institutions were largely centred on research laboratories for the investigation of epidemic diseases that were critical problems for colonial and commercial affairs throughout Africa and Asia. These diseases included sleeping sickness, malaria, yaws, filariasis, and other specific bacterial infections.

As colonial commercial interests of Britain, other European nations, and the United States transformed into a strategic need to expand economic development throughout their respective tropical holdings, major academic medical centres of these nations broadened their roles to foster public health and medical care for local and national populations. Also, there was growing awareness throughout the field of tropical medicine that poor diets contributed to infectious disease susceptibility among local populations. Therefore, the search for chemotherapies for tropical infectious diseases, as well as for methods for reducing nutritional disorders among local populations, encouraged Britain to expand its public health resources throughout its colonies, Jamaica included. [15]

In 1948, Britain established a medical school in Jamaica, the University College of the West Indies. Later (in 1967) this Faculty of Medical Sciences became the initial component of the University of the West Indies. Organized under the auspices of the University of London, the medical school graduated twenty-five physicians annually, who were then employed throughout Jamaica and the other Commonwealth Caribbean islands. By 1952, Jamaica was divided into forty-five medical districts, each with its own medical officer and central dispensary. The nation had thirty-one hospitals, some staffed by well-trained physicians, surgeons, nurses, and allied personnel. Kingston and the University of the West Indies were the sites of two large hospitals, one a university hospital. Also, that year there were 270 licensed physicians and surgeons, a tuberculosis hospital (in Slipe Road), and a chest clinic in operation since 1928. Jamaica also had an assortment of nursing homes and private physician practices. The government regulated midwives beginning in 1942. Given its recurrent encounters with epidemics in its history as a nation of slavery and international commerce, Jamaica's health authorities also were well versed in quarantine regulations and operations.[16]

During the 1940s and 1950s, the Jamaican population began to rise rapidly, and so did life expectancy. As a result, hospitals, clinics, physicians, and trained health personnel became inadequate for the primary health-care needs of this burgeoning population. For example, the physician pool was poorly distributed, with far too few of these professionals practicing in the nation's rural parishes. A study conducted by the International Bank for Reconstruction and Development in 1952 found that the leading causes of mortality in Jamaica were infectious diseases that were waning in modern nations. Pulmonary tuberculosis, syphilis, enteritis, malaria, and diarrhoea were still serious problems in Jamaica. The physician-to-population ratio was 1 to 4,000, and there were less than two general hospital beds per 1,000 citizens. The number of Jamaican hospitals was a respectable figure compared to other developing nations. However, on the whole, the hospitals were overcrowded and "still far below the requirements specified as desirable by professional bodies".[17]

After Jamaica gained independence, its specialized medical resources for disease control and nutritional problems were largely retained. In fact, medical research emanating from Jamaica after independence contributed to broader recognition that chronic diseases afflicted blacks and whites equally, regardless of the idea widely held in medicine that racial differences were behind the international disparities in chronic disease rates of blacks and whites. Noteworthy was the Tropical Metabolism Research Unit at the University College (later University) of the West Indies in Kingston. This centre was established by the Medical Research Council (MRC) of Britain in 1955. Throughout its first decades of operation, Unit researchers studied not only nutrition and infectious diseases, but also other health problems of rural and developing populations, such as heart disease, blood pressure, and diabetes.[18]

Pockets of highly competent clinical specialists could be found throughout hospitals, clinics, and public health agencies in Jamaica through the 1960s and early 1970s. However, the health-care system as a whole struggled to meet the medical needs of the rapidly growing rural and urban populations throughout Jamaica, including those communities affected by the spreading bauxite industry. By 1965, Jamaica had only 467 licensed physicians serving a national population of nearly two million. More than two-thirds of these practitioners were located in the metropolitan area of Kingston and St Andrew. This area had a ratio of practitioners to population of 1 to 1,600. However, throughout the rest of Jamaica, where 62 percent of the nation's population lived, the ratio of physicians to population was 1 to 16,000. In the rural parish of St Elizabeth, its 130,000 residents had only 8 physicians. The parish's government hospitals were insufficiently equipped and staffed.[19] Moreover, by the end of the 1960s, there was a serious problem of "brain drain" of Jamaican doctors and nurses emigrating from Jamaica.[20]

The thinly distributed supply of government and charity-sponsored physician- and hospital resources throughout Jamaica contrasted with the effective health-care centres at the bauxite–alumina company sites. The Kaiser Bauxite plant in Discovery Bay near the north coast, for example, provided top-notch medical care for its employees and their families. At this production site, Kaiser's medical building housed modern examination, surgery, and X-ray rooms, a laboratory, pharmacy, therapy equipment, and a laundry. Its staff of eight was headed by a full-time physician (medical director), and provided medical service to some 1,000 employees and their families. Medical service was available equally for both administrative and process worker personnel. In addition, the medical centre conducted vigilant preventive care, including screenings and immunizations for infectious diseases for both the employees and their families, particularly those workers involved in the shipping lines. The medical centre also promoted health through education and household hygiene initiatives.[21]

The Kaiser plant in the rural parish of St Elizabeth included buildings for bauxite mining and alumina processing. In its initial year, the company planned and implemented a medical centre for some 180 North American employees and their families. This centre also served other local plant employees, as well as 5,000 construction workers building various aspects of the plants and its roadways throughout St Elizabeth. The health centre provided the same services as the facilities at Kaiser Bauxite. However, the St Elizabeth centre also linked its personnel to local hospitals and health centres in Mandeville and Junction. Personnel from St Elizabeth served as affiliated specialists and medical teachers and reached into the larger community in support of the Jamaican government's hospital and public health initiatives.[22]

When bauxite mining began expanding in Jamaica, the nation's medical care institutions were not prepared to confront the industry's health impacts. By contrast, in developed nations, awareness among public health authorities and physicians that environmental pollution had significant and clinically measurable health effects was spreading. Fields such as occupational medicine, environment epidemiology, and toxicology began to equip these professionals to identify and attempt to reduce diseases, such as industrial lung diseases and occupational cancers. [23]

Despite shortcomings in providing public health and medical resources for major segments of Jamaican society, the research physicians and other specialists affiliated with the University of the West Indies or hospitals regularly contributed clinical articles and medical reports to major international journals. In the developed nations, many of the critical epidemiological and disease issues of the times—especially malaria, tuberculosis, yaws, and cancers—appeared to have a racial and climatic causal component. Thus, tropical medicine and disease research institutions located in the modern West considered studies originating from Jamaica and other parts of the Caribbean valuable.[24]

MEDICAL RESEARCH, RACE, AND THE CHANGING HEALTH ENVIRONMENT

In the decades following World War II, the influence of environmental pollution on disease in Jamaica and other developing nations received little consideration in Western medical research circles. As mentioned, specialty research relating to health effects of non-pathogenic exposures was still in its infancy and instead, a racialist paradigm dominated medical circles in Great Britain and the United States. This loose theoretical assumption emphasized that black racial traits tended to either protect black populations from the physiological effects of exposure to environmental toxins, or made these populations abnormally susceptible. The racialist paradigm was widely evident in the research published on lung diseases and cancers. During the 1960s, a growing interest in chronic lung disease emerged throughout the medical research sector of developed countries. Newer laboratory and clinical techniques for studying the physiology and morphology of lung disease were developed. Furthermore, the medical profession was becoming increasingly aware of the respiratory problems associated with cigarette smoking and heavy industry.[25]

However, most medical experts in developed nations believed that tropical nations like Jamaica had neither the cold, wet climates nor the industrial pollution that were the preconditions for environmentally induced respiratory disease. Moreover, the idea was still widespread throughout medical circles that the anatomical characteristics of the lungs of blacks or Negroes, wherever located geographically, were healthy for avoiding many respiratory disorders and diseases.[26]

In 1962, the prestigious *Journal of the American Medical Association* published a study supported by the US Public Health Service, "Is Emphysema a Disease Predominantly of the White Male?" The study answered this question in the affirmative. It was conducted by a group of research physicians connected with a US Veterans Administration (VA) hospital and medical school in the Washington, DC, area. The researchers collected patient data from three sources: a VA hospital, a large local public hospital, and records of discharged patients treated at all the nation's VA hospitals nationally. All three data sets had substantial proportions of black patients. According to their findings, the researchers reported, "the difference in incidence of emphysema between white and Negro is great". They pointed out that many variables influence emphysema rates, including "environmental exposure" and "smoking history". However, in their view, measurable variation in bronchial glands and secretions between the races most likely was the key to the racial differences in emphysema rates established in their study. The researchers cited another medical finding concerning children that bolstered their confidence in their judgment about racial differences in adult emphysema: "the strikingly greater incidence of mucoviscididosis in white than in Negro children".[27]

Also typical of medical interpretations that stressed racialism was a 1969 study in the respected journal *Thorax* titled "Bronchial Carcinoma in a Young Negro". The London researchers presented a case they considered unique—an occurrence of bronchial cancer in a 27-year-old Nigerian law student living in London. The purpose of their report was to highlight the broader, international implications of this case. The researchers asserted that bronchial cancer "is apparently rare in the native African, [however] it is much more common in the American of Negro stock". They gave two factors for the rates in American Negroes—"increasing longevity and increasing contact with external carcinogens, of which the most likely is cigarette smoke". As for bronchial cancer in Britain, this case study indicated that "the disease is, as yet, rare in the British Negro but may be expected to rise following the pattern [of Negroes] in the United States". The historical and familial health environments of black Americans and the Nigerians living in England had been distinct. Yet to these London researchers, a patient's racial membership based on visual racial categories was the overriding determinant that would cause the bronchial cancer rates of these two populations to converge.[28]

Despite the limited medical research infrastructure in Jamaica throughout the 1960s and 1970s, numerous clinical studies by researchers at Jamaican medical institutions appeared in leading international journals. Some studies were conducted by research teams that combined investigators living in Jamaica and Great Britain. The studies tried to cast doubt on the assumption that racial membership was the primary factor that appeared to deter respiratory disease and cancers in dark-skinned, African-descended populations. Most of these studies were surveys of cancer and respiratory disease cases in local hospital patients. Their findings ran against assumptions that people of an African background living in tropical climates, such as Jamaicans, did not contract these disorders in the same manner and at the same rates as white Americans and Europeans. This writer is going further and suggesting that these clinical studies were pointing toward histological evidence that environmental exposures associated with bauxite mining and other industrial materials may have contributed to respiratory and chronic disease patterns throughout the island nation.

One key Jamaican clinical study was a 1965 survey of malignant neoplasms in Jamaica by Bras, Watler, and Ashmeade-Dyer. They were members of the Pathology Department at the University of the West Indies, just outside of Kingston. Published in the *British Journal of Cancer*, the study was based on their compilation of clinical data from the Cancer Registry of Jamaica. The registry was maintained at the University, funded by the British Empire Cancer Campaign for Research, and highly organized. It recorded all cases diagnosed in the hospitals in Kingston and St Andrew, as well as the nursing homes and general practices located in these cities. The research analyzed 2,898 cases registered between 1958 and 1963. The authors compared cancer incidences of their Jamaican patient populations with similar cancer surveys that had been compiled for Denmark and South Africa (Bantu population). The authors did not state explicitly why they selected these two nations. They imply that these two nations had reliable cancer incidence figures based on actual diagnosis. Moreover, both nations had cancer data on large relatively homogenous racial populations—in the case of Denmark, a generally white national population; and, for South Africa's largest national population segment, the native African Bantu people. [29]

The researchers emphasized that it was essential to consider the demographic profile of the population from which the cancer data is derived. While census data for Jamaica and other nations was not always complete and reliable, it provided a basis for speculating about the contribution of social determinants to cancer rates. The Bras team described the occupational makeup of Jamaica's population as 5 percent professional, 14 percent domestic, 11 percent commercial, 44 percent agricultural, and 26 percent industrial. They underscored that, in Jamaica, "[i]ndustrialization is ... progressing rapidly and the agricultural labour force decreasing concurrently". Another demographic feature of their study population was its high literacy rate (90 percent of the adults), and "even in the most backward parishes [of Jamaica] the figure is not below 60 percent". [30]

The Bras study found that cancer incidence for several sites in Jamaica equalled or exceeded those of the Denmark population for roughly similar spans of time. For example, the number of oesophageal cancer cases (male) in Jamaica was over twice as high as those estimated for Denmark, and both lung and skin cancer cases in Jamaica slightly exceeded those estimated for Denmark. In sum, the study by Bras and colleagues offered empirical proof that many cancers were occurring at high levels in a predominantly black tropical nation and, moreover, these cancer cases were occurring in divergent sites. Cancer patterns likely reflected demographic, workforce, and economic development characteristics—in addition to racial group membership—more than just the reputed inherent racial tendencies of African-descended populations. [31]

Jamaica-based researchers analyzing data from their patients also questioned the heavy weight that racial determinants were given in Western research on respiratory diseases. In 1967, Walshe and J. A. Hayes published a study of respiratory symptoms and smoking habits in Jamaicans that appeared in the *American Review of Respiratory Disease*. The two researchers were in the Medical and Pathology Department at the University Hospital of the University of the West Indies, Mona, Kingston,

Jamaica. The researchers stated that they conducted their study since there was an "absence of documented evidence of respiratory symptoms in Jamaica" and an assumption that heavy smoking would not generate similar respiratory problems in populations of societies like Jamaica. They administered a questionnaire relating to specific bronchial symptoms (e.g., chronic coughing) and smoking habits to sixty-eight patients at their hospital. The patients selected were mostly from low socio-economic segments. Furthermore, to ensure some degree of randomness, the patients selected for the study had been admitted to the hospital for treatment of conditions other than chest and heart disease. [32]

Walshe and Hayes discovered that about two-thirds of the patients studied with moderate or severe cough and sputum were heavy smokers, while about one-third of the remaining patients with severe coughing and sputum production did not smoke or smoked moderately (according to criteria established by MRC). The bronchitis of these non- or moderately smoking patients was "typical of chronic bronchitis in temperate countries. Similarly, the frequency and severity of illness increased with age". Walshe and Hayes concluded their "finding of chronic bronchitis is unusual, as Jamaica does not have a cold, damp climate, and industrialization is minimal". Their result also "shows that the Jamaican Negro is subject to chronic bronchitis and that the frequency is much higher than had been the clinical impression". Walshe and Hayes took exception to the research by an American research group that asserted racial factors underlay Negro and white disparities in the incidence of chronic bronchitis."[33]

Another significant survey by researchers based in Jamaica concerned emphysema. It was published in *Thorax* in 1969. J. A. Hayes, mentioned earlier, and Joan Summerell, another member of the Pathology Department at the University Hospital at the University of the West Indies, coauthored this study.[34] They examined the lungs (about 1,600 necropsies) of a group of Jamaican adults comprised of "Negro (African)", "East Indian", and Chinese descent. They emphasized that these racial categories were descriptive of the social makeup of their patient study populations, not clearly delineated biological subpopulations. "These groups are [but] broad approximations due to the extensive intermarriage between the different racial groups". Their study revealed that "emphysema of the commonly recognized types occurs in the indigenous population of Jamaica". They conceded that some questions remained about the epidemiological factors underlying the emphysema cases. "Atmospheric pollution, as experienced in the industrialized areas of Britain, certainly does not exist in Jamaica, as industry is of recent origin and the number of automobiles has increased only lately". However, while they admitted that they had no definite answer as of yet, they suggested that "there is atmospheric pollution" in Jamaica, although "it is not likely to be of the conventional kind".[35]

J. A. Hayes teamed with Marigold Thorburn for a significant study that appeared in *Tropical and Geographical Medicine* in 1969. In this research piece, "Causes of Death in Jamaica, 1953 to 1964", they quantified patient records from the University College Hospital of the University of the West Indies. In the international medical community, the major cause of mortality in nations like Jamaica was believed to be infections "such as gastroenteritis, enteric fever, malaria, tuberculosis, or parasitic infestation". Their evaluation of autopsy records for 4,115 cases revealed otherwise. The most frequent cause of death was cancer, followed by cardiovascular disease, with "hypertensive heart disease the most common entity", chronic bronchitis, emphysema, and other respiratory diseases.[36]

In the early 1970s, more studies emerged from Jamaican researchers that focused on chronic diseases and their social—not just racial—patterning in the nation. A survey of lung cancer in Jamaica appeared in *Cancer* in 1972. The data for the study was derived from clinical and pathologic records of 105 patients spanning from 1952 to 1970 at the University Hospital of the West Indies. The cases and histological samples were from patients who had resided in the parishes of Kingston and St Andrews that contained about 555,000 of Jamaica's two million residents. The researchers analyzed their materials by age at the time of histological diagnosis, sex, lung affected, duration of symptoms attributable to lung cancer, and histological type. They found lung cancer was increasing as a trend. Moreover, the distribution of histological types of lung cancers in the cases they studied was highly differentiated. Comparing their findings with lung cancer data available for other nations, this study showed that the distribution of lung cancer types in Jamaica approximated that of "Norway, Venice, [and] colored South Africa, but [was] unlike that in Finland and in European South Africans".[37]

The studies in Jamaica using pathological surveys that had unveiled respiratory disorders associated with environmental exposures were small in number and survey scope. However, they were still significant for the medical research community of both developing and industrialized nations. Medical studies in industrial countries suspected an association between many kinds of industrial exposures and the development of chronic respiratory diseases. However, the effects of cigarette smoking were so heavily covered in epidemiological surveys that industrial workplace or environmental pollution exposures were difficult to causally delineate. Evidence from patholic studies such as those conducted in Jamaica were convincing enough to sustain strong interest in environmental factors throughout the clinical research community involved in respiratory diseases like silicosis, occupational health, and tuberculosis control.[38]

In the late 1970s, Jamaican researchers contributed a study on chronic disease linked to high blood pressure that appeared in *Lancet*. This research surveyed blood pressure and mortality among men and women aged 35 to 64 living in rural Jamaica. It analyzed records of 1,065 men and women who had examinations over the period of 1962 until 1976. The researchers found that the key determinant of differences in blood pressure and mortality in identical populations was the different profiles of cardiovascular pathology.[39] Research like this did much to chip away at the oversimplified assumptions in medical circles concerning environmental and genetic factors that appeared to stratify high blood pressure and heart disease differently in whites compared to blacks in Jamaica and other biracial societies.

NEW DILEMMAS IN THE MEDICAL HISTORY OF BAUXITE MINING IN JAMAICA

In the mid-1970s, world demand for aluminum plummeted. A worldwide economic recession most likely triggered this decline. The bauxite industry in Jamaica experienced increased layoffs and production cuts, and an increase in strikes and shutdowns. The glorious early period of the bauxite–alumina industry in Jamaica had ended.[40] Throughout these post-World War II decades, two apparently separate socio-economic worlds within Jamaica were merging into one socio-biological system. These worlds were the bauxite production sites and their transportation networks on one hand, and the larger Jamaican population and community environments on the other. This phenomenon was largely unrecognized by the medical researchers studying disease in nations like Jamaica.[41] However, today's medical historians can use current environmental epidemiology and toxicology as their lens. By so doing, they can see potential associations between the health problems of pre-1980 Jamaica and the frenetic early decades of bauxite production quite clearly. We will close by highlighting a few of the many future lines of investigation.

Experts have estimated that for each ton of bauxite produced, about five tons of caustic slurry is produced. This watery material known locally as "red mud" contains high concentrations of pollutants. Frequently, the highly alkali red mud was stored in lakes adjacent to the alumina plant. As a local geologist and professor stated, "they are not only an eyesore but a possible pollution hazard to underground water supplies".[42] Also, since the caustic waste is largely water (between 75 and 80 percent), when concentrated on a surface, it ponds, and these water bodies flow into the island's groundwater reserves.[43]

In the mid-1980s, university geologists described the magnitude of hazardous slurry in Jamaica's countryside. Studying Jamaica's bauxite industry, they found that, at the plant in Ewarton, 7,289 tons of red mud slurry was produced each day, 2.5 million tons annually. The slurry was pumped "to a large red mud lake . . . near Mt. Rosser". The researchers stated further:

> There is abundant evidence of contamination of ground and surface water both to the north and to the south of the red mud lake. To the south the tributaries of the Rio Cobre drain is a catchment area

(St. Thomas-Ye-Vale) which supplies the largest irrigation scheme in Jamaica and domestic water supplies for the second largest urban area.[44]

When other geologists studied the water contamination problem nationally, they found pollution from caustic waste in the groundwater near three of Jamaica's four bauxite–alumina plants.[45]

The bioavailability of the caustic red slurry waste opens a host of issues for medical historians seeking to trace the health and social effects of Jamaica's past in bauxite and alumina production. One such issue is the spread of heavy metals and minerals, such as silica, that is associated with bauxite and alumina production. Silica exposure has been documented in the handling of materials that contain aluminium, such as bauxite and corundum.[46] Furthermore, it is now clearly established from geological evidenced that in Jamaica, lead and other metal toxicants are widely dispersed and most heavily concentrated in bauxite soils. A recent geochemical survey of heavy metals in Jamaican surface soils was conducted with 200 sample sites across the island. The newest high-precision test instruments were employed: energy dispersive X-ray fluorescence analysis, instrumental neutron activation analysis, and atomic absorption spectrophotometry. The researchers were particularly interested in identifying metal levels in soils that would indicate human and animal health consequences. They discovered that lead, arsenic, cadmium, and mercury were significantly distributed and highly correlated with bauxite soils.[47]

Among these metals, lead's toxic effects on human health are the most well established in the medical sciences and toxicology. At high concentrations, it causes renal, neurological, and haematological damage. Absorbed in food, water, soil, and dust, lead is particularly harmful to fetal and infant neurological development. Numerous studies in environmental health and paediatrics have demonstrated conclusively the ante- and postnatal toxicity of lead. These studies demonstrated that children whose lead levels in their umbilical-cord blood were about 10 µg/dl developed measurable cognitive impairments at age 2. Other paediatric researchers (especially Herbert Needlemen) established that increased lead levels in children reduced IQ, decreased class performance, and increased behavioural problems in school-age children.[48] Future research building on such findings can contribute much to the historiography of the Caribbean by exploring environmental lead and the bauxite industry in Jamaica and neighbouring nations.

Another medical history hypothesis about the social impact of modern bauxite mining in Jamaica concerns another chemical found in red mud— sodium. In Jamaica, as in many other developing nations, hypertension and cardiovascular disease are pervasive health problems. Most researchers attribute these problems to diet, obesity, and genetics of populations in nations like Jamaica. However, the evidence of contamination of groundwater from red mud slurry raises interesting questions about environmental chemicals that may be associated with elevated levels of hypertension and cardiovascular disease in Jamaica's population.

Research on the possible health effects of high sodium content in drinking water, including an association with high blood pressure and cardiovascular disease, have been appearing since the 1940s.[49] Among the recent studies is one on water in the town of Gila Bend, Arizona, that has high sodium content. Local populations were surveyed for health risk factors, dietary sodium intake, and water consumption. No positive association between water sodium intake and blood pressure was found. However, the researchers cautioned that their study population was limited and did not include persons with health factors that possibly intensify due to water sodium consumption, such as hypertensives or cardiac patients.[50]

A few years later, another study of water with high sodium content appeared in England in the publication of the Royal Society of Chemistry. It suggested that sophisticated analytical techniques had uncovered water contamination, but attributing specific health effects to consumption of water with sodium and other contaminants still lacked evidence.[51] Nonetheless, evidence of a possible association between sodium content in water and health effects has grown. By the late 1990s, the US Environmental Protection Agency and the Centers for Disease Control and Prevention were debating the need to regulate sodium in water supplies, since evidence had grown suggesting a link between water with high sodium content and health problems.[52] The American movement to regulate sodium in water is suggestive of the potential health effects of this condition throughout Jamaica. Medical–historical, epidemiological, and toxicological exploration of this issue in Jamaica's past could yield important new hypotheses for other populations throughout the Caribbean as well.

This brief medical history of bauxite mining in Jamaica provided the reader with a glimpse at the immense tangle of medical, scientific, and social issues this episode entails. Commercial bauxite deposits have been mined and processed in other parts of the Caribbean and Latin America. Moreover, Asian, Middle Eastern, and European nations, as well as Australia, also have deep industrial stakes in this resource. As the medical history of this industry in Jamaica unfolds, social historians and the entire range of biological and ecological specialists in these other nations will have the Jamaican experience as an example to follow.

NOTES

1. C. E. Davis, *Jamaica in the World Aluminium Industry*, vol. 1 (Kingston: Jamaica Bauxite Institute, 1989), 96–97.
2. B. S. Young, "Jamaica's Bauxite and Alumina Industries," *Ann. Assoc. Am. Geogr.* 55, no. 3 (1965): 449–464.

3. Ibid.
4. R. W. Palmer, *The Jamaican Economy* (New York: Praeger, 1968), 15–23.
5. H.L. Geisert, *The Caribbean: Population and Resources* (Washington, DC: George Washington University, 1960), 96–97.
6. Ibid., 25–26; R. G. L. Grant, "Jamaica—Kaiser Bauxite Health Services," in *Health Care for Remote Areas: An International Conference*, ed. J. P. Hughes (Oakland, Calif.: Kaiser Foundation International, 1972), 100–102.
7. Palmer, *Jamaican Economy*.
8. "Mineral Wealth," *Directory of Jamaica 1962 Including Trade Index and Biographical Section* (London: The Diplomatic Press and Publishing Co., 1962), 30; Jamaica Information Service, *The Handbook of Jamaica for 1967* (Kingston, Jamaica: Government Printing Office, 1967), 879–881; B. Floyd, *Jamaica: An Island Microcosm* (New York: St. Martin's Press, 1979), 91–95; Palmer, *Jamaican Economy*, 19; Geisert, 96–97.
9. Floyd, *Jamaica*, 92.
10. Ibid., v, 92.
11. O. Jefferson, *The Post-War Economic Development of Jamaica* (1972; repr. Kingston, Jamaica: University of the West Indies, 1977), 162. Citation here refers to 1977 edition. Palmer, *Jamaican Economy*, 21–22.
12. A. Kuper, *Changing Jamaica* (London: Routledge & Kegan Paul, 1979), 129; E. LeClerc, "The Bauxite Labour Force in Jamaica: A High Wage Sector in a Dual Economy," *Social and Economic Studies* 36, no. 1 (1987): 217–266; Jefferson, *Post-War Economic Development*, 163–164.
13. W. T. Prout, "Malaria in Jamaica," in *The Prevention of Malaria*, ed. Ronald Ross (London: J. Murray, 1910), 377–378. The team discovered that about one-fifth of the nation's 680 annual deaths were attributed to malaria, as well as one-third of the estimated 19,000 annual admissions to the government hospitals.
14. See, for example, *The Report of the Jamaica Yaws Commission* published for the years 1932 through 1936 (Kingston, Jamaica: Government Printing Office).
15. Jennifer Beinart, "The Inner World of Imperial Sickness: The MRC and Research in Tropical Medicine," in *Historical Perspectives on the Role of the MRC: Essays in the History of the Medical Research Council of the United Kingdom and Its Predecessor, The Medical Research Committee, 1913–1953*, ed. J. Austoker and L. Bryder (Oxford: Oxford University Press, 1989), 109–135; David J. Bradley, "Tropical Medicine," in *The Oxford Companion to Medicine*, ed. S. Lock, J. M. Last, and G. Dunea (Oxford: Oxford University Press, 2001), http://www.oxfordreference.com/views/ENTRY.html?subview=Main&entry=t185.e490.
16. "Public Health and Social Welfare," *Directory of Jamaica 1952*, 52; W. A. Cover, *The Handbook of Jamaica for 1952* (Kingston, Jamaica: Government Printing Office, 1952), 489, 499–505.
17. International Bank for Reconstruction and Development, *The Economic Development of Jamaica* (Baltimore: The Johns Hopkins University Press, 1952), 121–122, quote on p. 122.
18. Beinart, "Inner World of Imperial Sickness," 130; George Miller, "William Enar Miall: Epidemiologist," *West Indian Med. J.* 54, no. 1 (2005): available online at http://caribbean.scielo.org.
19. G. G. Allen, "Jamaica—Health Affairs of ALPART," in *Health Care for Remote Areas*, 95; Grant, "Jamaica—Kaiser Bauxite Health Services," 100.
20. Allen, "Jamaica—Health Affairs," 94–96.
21. Grant, "Jamaica—Kaiser Bauxite Health Services."
22. Ibid.

23. For a summary of the state of these fields in the early1970s, see, for example, A. Blouhuys and J. M. Peters, "Control of Environmental Lung Disease," *New Engl. J. Med.* 283, no. 11 (1970): 573–582; M. M. Key and H. E. Ayer, "Silicosis in Hard Rock Mining," *Journal of Occupational Medicine* 14, no. 11 (1972): 863–865; M. X. FitzGerald, C. B. Carrington, and E. A. Gaensler, "Environmental Lung Disease," *Med. Clin. N. Am.* 57, no. 3 (1973): 593–622.
24. D. McBride, *Missions for Science: US Technology and Medicine in America's African World* (New Brunswick, NJ: Rutgers University Press, 2002).
25. J. A. Hayes and J. M. Summerell, "Emphysema in a Non-Industrialized Tropical Island," *Thorax* 24 (1969): 623–625.
26. E. R. Mays, "Pulmonary Diseases," in *Textbook of Black-Related Diseases*, ed. R. A. Williams (New York: McGraw-Hill, 1975), 415–435.
27. R. E. Murphy, S. Katz, D. J. Massaro, and P. C. Luchsinger, "Is Emphysema a Disease Predominantly of the White Male?" *JAMA* 181, no. 8 (1962): 140–141; quote on p. 141. Mucoviscididosis is a bronchopulmonary complication. This type of patient-based study has fundamental flaws in its statistical design. The emphysema distributions in the specific patient groups in the three data sources cannot be representative of population-level distributions of this disease. Also, the racial boundaries that these researchers assume define races are not biologically valid.
28. P. H. Kidner and H. O. Williams, "Bronchial Carcinoma in a Young Negro," *Thorax* 24 (1969): 472–475, quote on p. 472.
29. G. Bras, D. C. Watler, and A. Ashmeade-Dyer, "The Incidence of Malignant Neoplasms in Jamaica," *Bri. J. Cancer* 19 (1965): 681–694, figures on p. 694.
30. Ibid., 685.
31. Ibid.
32. M. H. Walshe and J. A. Hayes, "Respiratory Symptoms and Smoking Habits in Jamaica," *Am. Rev. Tuberc.* 96, no. 4 (1976): 640–644.
33. Ibid., 643. The US research Walshe and Hayes questioned was by D. Massaro, A. Cusick, and S. Natz, "Racial Differences in Incidence of Chronic Bronchitis," *Am. Rev. Respir. Dis.* 92 (1965): 94–97.
34. J. A. Hayes and J. M. Summerell, "Emphysema in a Non-Industrialized Tropical Island," *Thorax* 24 (1969): 623–625.
35. Ibid., quotes on pp. 623, 624, 625.
36. M. J. Thorburn and J. A. Hayes, "Causes of Death in Jamaica, 1953 to 1964: An Analysis of Post-Mortem Diagnosis at the University Hospital of the West Indies," *Trop. Geogr. Med.* 20 (1968): 35–49, quotes on pp. 35 and 49.
37. G. Bras, W. F. Whimster, A. L. Patrick, and M. Woo-Ming, "Aspects of Lung Cancer in Jamaica," *Cancer* 29 (1972): 1590–1596; quote on p. 1593.
38. T. Rodman and F. H. Sterling, *Pulmonary Emphysema and Related Lung Diseases* (St. Louis, MO: C. V. Mosby, 1969), 16–19; Mays, "Pulmonary Diseases."
39. M. T. Ashcroft and P. Desai, "Blood-Pressure and Mortality in a Rural Jamaican Community," *Lancet* 1, no. 8075 (1978): 1167–1170.
40. C. Stone, "Power, Policy and Politics in Independent Jamaica," in *Jamaica in Independence: Essays on the Early Years*, ed. R. Nettleford (Kingston, Jamaica: Heinemann, 1989), 19–53, esp. pp. 35–36; M. Kaufman, *Jamaica Under Manley: Dilemmas of Socialism and Democracy* (Westport, CT: Lawrence Hill & Co., 1985), 105–111.
41. L. B. Coke, C. C. Weir, and V. G. Hill, "Environmental Impact of Bauxite Mining and Processing in Jamaica," *Social and Economic Studies* 36, no. 1 (1987): 289–333.

42. One of the earliest occupational medicine studies I located was published in the leading Jamaican-based medical journal, *The West Indies Medical Journal*. The study was E. N. Harris and B. Rodney, "Arsenic-Poisoning in a Glass Factory in Kingston, Jamaica," *West Indian Med. J.* 31, no. 4 (1982): 213–216. Floyd, *Jamaica*, 93–94; quote on p. 94.
43. Coke et al., "Environmental Impact," *New Scientist* 110,no. 1502 (3 April 1986): 33-37; 297; J. Bell, "Caustic Waste Menaces Jamaica," *New Scientist* 3 April 1986, pp. 33–37; B. Fernandez, *Caustic Waste Pollution of Groundwater in Jamaica: Two Solutions* (Kingston, Jamaica: Water Resources Division, 1983), 27 pp; G. Pagano, et al., "Toxicity of Bauxite Manufacturing By-Products in Sea Urchin e\Embryos," *Ecotoxicol. Environ. Saf.* 51, no. 1 (2000): 28–34. Moreover, in the process of extracting alumina from a ground-up bauxite–lime mixture, caustic soda is added and cooked at high temperatures. Caustic aerosols result that have both a foul odour and negative health effects on humans who inhale them.
44. Coke et al., "Environmental Impact," 314.
45. C.-G. E. Fernandez, *Caustic Waste Pollution*.
46. B. Sjögren, C.-E., A. Iregen, , D. R. C.McLachlan, , and V. Riihimäki, "Occupational Aluminum Exposure and Its Health Effects," in *Research Issues in Aluminum Toxicity*, ed. R. A. Yokel and M. S. Golub (Washington, DC: Taylor & Francis, 1997), 165–183, esp. pp. 171–172.
47. A.H.M. Johnson, et al., "Heavy Metals in Jamaican Surface Soils," *Environ. Geochem. Health* 18, no. 3 (1996): 113–121.
48. M. Lippmann, *Environmental Toxicants: Human Exposures and Their Health Effects* (New York: John Wiley, 2000), 500–501; J. Grigg, "Environmental Toxins; Their Impact on Children's Health," *Arch. Dis. Child.* 89 (2004): 244–250.
49. On the earliest studies, see H. M. Perry, Jr., "Minerals in Cardiovascular Disease," *J. Am. Diet. Assoc.* 62 (1973): 631–637.
50. T.K. Weltyet al., "Effects of Exposure to Salty Drinking Water in an Arizona Community: Cardiovascular Mortality, Hypertension Prevalence, and Relationships Between Blood Pressure and Sodium Intake," *JAMA* 255, no. 5 (1986): 622–626.
51. R.F. Packham, "Water Quality and Health," in *Pollution: Causes, Effects and Control* (Cambridge: Royal Society of Chemistry, 1990), 83–97.
52. R.L. Hanneman, "Sodium Debate Continues," *Water Techno.* 21, no. 8 (1998): 51–53.

Contributors

Denise Challenger is a doctoral candidate in the Department of History at York University, Toronto, Canada. She is currently an Erskine Peters Dissertation Year Fellow at the University of Notre Dame, where she is working on her dissertation, "Constructing the Colonial Moral Order: Discourses on Sexuality in Post Slavery Barbados."

Juanita De Barros is an associate professor in the Department of History at McMaster University, Hamilton, Canada, where she teaches Atlantic, Caribbean, and African diasporic history. Her research focuses on the post-emancipation Anglophone Caribbean, particularly urban history, popular protest, and the history of health and health workers. She has, among other major publications, edited a special issue of *Caribbean Quarterly* that focuses on the history of public health in the Caribbean ("Colonialism and Health in the Tropics") and a collection of essays on recent Caribbean historiography (*Beyond Fragmentation: Perspectives on Caribbean History*, Marcus Weiner Publishers, 2006). Her current research project examines the role of health workers in the development of health and medical policies in the post-emancipation British Caribbean.

Jacques Dumont is a professor of history at the University of French Antilles and Guyane AIHP *(Archéologie industrielle, histoire et patrimoine)* Laboratory. He has written extensively on the history of the body in the French West Indies, including health, hygiene, sports, and physical education. His major publications include two books: *Sport et assimilation en Guadeloupe, les enjeux du corps performant de la colonie au département, 1914–1965* (Paris: L'Harmattan, 2002) and *Sport et formation de la jeunesse à la Martinique: Le temps des pionniers (fin XIXe années 1960)* (Paris: L'Harmattan, 2006).

Rosemarijn Hoefte is head of the Department of Collections and coordinator of the Caribbean Expert Center of the KITLV/Royal Netherlands Institute of Southeast Asian and Caribbean Studies in Leiden, the Netherlands. She is also the managing editor of the *New West Indian Guide*.

Currently, she is working on a book on the life and times of Grace Schneiders-Howard, the first female politician in Suriname.

Tara Inniss is currently a temporary lecturer in Caribbean History/ History of Medicine in the Department of History and Philosophy at the Cave Hill Campus of the University of the West Indies in Barbados. She also holds a Masters in Social Development from the University of New South Wales in Australia, and specializes in disability studies and human rights research.

Niklas Thode Jensen is a postdoctoral fellow and adjunct professor at the Department of History at the Saxo Institute, University of Copenhagen in Denmark. His research focuses on the medical history of the former Danish colonies in the Caribbean and in India, especially the enslaved population in the Danish West Indies. He is currently working on a post-doctoral project funded by the Carlsberg Foundation entitled: "Science without Empire: Science, Medicine, Scientific networks and the Danish Halle Mission in the Danish East Indies, 1770–1845". His PhD thesis is forthcoming, and is entitled (in English): "For the Health of the Enslaved: Slaves, Medicine and Power in the Danish West Indies, 1803–1848."

April Mayes received her PhD in history from the University of Michigan. She is currently an assistant professor of history at Pomona College, Claremont, California, where she teaches Latin American and Caribbean history. Professor Mayes is writing a book that examines Dominican national identity between 1870 and 1930.

David McBride received his BA from Denison University and his MPhil and PhD from Columbia University. He is a professor in the African and African-American Studies Department and Faculty Associate at the Center for Health Policy Research, Pennsylvania State University, University Park, Pennsylvania. His teaching areas include: African-American History, Health Issues of Minority Americans, Black Families, and Technology and Public Health Issues of US Minorities and in the Non-Western World. His research interests include: health and medical care of minority Americans and African diaspora populations; environmental issues and disadvantaged populations; science issues of disadvantaged populations.

Debbie McCollin began her Master of Philosophy degree at the University of the West Indies, St. Augustine, Trinidad and Tobago, where she is currently pursuing her PhD. Under the 2007/08 Commonwealth Split-Site programme, she spent a year as a visiting scholar at the Centre for the History of Science, Technology and Medicine at the University of Manchester. Her research is focused on the history of health of Trinidad and

Tobago, with particular emphasis on the Second World War and the pre-independence era.

Steven Palmer is Canada Research Chair in History of International Health and associate professor in the Department of History at the University of Windsor. He is the author of *From Popular Medicine to Medical Populism: Doctors, Healers and Public Power in Costa Rica, 1800–1940* (Durham, NC: Duke University Press, 2003), and *Launching Global Health: The Caribbean Odyssey of the Rockefeller Foundation* (University of Michigan Press, in press), and chief editor of the web-based research magazine, *Cultures of Health: A Historical Anthology* (hih. uwindsor.ca). Palmer is currently completing a book on the production of Cuban medical science in the nineteenth and early twentieth centuries.

Nicole Trujillo-Pagán has ten years of experience working with US Latinos' health in both academic and non-profit research settings. She earned her PhD in sociology from the University of Michigan-Ann Arbor. She is currently an assistant professor in the Sociology Department and the Center for Chicano-Boricua Studies at Wayne State University, Detroit, Michigan. Her dissertation examined the relationship between US colonialism and medicine in Puerto Rico. Her current research explores the relationship between immigrant incorporation and health outcomes, which includes a case study of Latino construction workers' occupational health in New Orleans, Louisiana.

David Sowell is a professor of History and International Studies at Juniata College, Huntingdon, Pennsylvania. After graduating from the University of Florida, he has focused on the social history of nineteenth-century Latin America. His book, *The Tale of Healer Miguel Perdomo Neira: Medicine, Ideologies, and Power in the Nineteenth-Century Andes* (2001) examined the clash between Hispanic medicine and biomedicine through the story of Perdomo's life. Sowell is currently working on a history of public health in Yucatan, Mexico.

David Wright holds the Hannah Chair in the History of Medicine at McMaster University, Hamilton, Canada. He is the former chair of the Society for the Social History of Medicine and teaches the history of nineteenth- and twentieth-century Anglo-American public health. A specialist in the history of mental health, he is the author and co-editor of seven books, including, most recently (with John Weaver, eds.), *Histories of Self-Destruction: International Perspectives on Suicide* (Toronto: University of Toronto Press, 2008).

Select Bibliography

Abel, Christopher. 1995. External Philanthropy and Domestic Change in Colombian Health Care: The Role of the Rockefeller Foundation, ca. 1920–1950," *Hispanic American Historical Review* 75 (3):339–376.

———. 1996. Health, Hygiene, and Sanitation in Latin America, c.1870 to c.1950. London: Institute of Latin American Studies Working Papers.

Allen, G. G. A. Jamaica—Health Affairs of ALPART," in *Health Care for Remote Areas*, ed. J. P. Hughes. Oakland: Kaiser Foundation International, 1972.

Amaro Méndez, Sergio. 1983. *Alas Amarillas: La Historia de Carlos J. Finlay y su Descubrimiento*. Havana: Científico-Técnica.

Anderson, Warwick. 1992. "Where Every Prospect Pleases and Only Man is Vile: Laboratory Medicine as Colonial Discourse." *Critical Inquiry* 18:506–529.

Anthony, Michael. 1978. *Port of Spain in a World at War*. Port of Spain: Ministry of Sport and Culture.

Arana-Soto, S. 1974. *Historia de la medicina puertorriqueña*. Barcelona: Artes Gráficas Medinaceli, S.A.

———. 1978. *La Sanidad en Puerto Rico hasta el 1898*. San Juan, Puerto Rico: Academia Puertorriqueña de la Historia.

Armus, Diego, ed. 2003. *Disease in the History of Modern Latin America: From Malaria to Aids*. Durham, NC: Duke University Press.

———. 2003. Disease in the Historiography of Modern Latin America. In *Disease in the History of Modern Latin America: From Malaria to Aids*, ed. Diego Armus, 7–24. Durham, NC: Duke University Press.

Arnold, David, ed. 1988. *Imperial Medicine and Indigenous Societies*. Manchester, UK: Manchester University Press.

———. 1993. *Colonizing the Body: State Medicine and Epidemic Disease in Nineteenth-Century India*. Berkeley: University of California Press.

———. 1994. Public Health and Public Power: Medicine and Hegemony in Colonial India. In *Contesting Colonial Hegemony: State and Society in Africa and India*, ed. Dagmar Engels and Shula Marks, 131–151. London: British Academic Press.

Atkins, P.J. 1992. White Poison? The Social Consequences of Milk Consumption, 1850–1930. *Social History of Medicine* 5(2):207–227.

Ayensu, E.S. 1981. *Medicinal Plants of the West Indies*. Algonac: Reference Publications.

Beardsley, E.H. 1983. Making Separate Equal: Black Physicians and the Problems of Medical Segregation in the Pre-World War II South. *Bulletin of the History of Medicine* 57(3):382–396.

Beckles, Hilary. 1990. *A History of Barbados*. Cambridge: Cambridge University Press.

Beckwith, Martha Warren. 1969. *Black Roadways: A Study of Jamaican Folk Life.* New York: Negro University Press.

Beldarraín Chaple, Enrique. 2006. *Los Médicos y los inicios de la antropología en Cuba.* La Habana: Fundación Fernando Ortíz.

———. 2006. La salud pública en Cuba y su experiencia internacional: 1959–2005. *História Ciências Saúde: Manguinhos* 13(3):709–716.

———. 2005. Cambio y revolución: El surgimiento del sistema nacional único de salud en Cuba, 1959–1970. *Dynamis* 25:257–278.

Bell, W.J. 1965. North American and West Indian Graduates of Glasgow and Aberdeen to 1800. *Journal of History of Medicine* 20:411–415.

Bergad, Laird. 1990. *Cuban Rural Society in the Nineteenth Century: The Social and Economic History of Monoculture in Matanzas.* Princeton, NJ: Princeton University Press.

Bergad, L.W. 1980. Toward Puerto Rico's Grito de Lares: Coffee, Social Stratification, and Class Conflicts, 1828–1868. *Hispanic American Historical Review* 60:617–642.

Beyan, Amos J. 1991. *The American Colonization Society and the Creation of the Liberian State: A Historical Perspective, 1822–1900.* Lanham, MD: University Press of America.

Birn, Anne-Emanuelle. 2006. *Marriage of Convenience: The Rockefeller International Health and Revolutionary Mexico.* Rochester, NY: University of Rochester Press.

———. 2003. Revolution, the Scatological Way: The Rockefeller Foundation's Hookworm Campaign in 1920s Mexico. In *Disease in the History of Modern Latin America: From Malaria to Aids,* ed. Diego Armus, 158–182. Durham, NC: Duke University Press.

Bissessar, Ann, et al. 2001. The Historical Development of the Health System in Trinidad and Tobago. In *Public Health and Policy Departmental Publication No. 34* London: London School of Hygiene and Tropical Medicine.

Blyden, Nemeta. 2000. *West Indians in West Africa, 1808–1880: The African Diaspora in Reverse.* Rochester, NY: Rochester University Press.

Boa, Sheena. 2001. Experiences of Women Estate Workers During the Apprenticeship Period in St. Vincent. *Women's History Review* 10(3):381–408.

Braithwaite, Lloyd. 2001. *Colonial West Indian Students in Britain.* Kingston, Jamaica: University of the West Indies Press.

Briggs, Laura. 2002. *Reproducing Empire. Race, Sex, Science, and U.S. Imperialism in Puerto Rico.* Berkeley: University of California Press.

Bronfman, Alejandra. 2002. "En Plena Libertad y Democracia": *Negros Brujos* and the Social Question. *Hispanic American Historical Review* 82(3):549–587.

———. 2004. *Measures of Equality: Social Science, Citizenship, and Race in Cuba, 1902–1940.* Chapel Hill: University of North Carolina Press.

Bruce-Chwatt, Leonard Jan, and Julian de Zulueta. 1980. *The Rise and Fall of Malaria in Europe: A Historico-Epidemiological Study.* Oxford: Published on behalf of the Regional Office for Europe of the World Health Organization (by) Oxford University Press.

Bryan, Patrick. 1991. *The Jamaican People 1880–1902: Race, Class and Social Control.* London: Macmillan Caribbean Ltd.

Burin, Eric. 2002. Envisioning Africa: American Slaves' Ideas about Liberia. *Liberian Studies Journal* 27(1):1–17.

Bush, Barbara. 1996. Hard Labor: Women, Childbirth, and Resistance in British Caribbean Slave Societies. In *More than Chattel: Black Women and Slavery in the Americas,* ed. David Barry Gaspar and Darlene Clark Hine, 83–99. Bloomington: Indiana University Press.

———. 1990. *Slave Women in Caribbean Society, 1650–1838.* London: James Curry Ltd.

Cabrera, Lydia. 1984. *La Medicina Popular de Cuba: médicos de antaño, curand-eros, santeros y paleros de hogaño*. Miami, FL: Ediciones Universal.

Calder, Bruce. 1984. *The Impact of Intervention: The Dominican Republic during the U.S. Occupation of 1916–1924*. Austin: University of Texas Press.

Castillo Canché, Jorge I. and José E. Serrano Catzín. 1994. Vigilar y normar el bur-del: Legalización de la prostitución femenina en Yucatán durante el porfiriato. *Revista de la Universidad Autónoma de Yucatán* 198:46–55.

de Castro y Bachiller, Raimundo. 1968. *Centenario del nacimiento del Dr. Jorge Le-Roy y Cassá*. Havana: Consejo Cientifico, Ministerio de Salud Publica.

Cervera Fernández, José Juan. 2002. Preceptos divinos y contradicciones raciona-les: el primer movimiento espiritista en yucatán, 1869–1879. In *Los Aguafies-tas: Desafíos a la Hegemonía de la Élite Yucateca, 1867–1910,* coord. Piedad Peniche Rivero and Felipe Escalante Tió, 193–238. Mérida: AGEY.

Chalhoub, Sidney. 1993. The Politics of Disease Control: Yellow Fever and Race in Nineteenth Century Rio de Janeiro. *Journal of Latin American Studies* 35:441–463.

Chamberlain, J. Edward and Sander L. Gilman, eds. 1985. *Degeneration: The Dark Side of Progress*. New York: Columbia University Press.

Chávez Alvarez, Ernesto. 1991. *El Crimen de la niña Cecilia: la brujería en cuba como fenómeno social, 1902–1925*. Havana: Editorial de Ciencias Sociales.

Christian, Mark, ed. 2002. *Black Identity in the Twentieth Century: Expressions in the US and UK African Diaspora*. London: Hansib.

Cirillo, Vincent J. 2004. *Bullets and Bacilli: The Spanish-American War and Mili-tary Medicine*. New Brunswick, NJ: Rutgers University Press.

———. 2000. Fever and Reform: The Typhoid Epidemic in the Spanish-American War. *Journal of the History of Medicine and Allied Sciences* 55(4):363–397.

Coke, L. B., C. C. Weir, and V. G. Hill. 1987. Environmental Impact of Bauxite Min-ing and Processing in Jamaica. *Social and Economic Studies* 36(1):289–333.

Collins, David. 1971. *Practical Rules for the Management and Medical Treatment of Negro Slaves in the Sugar Colonies*. London: Vernor, Hood, and Sharp.

Corbin, Alain. 1987. Commercial Sexuality in Nineteenth-Century France: A Sys-tem of Images and Regulations. In *The Making of the Modern Body: Sexuality and Society in the Nineteenth Century,* ed. Catherine Gallagher and Thomas Laquer, 209–219. Berkeley: University of California Press.

Craton, Michael. 1991. Death, Disease and Medicine on Jamaican Slave Planta-tion: The Example of Worthy Park 1767–1838. In *Caribbean Slave Society and Economy,* ed. Hilary Beckles and Verene Shepherd, 183–196. Kingston, Jamaica: Ian Randle Publishers.

Crosby, Alfred W. 1989. *America's Forgotten Pandemic: The Influenza of 1918*. Cambridge: Cambridge University Press.

Cubano-Iguina, A. 1998. Political Culture and Male Mass-Party Formation in Late-Nineteenth-Century Puerto Rico. *The Hispanic American Historical Review* 78(4):631–662.

Cueto, Marcos. 1997. *El regreso de las epidemias: salud y sociedad en el Perú del siglo XX*. Lima, Peru: Instituto de Estudios Peranos.

———. 1994. Introd. to *Missionaries of Science: The Rockefeller Foundation and Latin America,* ed. by Marcus Cueto, ix–xx. Bloomington: Indiana University Press.

———. 1994. Visions of Science and Development: The Rockefeller Foundation's Latin American Surveys of the 1920s. In *Missionaries of Science: The Rock-efeller Foundation and Latin America,* ed. Marcus Cueto, 1–22. Bloomington: Indiana University Press.

Cueto, Marcos, ed. 1994. *Missionaries of Science: The Rockefeller Foundation and Latin America*. Bloomington: Indiana University Press.

Cummings, James Damian. 2004. *Barrack Yard Dwellers*. St. Augustine, Trinidad and Tobago: The University of the West Indies.

Dabydeen, David and Brinsely Samaroo, eds. 1987. *India in the Caribbean*. London: Hansib.

Danielson, Ross. 1979. *Cuban Medicine*. New Brunswick, NJ: Transaction Books.

Deacon, Harriet. 1997. Cape Town and "Country" Doctors in the Cape Colony During the First Half of the Nineteenth Century. *Social History of Medicine* 10(1):25–52.

———. 1998. Midwives and Medical Men in the Cape Colony Before 1860. *Journal of African History* 39:271–292.

De Barros, Juanita. 2001. Congregationalism and Afro-Guianese Autonomy. In *Nation Dance: Religion, Identity, and Cultural Difference in the Caribbean*, ed. Patrick Taylor, 89–103. Bloomington: Indiana University Press.

———. 2002. *Order and Place in a Colonial City: Patterns of Struggle and Resistance in Georgetown, British Guiana 1889–1924* (Montreal, Canada: McGill-Queens University Press.

———. 2003. Sanitation and Civilization in Georgetown, British Guiana. *Caribbean Quarterly* 49(4):65–86.

———. 2004. "Setting Things Right": Medicine and Magic in British Guiana, 1803–1834. *Slavery and Abolition* 25:28–50.

———. 2003. "Spreading Sanitary Enlightenment": Race, Identity, and the Emergence of a Creole Medical Profession in British Guiana. *Journal of British Studies* 42:483–504.

De Barros, Juanita and Sean Stilwell, eds. 2003. Colonialism and Health in the Tropics. Special issue, *Caribbean Quarterly* 49:4.

Delaporte, Francois. 1991. *The History of Yellow Fever: An Essay on the Birth of Tropical Medicine*. Cambridge, MA: MIT Press.

Delgado García, Gregorio. 1983. Los Estudios de la historia de la medicina en Cuba. *Cuadernos de la Historia de la Salud* 66.

Devin, Anna. 1975. Imperialism and Motherhood: Population and Power. *History Workshop Journal* 5:7–65.

Diaz, José F. and Benjamín Gongora Triay. 1977. La Higiene. In *Enciclopedia Yucatanese*, tomo VI, 2nd ed., 377–421. Mérida, Mexico: Edición Oficial del Gobierno de Yucatán.

Díaz-Briquets, Sergio. 1983. *The Health Revolution in Cuba*. Austin: University of Texas Press.

Duarte Nunes, Everardo, ed. 1989. *Juan César Garcia: Pensamento social em saúde na América Latina*. São Paulo, Brazil: Cortez Editora.

Dumont, J. 2006. Antilles Conscription and the Demand for Citizenship [*Conscription antillaise et citoyenneté revendiquée*]. *Vingtième siècle Revue d'histoire* 92:101–116.

———. 2007. Health and Creole Conscription: The Watershed of the First World War [*Santé et conscription créole: le tournant de la première guerre mondiale*]. *Outre-mers (revue du SFHOM)* 95:223–241.

———. 2002. *Sport and Assimilation in Guadeloupe* [*Sport et assimilation à la Guadeloupe*]. Paris: L'Harmattan.

———. 2006. *Sport and the Training of Youth in Martinique from the end of the Nineteenth Century to the 1960s* [*Sport et formation de la jeunesse à la Martinique, le temps des pionniers (fin XIXe-années 1960)*]. Paris: L'Harmattan.

Dunn, Frederick L. 1993. Malaria. In *The Cambridge World History of Human Disease*, ed. Kenneth F. Kiple, 855–862. Cambridge: Cambridge University Press.

Du Toit, Brian M. 1997. Ethnomedical (Folk) Healing in the Caribbean. *Journal of Caribbean Studies* 12(1).

Engelstein, Laura. 1987. Morality and the Wooden Spoon: Russian Doctors View Syphilis, Social Class, and Sexual Behavior. In *The Making of the Mod-*

ern Body. Sexuality and Society in the Nineteenth Century, ed. Catherine Gallagher and Thomas Laquer, 169–208. Berkeley: University of California Press.

Erosa Barbachano, Arturo. 1997. *La Escuela de Medicina de Mérida, Yucatán.* Mérida, Mexico: Ediciones de la Universidad Autónoma de Yucatán.

Ettling, John. 1981. *The Germ of Laziness: Rockefeller Philanthropy and Public Health in the New South.* Cambridge MA: Harvard University Press.

Farley, John. 2004. *To Cast Out Disease: A History of the International Health Division of the Rockefeller Foundation (1913–1951).* Oxford: Oxford University Press.

Farmer, Paul. 1992. *AIDS and Accusation: Haiti and the Geography of Blame.* Berkeley: University of California Press.

Fauché, S. 1996. Childhood Hygiene and Physical Education [*Hygiène de l'enfance et de l'éducation physique*]. *Revue STAPS* 40:39–52.

Fett, Sharla M. 2002. *Working Cures: Healing, Health, and Power on Southern Slave Plantations.* Chapel Hill: University of North Carolina Press.

Figueroa Mercado, L. 1972. *History of Puerto Rico from the beginning to 1892.* New York: Anaya Book Co., Inc.

Findlay, Eileen. 1999. *Imposing Decency. The Politics of Sexuality and Race in Puerto Rico, 1870–1902.* Durham: Duke University Press.

Finlay, Carlos E. 1940. *Carlos Finlay and Yellow Fever.* New York: Published under the auspices of the Institute of Tropical Medicine of the University of Havana by Oxford University Press.

Fleitas, Carlos Rafael, comp. 2003. *Medicina y Sanidad en la Historia de Santiago de Cuba, 1515–1898.* Santiago: n. p. .

Floyd, B. 1979. *Jamaica: An Island Microcosm.* New York: St. Martin's Press.

Fraser, Gertrude Jacinta. 1998. *African American Midwifery in the South: Dialogues of Birth, Race and Memory.* Boston: Harvard University Press.

Funes Monzote, Reinaldo. 2003. *Despertar del asociacionismo científico en Cuba, 1876–1920.* Madrid: CSIC.

Gamble, V. 1995. *Making a Place for Ourselves: The Black Hospital Movement, 1920–1945.* New York: Oxford University Press.

Games, Alison. 1999. *Migration and the English Atlantic World.* Cambridge, MA: Harvard Univ Press.

García González, Armando and Raquel Alvarez Peláez. 1991. *En Busca de la raza perfecta: eugenesia e higiene en Cuba (1898–1958).* Madrid: Consejo Superior de Investigaciones Cientificas.

Garver, E.S. and E.B. Fincher. 1945. *Puerto Rico: Unsolved Problem.* Elgin: Brethren Publishing House.

Geisert, H.L. 1960. *The Caribbean: Population and Resources.* Washington, DC: George Washington Univ. .

Gillett, M.C. 1995. *The Army Medical Department, 1865–1917.* Washington, DC: Center of Military History.

Gillet, Mary C. 1990. U.S. Army Medical Officers and Public Health in the Wake of the Spanish-American War, 1898–1905. *Bulletin of the History of Medicine* 64(4):567–587.

Gilroy, Paul. 1993. *The Black Atlantic: Modernity and Double Consciousness.* Cambridge: Harvard University Press.

González, Raymundo. 2003. Hostos y la conciencia moderna en República Dominicana. In *Política, identidad y pensamiento social en la República Dominicana (Siglos XIX y XX),* ed. Raymundo González, et al. Madrid: Doce Calles.

Goodyear, J.D. 1978. The Sugar Connection: A New Perspective on the History of Yellow Fever. *Bulletin of the History of Medicine* 52(1):5–21.

Gorgas, William Crawford. 1915. *Sanitation in Panama.* New York: Appleton.

278   Bibliography

Güémez Pineda, Miguel A. 1997. De Comadronas a promotoras de salud y planificación familiar: proceso de incorporación de las parteras empíricas yucatecas al sistema institucional de salud. In *Cambio Cultural y Resocialización en Yucatán*, coord. Estebán Krotz, 117–145. Mérida, Mexico: Ediciones de la Universidad Autónoma de Yucatán.

Guerra, F. 1998. *La Educacion medica en Hispanoamerica y Filipinas durante el dominio español*. Madrid: University de Alcalá.

Guillaume, P. 2001. Antilles Pathologies and the Politics of Public Health at the Beginning of the Twentieth Century [*Pathologies antillaises et politiques de santé publique au début du XXᵉ siècle*]. In *Identités caraïbes,* ed. P. Guillaume, 161–169. Paris: Editions du CTHS.

Hallewas, Geert-Jaap. 1981. *De gezondheidszorg in Suriname*. Meppel, the Netherlands: Krips.

Handler, Jerome S. and Frederick W. Lange. 1999. *Plantation Slavery in Barbados: An Archaeological and Historical Investigation*. San Jose: ToExcel.

Hansen, Asael T. and Juan R. Bastarrachea M. 1984. *Mérida: su transformación: de capital colonial a naciente metrópolis*. Mexico: Instituto Nacional de Antropología e Historia.

Harris, Joseph. 1982. Introd. to *Global Dimensions of the African Diaspora*, ed. by Joseph Harris, 3–8. Washington, DC: Howard University Press, 1993.

Harrison, Gordon. 1978. *Mosquitoes, Malaria and Man: A History of the Hostilities Since 1880*. New York: Dutton.

Helg, Aline. 1990. Race in Argentina and Cuba, 1880–1930: Theory, Policies, and Popular Reaction. In *The Idea of Race in Latin America, 1870–1940*, ed. Richard Graham, 38–70. Austin: University of Texas Press.

Hernández Sáenz, Luz María. 1997. *Learning to Heal: The Medical Profession in Colonial Mexico, 1767–1831*. New York: Peter Lang.

Hernández, Luz María and George M. Foster. 2001. Curers and Their Cures in Colonial New Spain and Guatemala: The Spanish Component. In *Mesoamerican Healers*, ed. Brad R. Huber and Alan R. Sandstrom, 19–46. Austin: Texas University Press.

Higman, Barry. 1995. *Slave Populations of the British Caribbean 1807–1834* (Kingston, Jamaica: University of the West Indies Press.

———. 1976. *Slave Population and Economy in Jamaica, 1807–1834*. Cambridge: Cambridge University Press, 1979.

Hine, Darlene Clark. 1989. *Black Women in White. Racial Conflict and Cooperation in the Nursing Profession 1890–1950*. Bloomington: Indiana University Press.

Hoefte, Rosemarijn. 1998. *In Place of Slavery: A Social History of British Indian and Javanese Laborers in Suriname*. Gainesville: University Press of Florida.

———. 2007. The Lonely Pioneer: Suriname's First Female Politician and Social Activist, Grace Schneiders-Howard. *Wadabagei,* 10(3):84–103.

Hoemel, Robert B. 1976. Sugar and Social Change in Oriente, Cuba, 1898–1946. *Journal of Latin American Studies* 8(2):215–249.

Hoetink, H. 1986. *El pueblo dominiceno*. Santo Domingo: Editora de Colores.

———. 1965. Materiales para el estudio de la República Dominicana en la segunda mitad del siglo XX. *Caribbean Studies* 5(3):3–21.

Holt, Thomas. 1999. Slavery and Freedom in the Atlantic World: Reflections on the Diasporan Framework. In *Crossing Boundaries: Comparative History of Black People in Diaspora*, ed. Darlene Clarke Hine and Jacqueline McLeod, 3–32. Bloomington: Indiana University Press.

Honychurch, Penelope. 1986. *Caribbean Wild Plants and Their Uses*. London: Macmillan Caribbean.

Howe, G. 2002. *Race, War and Nationalism: A Social History of West Indians in the First World War.* Kingstown/Oxford: Ian Randle/James Curey.

Huber, Brad R. and Alan R. Sandstrom, eds. 2001. *Mesoamerican Healers.* Austin: Texas University Press.

Ibarra, Jorge. 1992. *Cuba: 1898–1921. Partidos políticos y clases sociales.* Havana: Editorial de Ciencias Sociales.

Iliffe, John. 1998. *East African Doctors: A History of the Medical Profession.* Cambridge: Cambridge University Press.

Inniss, Tara. 2006. "Fed with the Bread of Slavery": Children's Health in Barbados During Slavery and the Apprenticeship Period, 1790–1838. PhD diss., University of the West Indies.

Jacobs, Sylvia. 1987. Afro-American Women Missionaries Confront the African Way of Life. In *Women in Africa and the African Diaspora,* ed. Rosalyn Terborg-Penn, et al., 121–132. Washington, DC: Howard University Press.

James, Winston. 1998. *Holding Aloft the Banner of Ethiopia: Caribbean Radicalism in Early Twentieth-Century America.* London: Verso.

James, Winston and Clive Harris, eds. 1993. *Inside Babylon: The Caribbean Diaspora in Britain.* London: Verso.

Jenkins, David. 1975. *Black Zion: Africa, Imagined and Real, as Seen by Today's Blacks.* New York: Harcourt Brace Jovanovich.

Johnson, Michele A. and Brian L. Moore. 2004. *Neither Led nor Driven: Contesting British Cultural Imperialism in Jamaica, 1865–1920.* Kingston, Jamaica: University Press of the West Indies.

Johnson, T. 1982. The State and the Professions: Peculiarities of the British. In *Social Class and the Division of Labor,* ed. A. Givens and G. MacKenzie, 186–208. Cambridge: Cambridge University Press.

Jones, Zeina Omisola. 2004. Knowledge Systems in Conflict: The Regulation of African American Midwifery. *Nursing History Review* 12:167–184.

Killingray, David. 1994. The Influenza Pandemic of 1918–1919 in the British Caribbean. *Social History of Medicine* 7(1):59–87.

———. 2003. "A New Imperial Disease": The Influenza Pandemic of 1918–1919 and Its Impact on the British Empire. In *Colonialism and Health in the Tropics,* ed. Juanita De Barros and Sean Stilwell, Special issue, *Caribbean Quarterly* 49(4):30–49.

———. 2003. "To Do Something for the Race": Harold Moody and the League of Coloured Peoples. In *West Indian Intellectuals in Britain,* ed. Bill Schwarz, 51–70. Manchester, UK: Manchester University Press.

King, Wilma. 1996. "Suffer with Them Till Death": Slave Women and Their Children in Nineteenth Century America. In *More than Chattel: Black Women and Slavery in the Americas,* ed. David Barry Gaspar and Darlene Clark Hine, 147–168. Bloomington: Indiana University Press.

Kiple, Kenneth. 1987. A Survey of Recent Literature on the Biological Past of the Black. In *The African Exchange: Toward a Biological History of Black People,* ed. Kenneth F. Kiple. Durham, NC: Duke University Press

———. 1976. *Blacks in Colonial Cuba, 1774–1899.* Gainesville: University Press of Florida.

———. 1984. *The Caribbean Slave: A Biological History.* New York: Cambridge University Press.

———. 1985. Cholera and Race in the Caribbean. *Journal of Latin American Studies* 17:157–177.

———. 1993. Disease Ecologies of the Caribbean. In *The Cambridge World History of Human Disease,* ed. Kenneth F. Kiple. Cambridge: Cambridge University Press.

Kiple, Kenneth and Brian T. Higgins. 1991. Cholera in Mid-Nineteenth Century Jamaica. *Jamaican Historical Review* 17:31–47.

Kiple, Kenneth and Virginia Kiple. 1991. Deficiency Diseases in the Caribbean. In *Caribbean Slave Society and Economy*, ed. Hilary Beckles and Verene Shepherd, 173–182. Kingston, Jamaica: Ian Randle Publishers.

Kraut, Alan M. 1995. *Silent Travelers: Germs, Genes, and the "Immigrant Menace."* New York: Johns Hopkins University Press.

Kunow, Marianna Appel. 2003. *Maya Medicine: Traditional Healing in Yucatán.* Albuquerque: University of New Mexico Press.

Laurence, K. O. 1964. The Development of Medical Services in British Guiana and Trinidad 1841–1873. *Jamaica Historical Review* 4:59–67.

———. 1994. *A Question of Labour: Indentured Immigration into Trinidad and British Guiana 1875–1917.* Kingston, Jamaica: Ian Randle Publishers.

Le Roy y Gálvez, Jorge F. 1975. *Dos Conferencias Sobre el 27 de Noviembre de 1871.* La Habana: Centro de Información Científica y Técnica, Universidad de la Habana.

———. 1971. *La inocencia de los estudiantes fusilados en 1871.* La Habana: Centro de Información Científica y Técnica, Universidad de la Habana.

LeRoy y Gálvez, Luis Felipe. 1976. *Bio-bibliografía del Doctor Jorge LeRoy y Cassá* Havana: Orbe.

Levine, Philippa. 2003. *Prostitution, Race and Politics: Policing Venereal Disease in the British Empire.* London: Routledge.

Lewis, Earle. 1999. To Turn as if on a Pivot: Writing African Americans into a History of Overlapping Diasporas. In *Crossing Boundaries: Comparative History of Black People in Diaspora*, eds. Darlene Clarke Hine and Jacqueline McLeod, 3–32. Bloomington: Indiana University Press.

Lignon, Richard. 1998. *A True & Exact History of the Island of Barbadoes.* London: Frank Cass Publishers.

Lindskog, Bengt I. 2004. *Medicinsk Ordbog.* København, Denmark: Gyldendalske boghandel, Nordisk Forlag A/S.

Linebaugh, Peter and Marcus Rediker. 2000. *The Many-Headed Hydra: The Hidden History of the Revolutionary Atlantic.* Boston, MA: Beacon Press.

Løkke, Anne. 2002. Did Midwives Matter? 1787–1845. In *Pathways of the Past. Essays in Honour of Sølvi Sogner*, ed. Hilde Sandvik, Kari Telste, and Gunnar Thorvaldsen, 71–72. Oslo, Norway: Novus Forlag.

———. 1988. *Døden i Barndommen. Spædbørnsdødelighed og Moderniseringsprocesser i Danmark 1800 til 1920.* København, Denmark: Gyldendal.

López Denis, Adrián. 2007. Disease and Society in Colonial Cuba. PhD diss., University of California at Los Angeles.

———. 2005. Melancholia, Slavery, and Racial Pathology in Eighteenth-Century Cuba. *Science in Context* 18(2):179–199.

———. "Sugar in the Times of Cholera," http://en.wikiversity.org/ wiki/Sugar-in-the-times-of- cholera.

López Sánchez, José. 1999. *Carlos J. Finlay: His Life and Work.* Havana: Editorial José Martí.

Lord, Ann. 2002. "An Imperative Obligation": Public Health and the United States Military Occupation of the Dominican Republic, 1916–1924. PhD diss., University of Maryland, College Park.

Loudon, Irvine. 1992. *Death In Childbirth: An International Study of Maternal Care and Maternal Mortality 1800–1950.* Oxford: Clarendon Press.

Lovejoy, Paul. 1997. Biography as Source Material: Towards a Biographical Archive of Enslaved Africans. In *Source Material for Studying the Slave Trade and the African Diaspora*, ed. Robin Law, 119–140. Stirling: Centre of Commonwealth Studies.

Lozoya, X. 1987. La medicina tradicional en México: Balance de una década y perspectivas. In *El futuro de la medicina tradicional en la atención a la salud de los paises latinoamericanos*, 65–74. Mexico: CIESS.

Luker, Kristen. 1998. Sex, Social Hygiene, and the State: The Double-Edged Sword of Social Reform. *Theory and Society* 27:601–634.

Lyons, Maryinez. 1994. The Power to Heal: African Medical Auxiliaries in Colonial Belgian Congo and Uganda. In *Contesting Colonial Hegemony: State and Society in Africa and India*, ed. Dagmar Engels and Shula Marks, 202–223. London: British Academic Press.

Macpherson, Anne. 2003. Citizens v. Clients: Working Women and Colonial Reform in Puerto Rico and Belize, 1932–45. *Journal of Latin American Studies* 35:279–310.

———. 2003. Colonial Matriarchs: Garveyism, Maternalism, and Belize's Black Cross Nurses, 1920–1952. *Gender and History* 15(3):507–527.

Markel, Howard. 1997. *Quarantine! East European Jewish Immigrants and the New York City Epidemics of 1892*. Baltimore: John's Hopkins University Press.

Marks, Shula. 1994. *Divided Sisterhood: Race, Class and Gender in the South African Nursing Profession*. London: St. Martin's Press.

Martin, Tony. 1983. *The Pan-African Connection: From Slavery to Garvey and Beyond*. Dover: The Majority Press.

Martínez-Fortún Foyo, José A. y. 1958. *Historia de la Medicina en Cuba*. Havana: publisher.

Martínez-Vergne, Teresita. 2005. *Nation and Citizen in the Dominican Republic, 1880–1919*. Chapel Hill: University of North Carolina Press.

———. 1999. *Shaping the Discourse on Space: Charity and its Wards in Nineteenth-Century San Juan, Puerto Rico*. Austin: University of Texas Press.

Mayes, April. 2003. Sugar's Metropolis: The Politics and Culture of Progress in San Pedro de Macorís, Dominican Republic, 1870–1930. PhD diss., University of Michigan.

McBride, D. 2002. *Missions for Science: US Technology and Medicine in America's African World*. New Brunswick, NJ: Rutgers University Press.

McBride, David. 1989. *Integrating the City of Medicine: Blacks in Philadelphia Health Care, 1910–1965*. Philadelphia: Temple University Press.

McLean, N.T. 1922. Public Health Problems of the Southern Countries. *The United States Naval Medical Bulletin* 2(1):25–39.

McLeod, James Angus. 1990. Public Health, Social Assistance and the Consolidation of the Mexican State: 1888–1940. PhD diss., Tulane University.

Menéndez, Eduardo L. 1981. *Poder, estratificación y salud: Analisis de las condiciones sociales y económicas de la enfermedad en Yucatán*. Mexico City: Ediciones de la Casa Chata.

Millington, Claire. 1995. Maternal Health Care in Barbados, 1880–1940. History Forum Seminar Paper, University of the West Indies.

Moitt, Bernard. 1996. Slave Women and Resistance in the French Caribbean. In *More than Chattel: Black Women and Slavery in the Americas*, ed. David Barry Gaspar and Darlene Clark Hine, 239–258. Bloomington: Indiana Univ. Press.

Moore, Brian L. 1995. *Cultural Power, Resistance, and Pluralism: Colonial Guyana, 1838–1900*. Montreal: McGill-Queens University Press.

Moreno Fraginals, Manuel. 1976. *Sugarmill: The Socioeconomic Complex of Sugar in Cuba, 1760–1860*. New York: Monthly Review.

Mort, Frank. 1987. *Dangerous Sexualities: Medico-Moral Politics in England since 1830*. London: Routledge and Kegan Paul.

Mott, Maria Lucia. 2003. Midwifery and the Construction of an Image in Nineteenth-Century Brazil. *Nursing History Review* 11:31–49.

282   Bibliography

Mumford, Kevin. 1997. *Interzones. Black/White Sex Districts in Chicago and New York in the Early Twentieth Century*. New York: Columbia University Press.

Naranjo Orovio, Consuelo and Armando García González. *Medicina y racismo en Cuba. La ciencia ante la lenmigración canaria en el siglo XX*. Tenerife: La Laguna. .

Negrón-Portillo, M. 1990. *Las Turbas Republicanas, 1900–1904*. Rio Piedras: Ediciones Huracan.

Nigenda, Gustavo. 2001. La Práctica de la Medicina Tradicional en América Latina y el Caribe. *Salud Pública de México* 43:1.

Nigenda-López, Gustavo. 1995. The Medical Profession, the State and Health Policy in Mexico. 1917–1988. Thesis. London School of Economics and Political Science.

Nouzeilles, G. 1996. Modernization and Racial Economy in Manuel Zeno Gandía's *La Charca*. Paper presented at the 5th International Conference on Emile Zola, New York.

Nouzeilles, G. 1997. La Espinge De Monstruo: Modernidad e Higiene Racial en La Charca de Zeno Gandia. *Latin American Literary Review* 25:50, 89–107.

Nyland, Nick. 2000. *De praktiserende læger i Danmark, 1800–1910. Træk af det historiske grundlag for almen medicin*. Odense: Syddansk University

Obregón, Diana. 2005. Building National Medicine: Leprosy and Power in Colombia, 1870–1910. *Social History of Medicine* 15(1):89–108.

Ortiz de Montellano, Bernard R. 1990. *Aztec Medicine, Health, and Nutrition*. New Brunswick, NJ: Rutgers University Press.

Palmer, Steven. 1998. Central American Encounters with Rockefeller Public Health, 1914–1921. In *Close Encounters of Empire: Writing the Cultural History of U.S.–Latin American Relations*, ed. Gilbert M. Joseph, Catherine C. LeGrand, and Ricardo D. Salvatore, 311–332. Durham, NC: Duke University Press.

———. 2003. *From Popular Medicine to Medical Populism: Doctors, Healers and Public Power in Costa Rica, 1800–1940*. Durham, NC: Duke University Press.

———. 2006. "O Demônio que se transformou em vermes": a tradução da saúde pública no Caribe Britânico, 1914–1920. *História Ciências, Saúde-Maguinhos* 13(5):571–589.

Palmié, Stephan. 2002. *Wizards and Scientists: Explorations in Afro-Cuban Modernity and Tradition*. Durham, NC: Duke Univ Press.

Patterson, K. David and Gerald F. Pyle. 1991. The Geography and Mortality of the 1918 Influenza Pandemic. *Bulletin of the History of Medicine* 65(1):4–21.

Patton, Adell. 1982. Howard University and Meharry Medical Schools in the Training of African Physicians, 1868–1978. In *Global Dimensions of the African Diaspora*, ed. Joseph Harris, 109–135. Washington, DC: Howard University Press, 1983.

———. *Physicians, Colonial Racism, and Diaspora in West Africa*. Gainesville: University Press of Florida.

Peard, Julyan G. 1999. *Race, Place, and Medicine: The Idea of the Tropics in Nineteenth-Century Brazilian Medicine*. Durham, NC: Duke University Press.

Pemberton, Rita. 2003. A Different Intervention: The International Health Commission/Board, Health, Sanitation in the British Caribbean, 1914–1930. In *Colonialism and Health in the Tropics*, ed. Juanita De Barros and Sean Stilwell, Special issue, *Caribbean Quarterly* 49(4):87–103.

Pérez, Louis A., Jr. 1999. *On Becoming Cuban: Identity, Nationality, and Culture*. Chapel Hill: University of North Carolina Press.

Piqueras, José A. 2005. El mundo reducido a una isla. La unión cubana a la metrópoli en un tiempo de Tribulaciones. In *Las antillas en la era de la revolución*, ed. José A. Piqueras, 319–342. Madrid: Iglo XXI.

Porter, Dorothy. 1999. *Health, Civilization and the State: A History of Public Health from Ancient to Modern Times.* London: Routledge University Press.

Power, Helen. 1996. The Calcutta School of Tropical Medicine: Institutionalizing Medical Research in the Periphery. *Medical History* 40:197–214.

Prout, W. T. 1910. Malaria in Jamaica. In *The Prevention of Malaria*, ed. Ronald Ross. London: Murray.

Pruna Goodgall, Pedro M. 2002. *La Real Academia de Ciencias de la Habana, 1861–1898.* Madrid: CESIC.

———. 1994. National Science in a Colonial Context: The Royal Academy of Sciences of Havana, 1861–1898. *Isis* 85(3):412–426.

Quevedo Báez, M. 1946. *Historia de la medicina y cirugia en Puerto Rico.* 2 vols. Asociación Médica de Puerto Rico.

Quezada, Noemí. 1991. The Inquisition's Repression of *Curanderos*. In *Cultural Encounters: The Impact of the Inquisition in Spain and the New World*, ed. Mary Elizabeth Perry and Anne J. Cruz. Berkeley: University of California Press.

Rago, Margareth. 1991. *Os prazeres da noite. Prostituição e códigos da sexualidade feminine em São Paolo, 1890–1930.* Rio de Janeiro: Paz e Terra.

Ramsey, Frank C. 1995. Child Care in Barbados: Past Achievements and Future Needs. *The Barbados Association of Medical Practitioners* 135:2–6.

Ramsey, M. 1984. The Politics of Professional Monopoly in Nineteenth-Century Medicine: The French Model and Its Rivals. In *Professions and the French State, 1700–1900*, ed. G. L. Geison, 225–305. Philadelphia: University of Pennsylvania Press.

Reiser, S. J. 1978. *Medicine and the Reign of Technology.* Cambridge: Cambridge University Press.

Renda, Mary. 2001. *Taking Haiti. Military Occupation and the Culture of U.S. Imperialism, 1915–1940.* Chapel Hill: University of North Carolina Press.

Richardson, Bonham. 1983. *Caribbean Migrants: Environment and Human Survival on St. Kitts and Nevis.* Knoxville: The University of Tennessee Press.

Richardson, Bonham C. 1985. *Panama Money in Barbados, 1900–1920.* Knoxville: The University of Tennessee Press.

Richardson, Bonham C. and Joseph L. Scarpaci. 2004. The Quality of Life in the Twentieth Century Caribbean. In *General History of the Caribbean*, vol. 5, *The Caribbean in the Twentieth Century*, ed. Bridget Brereton (Paris: UNESCO Publishing.

Rigau-Perez, J. G. 1989. The Introduction of Smallpox Vaccine in 1803 and the Adoption of Immunization as a Government Function in Puerto Rico. *Hispanic American Historical Review* 69:393–323.

Riley, James C. 2005. *Poverty and Life Expectancy: The Jamaica Paradox.* Cambridge: Cambridge University Press.

Ríos-Font, W. 2005. El Crimen de la Calle de San Vicente: Crime Writing and Bourgeois Liberalism in Restoration Spain. *MLN* 120(2):335–354.

Rodney, Walter. 1982. *A History of the Guyanese Working People, 1881–1905.* Baltimore: Johns Hopkins University Press, 1981.

Rodriguez-Trias, H. 1984. The Women's Health Movement: Women Take Power. In *Reforming Medicine: Lessons of the Last Quarter Century*, ed. V.W. Sidel and R. Sidel, 107–126. New York: Pantheon Books.

Rollet, Catherine. 1997. The Fight against Infant Mortality in the Past: An International Comparison. In *Infant and Child Mortality in the Past*, ed. Alain Bideau, Bertrand Besjardins, and Héctor Pérez Brignoli, 38–60. Oxford: Clarendon Press.

Román, Reinaldo Luis. 2000. Conjuring Progress and Divinity: Religion and Conflict in Cuba and Puerto Rico, 1899–1956. PhD diss., University of California, Los Angeles.

Rosenberg, Charles E. and Janet Golden, eds. 1992. *Framing Disease: Studies in Cultural History*. New Brunswick, NJ: Rutgers University Press.

Sandstrom, Alan R. 2001. Mesoamerican Healers and Medical Anthropology: Summary and Concluding Remarks. In *Mesoamerican Healers*, ed. Brad R. Huber and Alan R. Sandstrom, 307–330. Austin: Texas University Press.

Santiago-Valles, Kelvin. 1994. *"Subject People" and Colonial Discourses, Economic Transformation and Social Disorder in Puerto Rico, 1898–1947*. Albany: State University of New York Press.

Savitt, Todd L. 1982. The Use of Blacks for Medical Experimentation and Demonstration in the Old South. *The Journal of Southern History* 48(3):331–348.

Scarano, F. A. 1996. The Jibaro Masquerade and the Subaltern Politics of Creole Identity Formation in Puerto Rico, 1745–1823. *The American Historical Review* 101:1398–1431.

Schmidt, Johan Christian. 1998. *Various Remarks Collected on and about the Island of St. Croix in America*. St. Croix, US Virgin Islands: The Virgin Islands Humanities Council.

Scobie, Edward. 1972. *Black Britannia: A History of Blacks in Britain*. Chicago: Johnson Publishing Company.

Seecharan, Clem. 1997. *'Tiger in the Stars': The Anatomy of Indian Achievement in British Guiana 1919–29*. London: Macmillan Caribbean Publishers.

Seoane Gallo, José. 1984. *El Folclor Médico de Cuba: Provincia de Camagüey*. Havana: Editorial de Ciencias Sociales.

Shapiro, Karin. 1987. Doctors or Medical Aids—The Debate over the Training of Black Medical Personnel for the Rural Black Population in South Africa in the 1920s and 1930s. *Journal of Southern African Studies* 13(2):234–255.

Shepperson, George. 1982. African Diaspora: Concept and Context. In *Global Dimensions of the African Diaspora*, ed. Joseph Harris, 41–49. (Washington, DC: Howard University Press, 1993.

Sheridan, Richard. 1991. Mortality and the Medical Treatment of Slaves in the British West Indies. In *Caribbean Slave Society and Economy*, ed. Hilary Beckles and Verene Shepherd, 197–208. Kingston, Jamaica: Ian Randle Publishers.

Sheridan, Richard B. 1985. *Doctors and Slaves: A Medical and Demographic History of Slavery in the British West Indies, 1680–1834*. Cambridge: Cambridge University Press.

Shortt, S. E. D. 1983. Physicians, Science, and Status: Issues in the Professionalization of Anglo-American Medicine in the Nineteenth Century. *Medical History* 27:51–68.

Skinner, Elliott P. 1982. The Dialectic between Diasporas and Homeland. In *Global Dimensions of the African Diaspora*, ed. Joseph Harris, 11–40. Washington, DC: Howard University Press, 1993.

Solórzano, Armando. 1994. The Rockefeller Foundation in Revolutionary Mexico: Yellow Fever in Yucatan and Veracruz. In *Missionaries of Science: The Rockefeller Foundation and Latin America*, ed. Marcos Cueto, 52–71. Bloomington: Indiana Univ. Press.

Soloway, Richard. 1990. *Demography and Degeneration: Eugenics and the Declining Birthrate in Twentieth-Century Britain*. Chapel Hill: The University of North Carolina Press.

Spongberg, Mary. 1997. *Feminizing Venereal Disease: The Body of the Prostitute in Nineteenth-Century Medical Discourse*. New York: New York University Press.

Starr, P. 1982. *The Social Transformation of American Medicine*. New York: Basic Books.

Steckel, Richard. 1996. Women, Work, and Health under Plantation Slavery in the United States. In *More than Chattel: Black Women and Slavery in the Americas,* ed. David Barry Gaspar and Darlene Clark Hine. Bloomington: Indiana University Press.

Stepan, Nancy Leys. 1991. *"The Hour of Eugenics": Race, Gender, and Nation in Latin America.* Ithaca, NY: Cornell University Press.

Stepan, Nancy. 1978. The Interplay between Socioeconomic Factors and Medical Science: Yellow Fever Research, Cuba, and the United States. *Social Studies of Science* 8(4):397–423.

Stone, C. 1989. Power, Policy and Politics in Independent Jamaica. In *Jamaica in Independence: Essays on the Early Years,* ed. R. Nettleford, 19–53. Kingston, Jamaica: Heinemann, 1989.

Svend E. 1981. Green-Pedersen: Slave Demography in the Danish West Indies and the Abolition of the Danish Slave Trade. In *The Abolition of the Atlantic Slave Trade: Origins and Effects in Europe, Africa and the Americas,* ed. David Eltis and James Walvin, 231–255. Madison: University of Wisconsin Press.

Temperley, Howard. 2000. African-American Aspirations and the Settlement of Liberia. In *After Slavery: Emancipation and Its Discontents,* ed. Howard Temperly, 150–168. London: Frank Cass Publishers.

TePaske, John Jay. 2000. Regulation of Medical Practitioners in the Age of Francisco Hernández. In *Searching for the Secrets of Nature: The Life and Works of Dr. Francisco Hernández,* ed. Simon Varey, Rafael Chabrán, and Dora B. Weiner, 55–64. Stanford, CA: Stanford University Press,.

Thompson, Vincent Bakpetu. 1993. Leadership in the African Diaspora in the Americas Prior to 1860. *Journal of Black Studies* 24:42–76.

Thorburn, M. J., and J. A. Hayes. 1968. Causes of Death in Jamaica, 1953 to 1964: An Analysis of Post-Mortem Diagnosis at the University Hospital of the West Indies. *Tropical and Geographical Medicine* 20:35–49.

Trigo, B. 1999. Anemia and Vampires: Figures to Govern the Colony, Puerto Rico, 1880–1904. *Comparative Studies in Society and History* 41(1):104–123.

Van Drenth, Annemieke and Francisca De Haan. 1999. *The Rise of Caring Power: Elizabeth Fry and Josephine Butler in Britain and the Netherlands.* Amsterdam: Amsterdam University Press.

Van Heyningen, E. B. 1989. Agents of Empire: The Medical Profession in the Cape Colony, 1880–1910. *Medical History* 33:450–471.

Vaughan, Megan. 1991. *Curing Their Ills: Colonial Power and African Illness.* Cambridge: Cambridge University Press.

———. 1994. Healing and Curing: Issues in the Social History and Anthropology of Medicine in Africa. *Social History of Medicine* 7(2):283–295.

———. 1992. Syphilis in Colonial East Central Africa: The Social Construction of an Epidemic. In *Epidemics and Ideas: Essays on the Historical Perception of Pestilence,* ed. Terence Ranger and Paul Slack, 269–302. Cambridge: Cambridge University Press.

Vertovec, Steven. 2000. *The Hindu Diaspora: Comparative Patterns.* London: Routledge.

Vibæk, Jens. 1966. Dansk Vestindien, 1755–1848. Vestindiens Storhedstid. In *Vore Gamle Tropekolonier,* Vol. 2ed. Johannes Brøndsted, 271–273. København, Denmark: Fremad.

Viesca Treviño, Carlos. 2001. *Curanderismo* in Mexico and Guatemala: Its Historical Evolution from the Sixteenth to the Nineteenth Century. In *Mesoamerican Healers,* eds. Brad R. Huber and Alan R. Sandstrom, 47–65. Austin: Texas University Press.

Von Eschen, Penny. 1997. *Race Against Empire: Black Americans and Anticolonialism, 1937–1957.* Ithaca, NY: Cornell University Press.

Walkowitz, Judith R. 1980. *Prostitution and Victorian Society: Women, Class, and the State.* London: Cambridge University Press.

Watkins-Owens, Irma. 1996. *Blood Relations: Caribbean Immigrants and the Harlem Community, 1900–1930.* Bloomington: Indiana University Press.

Watson, Karl. 2000. *A Kind of Right to be Idle: Old Doll Matriarch of Newton Plantation.* Bridgetown, Barbados: University of the West Indies and the Barbados Museum and Historical Society.

Watts, Sheldon. 1997. *Epidemics and History: Disease, Power, and Imperialism.* New Haven, CT: Yale University Press.

Welch, Pedro and Richard Goodridge. 2000. *"Red" & Black Over White: Free-Coloured Women in Pre-Emancipation Barbados.* Bridgetown, Barbados: Carib Research and Publications Inc. .

Index